Bio-Replenishment
for
BONE
HEALTH

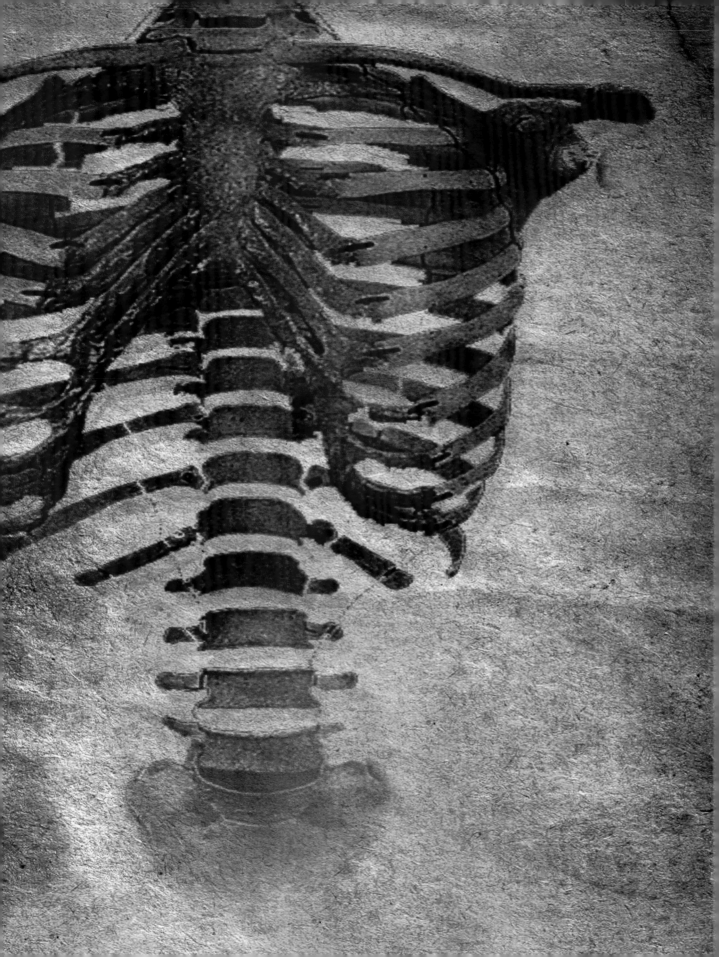

Bio-Replenishment

for

BONE
HEALTH

A S NAIDU

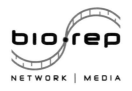

bio·rep
NETWORK | MEDIA

Published by:
Bio-Rep Network | Media
Pomona, California, USA

www.biorepnetwork.com

DISCLAIMER: All reasonable precautions have been taken to verify the information contained in this publication. However, the published material is being distributed without warranty of any kind, either expressed or implied. The responsibility for the interpretation and use of the material lies with the reader. In no event shall the publishers be liable for damages arising from its use. Always consult your primary health care provider before starting any major change in your diet, health programs, or any course of supplementation or treatment, particularly if you are currently under medical care. If you have or suspect you may have a health problem, you should talk to your healthcare provider immediately. Only your physician should evaluate your health problems and prescribe treatment. Statements about theories and health conditions have not been evaluated by the U.S. Food & Drug Administration. The FDA has not reviewed or approved the Bio-Replenishments to diagnose, treat, cure or prevent any disease.

Design : Neha Madan

Layout : Digital Spice Studios (P) Limited & Bio-Rep Network | Media

Printed and Bound at Pragati Offset

First Printing : August 2009

10 9 8 7 6 5 4 3 2 1

ISBN 978-0-9824451-0-5

Printed in India

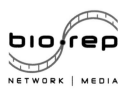

to

SMITA
smile of my life

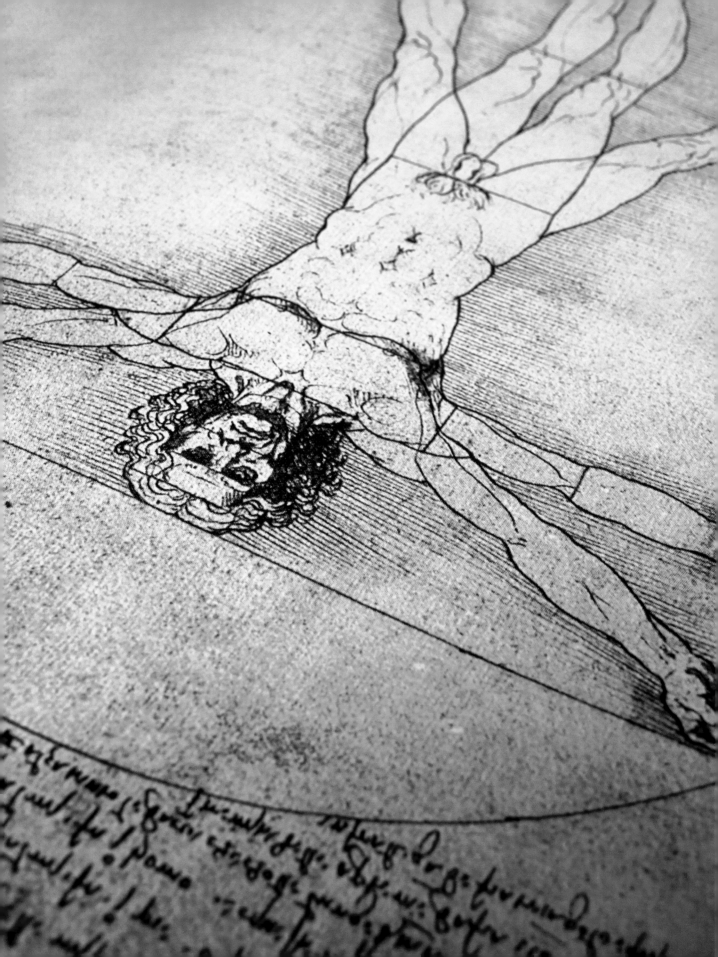

Contents

Archives

Those tons of bread, gallons of water
Churned for that power, I could never see
Transacted for this flesh and blood
To the saturation of a useless mass
Yet, I believe in my work and myself
What will happen dear Einstein
To my Mass-Energy equation
Conserved in the Grand Universe?

A S 'Narain' Naidu
January 17, 1980
(poem from the journal: **Molecular and Cellular Biochemistry 32:115, 1980**)

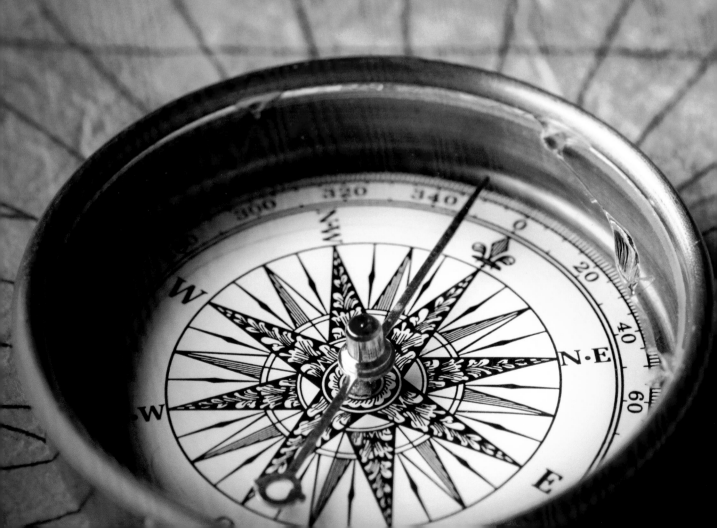

Preface

ARCHIVES - penning down the poem in 1979 was just a tiny seed of curiosity sowed in my mind when I was a young research graduate. The following three decades of scientific quest for logical explanations harvested a wealth of knowledge and simultaneously unleashed a flood gate of questions into the abyss of my ignorance. What is life? What is the need for life to evolve from a simple single cell to a complex multi-cellular form? If living organisms are self-constructed from raw organic chemicals, why can't they maintain a steady-state of immortality? *(Repair and maintenance certainly seems much easier than self-construction!)* Is aging purposely programmed into the design of life? Since the antiquity of human civilization, these questions bogged both philosophers and scientists.

Which chemical processes could possibly have created LIFE – the self-duplicating energy management system? Rudolf Clausius (1822-1888 AD), the German physicist who formulated the 2nd law of thermodynamics stated that "the energy of the universe is constant and its entropy tends toward a maximum". The universe is programmed to shift *from order to disorder*, and step down the complexity to simplicity. However, in a sheer contradiction to the 2nd law of thermodynamics, the biological evolution is a hierarchical progression of highly complex forms of living systems. The critical biochemicals of living systems (i.e. DNA, proteins) are more energy rich than their precursors (amino acids, heterocyclic bases, phosphates, and sugars).

What is Life? The question, entitled as a classic volume of Nobel Laureate Erwin Schrödinger (1887-1961 AD), elucidates an important question: *how can the events in space and time, which take place within the spatial boundary of a living organism are accounted for by physics and chemistry?* Schrödinger explains that living matter evades the decay to thermodynamic equilibrium by feeding on negative entropy, in other words, life is based on a different principle – *order-from-order*. Schrödinger's prophetic concept of an "aperiodic crystal" that contained hereditary information in its configuration of covalent chemical bonds stimulated enthusiasm in 1950s for discovering DNA – the genetic molecule.

What operates LIFE – the intricate biochemical system? The smallest single-cell organism has millions of molecules that must each be arranged in an exact pattern to provide the required functions. The cell has an energy-generating system, a protective housing, a security system to let molecules in and out of the housing, a reproductive system and a central control system. This complexity requires an intelligent design.

What is aging? Aging refers to the time-sequential deterioration that occurs in most animals including weakness, increased susceptibility to disease and adverse environmental conditions, loss of mobility and agility, and age-related bodily changes. Aging is usually understood to include reductions in reproductive capacity.

Scientific theories regarding the cause of aging are closely related to theories of evolution, particularly those of Charles Darwin (1809-1882 AD). According to the *Darwin's Theory of Natural Selection*, any evolved trait benefits the survival and reproductive fitness of an organism. If so - *is aging a feature of an organism's design that evolved because it confers some benefit, or, a defect with no benefit?*

Although Darwin believed that longevity was an evolved trait, and assumed that a limited life span was of benefit to some species, he did not suggest any mechanism for a trait that was adverse to fitness could evolve or propose a specific benefit for aging. It was apparent that human characteristics regarding aging and longevity did not fit the rules set forth by Darwin for natural selection.

August Weismann's (1834-1914 AD) *Programmed Death Theory* suggested that physical deterioration and death due to aging is genetically programmed characteristic (an adaptation) evolved through natural selection. Nobel Laureate Peter Medawar (1915-1987 AD) theorized that aging was due to random mutations, each of which has adverse symptoms. These programmed theories imply that aging is regulated by biological clocks operating throughout the life span. *Is aging process induced by evolution into an organism's genetic make up so that it may live to its healthiest potential until its reproductive age, die slowly and gradually thereafter?*

Stochastic theories blame environmental impacts on living organisms that induce cumulative damage at various levels as the cause of aging, examples which range from damage to DNA, tissues and cells by free radicals, and toxins. Living organism, as a reactive entity, is naturally designed to interact with a plethora of chemicals in its milieu through food, contact, inhalation and administration. Such interactions recalibrate the biochemical matrix of a life form, for instance, *actinolite* (from asbestos), *nicotine* (from tobacco), and vinyl chloride (from plastic) are carcinogens and their exposure could induce cancer. *Thiomerosal* (mercury-based preservative in certain vaccines) could bind to brain cells and cause *autism*. Estrogen overload in water supplies (flush following the use of birth control pills and HRT) could react with the reproductive system and bring down human sperm counts. Though, human body is a bio-engineering marvel with an efficient detoxification system (i.e. liver, kidney), the physiological turnover of certain synthetic chemicals is unknown. For example, the half-life of insecticide DDT, the endocrine disrupting chemical, is estimated at about 100 years! *Is there any general limit on the ability of an organism to perform self-repair? Theoretically if such limit is reached, what are the consequences of such damage?* Put together, aging appears to be a progressive failure of (i) homeostasis involving genes for the maintenance and repair; (ii) stochastic events leading to molecular damage and molecular heterogeneity; which cumulatively increases the probability of death. Undoubtedly, WE, the *Homo sapiens* are the fittest species surviving on the *Blue Planet*. Indeed, our *bipedal* population tripled beating the odds during the past century alone! The human life expectancy has improved significantly for individual biological years. *Consequently, what is the likelihood of natural selection playing a role in restraining the human race (enforcing the basic rule of self containment with population growth kinetics)?*

A number of existing laws of nature – from *Clausius's 2nd Law of Thermodynamics to Mendel's Laws of Heredity*; several classic theories, ranging from the *Darwin's Theory of Natural Selection to Medawar's Mutation Accumulatio Theory*; provided an invaluable collateral to the realty of my new **BIO-REPLENISHMENT THEORY.**

Bio-Replenishments comprise a class of molecules critical for the regulation of homeodynamics in mammalian species. Bio-Replenishments are genetically programmed to appear in a structured sequence during the development of embryonic, puberty and reproductive phases. These revitalizers are also programmed to disappear gradually in a specific manner with the progression of natural (chronological) aging. Bio-Replenishments are produced, utilized and replenished inside the body on a regular-basis in response to metabolic demand. Genetic mutations, environmental toxicity, stress, physical 'wear and tear' can negatively impact the production, utilization and repletion of Bio-Replenishment levels in the body; and such depleted conditions may lead to rapid aging, dysfunction, disease, or death. The functional properties and the underlying mechanisms of these fundamental molecules will be elucidated in the BIO-REPLENISHMENT THEORY.

Why Bone Replenishment? With the emergence of terrestrial vertebrates, bone acquired a new challenge in supporting a heavy body on land. Bone may appear inert, but it is a living tissue that performs several important functions – well beyond providing locomotion, shape and a beautiful face. It serves as a mineral bank for deposits and withdrawals of essential alkalizing compounds on a minute-to minute-basis to maintain blood calcium homeostasis and pH (acid-alkaline) balance. Survival is contingent upon these regular transactions of bone mineral bank with body's internal systems, which are so "interconnected" that poor health in one part of the body can quickly compromise the integrity and wellness of other areas. Skeleton and all its individual bones have a unique ability to self-repair (model and remodel) and remain strong to take us through every walk of life. If this is true – and it is – *how come we are finding ourselves in the midst of a global bone health crisis?* Low calcium intake, the natural lowering of estrogen levels at menopause, and low bone density are not the only reasons for the sprawling osteoporosis "pandemic", particularly among women. Our fixation on these factors has been keeping us away from uncovering the true causes of this monumental health issue. The BIO-REPLENISHMENT THEORY and this publication is an attempt to fill that void.

This endeavor is a cumulative outcome of several contributors to my professional career. I am truly indebted to my professors, research colleagues, and those premier institutes of higher learning across six continents that stimulated and channeled my scientific curiosity. I thank Sreus Naidu *(Bio-Rep Media | Network, Pomona)* for undertaking the task of publishing the BioRep Book Series ; Tezus Naidu and Dr. S. Bharadwaj *(N-terminus Research Laboratories, Pomona)*; Dr. P. Nemani *(Children's Hospital, University of Southern California, Los Angeles)*; Dr. G. Betagiri *(School of Pharmacy, Western University of Health Sciences, Pomona)* for being my critics and integral part of my clinical research team. I am also grateful to Binoy Samuel and Neha Madan *(Digital Spice)* ; Narendra Paruchuri and Mahendra Paruchuri *(Pragati Offset)*; Ravi Kola *(Srinivasa Lithographics);* and Prof. Ashutosh Muchrikar *(Pune University)* for their publishing efforts.

In my struggle to simplify a complex array of scientific concepts and ideas, I thought it would be helpful to provide various analogies from day-to-day life. Despite all the good intentions, however, I stand alone to accept responsibility for any inaccuracies and idiosyncrasies. *A living organism continuously reverses entropy by creating new structures from random components.* In analogy, this preamble to the BIO-REPLENISHMENT THEORY is a humble attempt to reverse my academic entropy – a modest sum up of my random scientific thoughts!

July 5, 2009
Pomona, California

A S Naidu

XIV

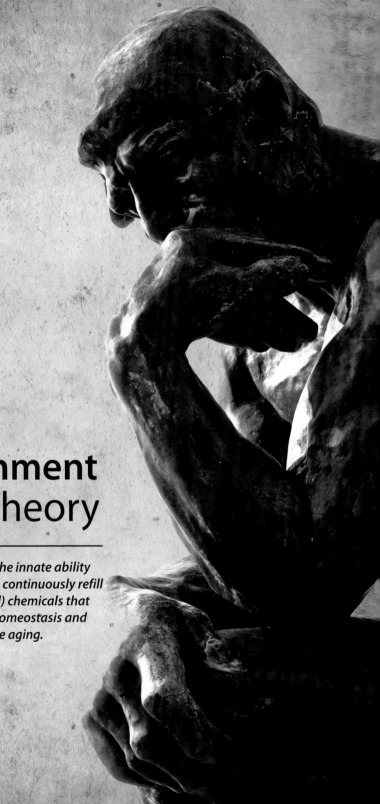

Bio-Replenishment
Theory

---

1 *Bio-Replenishment is the innate ability of a living organism to continuously refill its expended (depleted) chemicals that are vital to maintain homeostasis and negative entropy, while aging.*

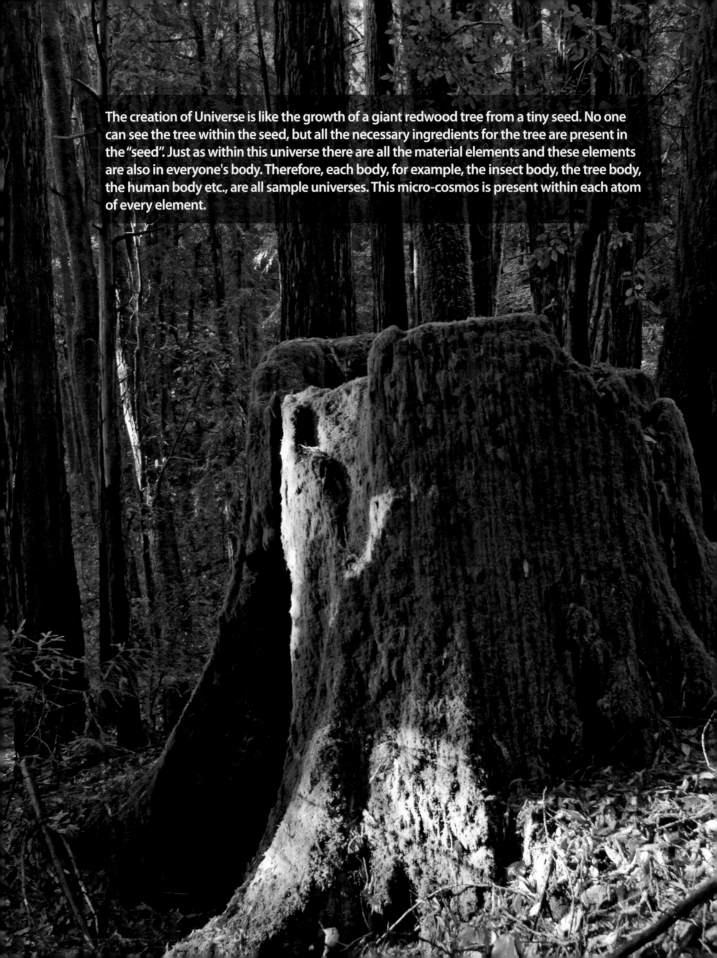

The creation of Universe is like the growth of a giant redwood tree from a tiny seed. No one can see the tree within the seed, but all the necessary ingredients for the tree are present in the "seed". Just as within this universe there are all the material elements and these elements are also in everyone's body. Therefore, each body, for example, the insect body, the tree body, the human body etc., are all sample universes. This micro-cosmos is present within each atom of every element.

1

1.1 | What is a **Theory?**

THEORY is a systematic review process that summarizes what is already known, adds to existing knowledge, and provides guidance for what is yet to be understood. Theory is the compass that helps navigate through an ocean of data. It is a method that transforms data into meaningful explanation(s).

In science, a theory is considered as a *logical explanation*, or a testable model for a given set of natural phenomena; able to predict future occurrences or observations of the same kind and capable of being tested through experiment or otherwise falsified through empirical observation.

For a scientist, theory is an *extrapolation of fact(s)* that do not necessarily contradict. For example, it is a fact that an apple dropped on earth. The extrapolation was that the apple fell towards the center of the planet. However, Newton explained this phenomenon beyond the planet Earth through the theories of *Universal Gravitation*, and *General Relativity*.

Furthermore, a theory may contain interrelated, coherent set of *assumptions*. Albert Einstein has considered two previously postulated phenomena that the 'addition of velocities' is valid *(Galilean transformation)*, and that light did not appear to have any 'addition of velocities' *(Michelson-Morley experiment)*. Einstein assumed both observations to be correct, and formulated the *Special Theory of Relativity*, by simply altering the Galilean transformation to accommodate the lack of addition of velocities with regard to the speed of light. The model created in his theory, therefore, was based on the assumption that light maintains a constant velocity.

In human quest for knowledge, THEORY has proven to be extremely useful, sometimes a ground-breaking tool

In addition to the depth of understanding that theoretically based research provides, the breadth of pragmatic justifications for a theory can be seen in 4 ways:

i) Integration: A good theory summarizes the many discrete findings from empirical studies and puts them into a brief statement to describe the relationship among the crucial observations, variables and theoretical constructs.

ii) Explanation: A useful theory provides not only description of the ways of empirically observed phenomena are related (this is what models reflect) but also *how* and especially *why* they are related.

iii) Prediction: Research based on a theory can lead to subsequent discoveries based on earlier theories. Historical examples from science include Charles Darwin's theory of natural selection in biology; Dimitri Mendeleev's theory leading to the periodic table of elements in chemistry; and Albert Einstein's theory of relativity in physics.

iv) Intervention: A theory is valuable only when applied to advance the existing knowledge to solve problems or alleviate undesirable conditions. Applications of the "Germ Theory", for instance, led to the virtual elimination of childhood infectious diseases. As biological pathogens were identified and controlled by modern medicine and for the first time in human history parents could take for granted that most of their children would survive infancy and grow up into adulthood.

A good THEORY prompts a simple question: "If the problem is not understood, how can it be fixed?"

Germ Theory of Disease, the most important milestone in the medical history, was first proposed by the French chemist and microbiologist Louis Pasteur, in the 1850s. This theory postulates that certain diseases are caused by the invasion of the body by microorganisms ("germs too small to be seen by a naked eye, except through a microscope"). In the 1860s, English surgeon Joseph Lister revolutionized surgical practice by utilizing carbolic acid (phenol) to exclude atmospheric germs and thus prevent putrefaction in compound fractures of bones. In the 1870s, German physician Robert Koch devised a series of proofs to verify the germ theory of disease. Koch's postulates were first used in 1875 to demonstrate anthrax was caused by the bacterium *Bacillus anthracis*, and later identified the organisms that cause tuberculosis and cholera. Koch's postulates are still in use to help determine if a newly discovered disease is caused by a microorganism.

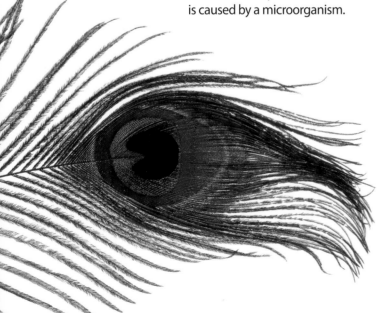

The Atharvaveda, an ancient scripture (corresponding to the 12th to 10th centuries BC or the early Kuru kingdom) is the first text that dealt with medicine. It identifies the causes of disease as living agents such as the "krimi" (germ) and the "durnama" (microorganism). It also teaches several ways to contain these germs with natural interventions, thereby prevent or cure any disease through 'sanhita' (therapy)

1.2 | What is **Life?**

LIFE is a distinct trait that sets apart our *Blue Planet* from everything else in the Universe. Human species is a unique life form and amongst the few dominating organisms on the earth; therefore, understanding the nature of life is an important step towards knowing ourselves.

Nobel Laureate Erwin Schrödinger's theory on 'Life' is one of the greatest science classics of the 20th century. Schrödinger postulated that a living organism continuously increases its *entropy* (or produces 'positive entropy') and tends to approach a dangerous state of 'maximum entropy' (or 'death'). A living organism can only avoid this detrimental condition and stay alive, by steady withdrawal of 'negative entropy' from its environment. Accordingly, living organisms are defined as open systems that respond to internal and external changes, in specific ways to promote their own continuation. It is a self-perpetuating open system of organic reactions propelled by complex chemicals.

Schrödinger's theory has created one of the major spurs in establishing the field of molecular biology. He also speculated the heredity material to be a molecule, which unlike a normal crystal does not repeat itself. This *aperiodic crystal* facilitates encoding an almost infinite number of possibilities with a small number of atoms. This idea led to the subsequent discovery of DNA, the genetic molecule, and won the 1962 Nobel Prize for James Watson, Francis Crick and Maurice Wilkins.

What is the characteristic feature of life? When a piece of matter is said to be alive? These questions can be addressed by considering that a living organism exhibits all or most of the following characteristic features:

i) Metabolism: Life requires energy to maintain the balance of its internal organization ('homeostasis') in a survival mode. Life consumes energy by breaking down the chemicals and converting them into cellular components ('anabolism'); it also decomposes the internal organic matter ('catabolism'). These vital processes are collectively known as 'metabolism'. Metabolism creates waste, when the underlying processes cease with no prospect of restarting, life is terminated resulting in death.

The role of metabolism in a living organism can be exemplified with a steam locomotive that feeds on coal or some other fuel. A locomotive burns the fuel, which enables it to perform work (moving forward). Like living things, the locomotive degrades the coal and exhausts heat into the environment.

ii) Homeostasis: The body expends its internal chemicals during metabolism and eventually 'replenishes' them back. However, the overall concentration of vital (species-specific) biochemicals in the body stays about the same or changes only in a gradual manner (eg. aging). Such internal maintenance of biochemicals at a steady state is referred to as *homeostasis* – the sign of a healthy body. Any significant deviation from the homeostasis, with chemical levels either above ('hyper') or below ('hypo') the steady state can trigger malfunction of several internal systems, which could lead to disorders, diseases and even dealth.

Therefore, homeostasis is a chemical monitoring system that keeps life in check from the inside. A living organism requires round the clock monitoring of the internal environment to maintain a constant metabolic state; for example, calcium levels are regulated in the body fluids or its excretion through urine to avoid *hypercalcemia*; melatonin levels are maintained to aid sleep and soothe the nerves; electrolyte concentration is balanced through various mechanisms (eg. sweating) to maintain body temperature.

iii) Growth: The quality of life also depends on the degree of variations that occur in an organism on a daily basis, which is simply known as 'growth'. Life needs to sustain a higher rate of biochemical (protein) synthesis than catabolism. A growing organism increases in size with all of its parts, rather than simply accumulating organic matter. An individual species begins to multiply and expand its own existence as the evolution continues to thrive.

More significant changes occur in the insect world, when a caterpillar acquires beautiful wings and alights on wild flora as a butterfly

In humans, a wide range of variation begins when life starts from a tiny single celled, 'fertilized egg' to reach a progressive growth phase with trillions of cells to form a multiple systems called – the physical body. Even in a simple bacterial cell, about a million functional molecules of 3,000 different types exist. Each of these molecular types perform a specialized function critical for sustaining life.

iv) Organization: Every life form, a tiny bacterium or a gigantic sperm whale, is structurally composed of one or more cells, which are the basic units of life. These cells need to communicate with each other and at the same time also check their milleu. These cellular efforts require tremendous networking, management and organization. Life evolves in an organized manner. Notably, simpler forms are succeeded by complex forms with greater organization.

v) Reproduction: The property of self-replication is the most fundamental aspect of life. Living organisms replicate either individually or in sexual pairs. Organisms have encoded set of instructions and a well geared up machinery to accomplish this replication. Reproduction can be the division of one cell to form two new cells for growth or creating a totally new offspring to propagate its own species. Usually the term is applied to the production of a new individual (*asexually*, from a single parent organism, or *sexually*, from at least two different parent organisms).

Evolution has provided each life form with reproductive instincts, despite ignorance about its own individual extinction through death, and that the partial extension of life through offspring is its only long term chance for survival. However, due to the randomness in sexual reproduction, the offspring resemble each parent only in certain attributes. Therefore, survival through children is only a partial and limited means of survival. Ultimately, everyone dies and limited survival through children is the best backup plan available.

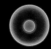

The lifespan of an organism widely differ from species to species. The quality of life is proportional to the average lifespan of an organism within a species. Since organisms always die eventually, and have continuance beyond death primarily only through offspring, the reproductive pattern of a species is of prime importance. Therefore, the quality of life might be proportional to the degree of resemblance between a parent and its offspring. Bacteria and viruses can reproduce their own copy more or less exactly. Since, higher organisms (eg. humans) reproduce sexually; none of the offspring exactly resembles either parent. Based on this criterion, it may appear that a virus is more alive than a human.

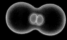

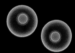

Do Automobiles Reproduce? Viruses are similar to automobiles in many ways. Automobiles contain a great deal of information and their body parts are put together in an assembly line; in a sense, to reproduce an exact copy. The assembly line of an automobile is what a living cell's biochemical machinery to a virus. The model of automobiles in the environment is driven by natural selection; basis for the evolution of electric, hybrid, fuel efficient diesel and gasoline engines. A fierce struggle for existence is also evident between different makes of automobiles; survival of the fittest, ultimately results in the mass production of Japanese, German or American cars in the environment.

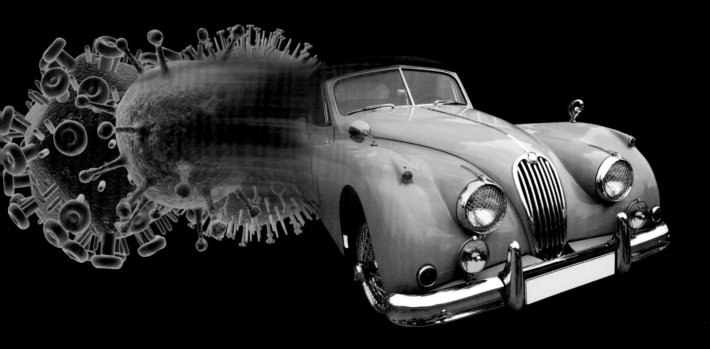

vi) Response to stimuli: A response to stimuli can take many forms, from the contraction of a unicellular organism to external chemicals, to complex reactions involving all the senses of a higher animal. A response is often expressed by motion, for example, the leaves of a plant turning toward the sun *(phototropism)* and a male sperm swimming towards the female egg *(chemotaxis)*.

Most plants react to light by bending toward it, and roots grow toward the pull of the earth's gravitational field, while stems preferentially grow away from it. Some plants move their leaves in response to touch. This is true of the 'Venus fly trap', which rapidly closes a pair of hinged leaves to trap insects.

Unicellular organisms show several kinds of behavioral responses to specific stimuli. For example, certain species of bacteria that contain particles of iron oxides in their cytoplasm preferentially orient themselves in certain directions when placed in weak magnetic fields.

vii) Adaptation: The ability to change over a period of time in response to the environmental influence is called 'adaptation'. This ability is fundamental to segway a living organism through the best possible evolutionary pathway. Adaptation is determined by the organism's heredity as well as the composition of metabolized substances, and external factors present.

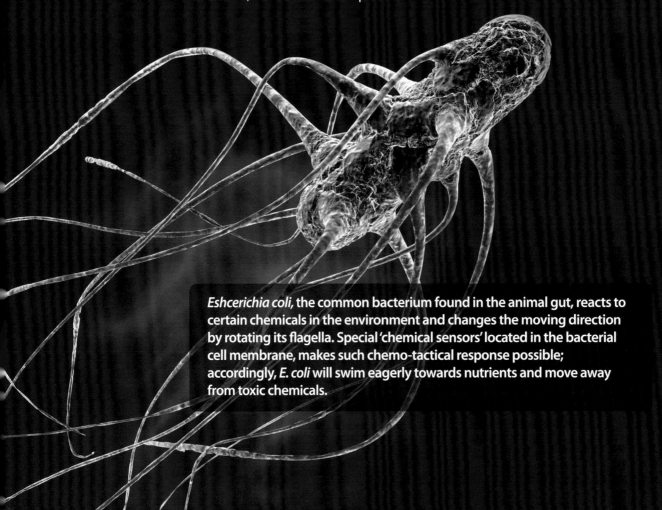

Eshcerichia coli, the common bacterium found in the animal gut, reacts to certain chemicals in the environment and changes the moving direction by rotating its flagella. Special 'chemical sensors' located in the bacterial cell membrane, makes such chemo-tactical response possible; accordingly, *E. coli* will swim eagerly towards nutrients and move away from toxic chemicals.

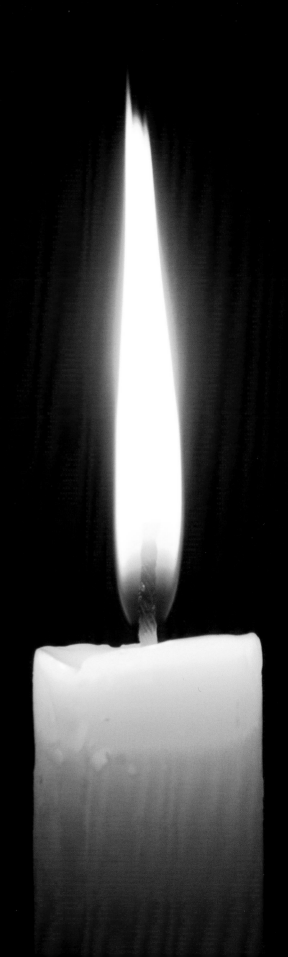

Flames
Are they alive?

If the systematic phenomenon of reproduction is removed from the list of vitality, then it may seem like the candle flames are living organisms! Flames 'eat' or consume fuel (candle tallow), and 'breathe' oxygen just like we do. The oxygen and fuel are burned (or rather metabolized) in a process similar to the underlying oxidation reaction that supplies humans with their energy. Flames can also grow in size, if the fuel is available in the nearby space and can move from place to place. There is something self-sustaining about flames, in the sense that, as the fuel burns, new fuel is continuously supplied and heated to the point where it can also burn. Schrödinger's definition, by itself, does not appear to exclude flames from the list of life.

Then why a candle flame can not be considered alive? Let the candle flame be compared with a living mouse. Both need fuel, however, when the candle runs out of wax, it is doomed. Whereas, the mouse when runs out of food, it just starts exploring until it finds some. This behavior is possible because the mouse doesn't have to feed at every moment, as the flame does. It can store up energy inside and use it to survive until it finds more food. Besides the risk of running out of fuel, there are other hazards that can affect the candle flame and the mouse. One can walk up to the candle flame and blow it out. But if one decides to trap the mouse from the enemy, it is a bit more difficult. Most likely, the mouse will run for cover to protect itself.

Living Cell (versus) Computer

The structural and functional features of a living cell can be explained at a basic level by drawing certain analogies with a computer – the most popular instrument of our modern times.

- Computers have coded instructions inside called 'programs'; which can be compared to genetic program *(code)* of the DNA within cells. The DNA is subdivided into functional units called 'genes'; these would correspond to 'files' in the computer.

- The programs in a cell and computer can both be copied and executed. The execution of protein synthesis by the genetic program would loosely match with the computer's paper printout.

- A cell can make a complete copy of itself; it contains the complete instructions *(software)* and the cellular machinery *(hardware)* necessary to duplicate itself. Nothing about the computer is even close to such cellular self replication. However, a computer may be able to reproduce its files by 'automatic full backup'. A computer that could clone itself would be more properly described as a 'self-replicating robot' - which is conceivable, but none exists today.

- Upgrading or changing a computer's format requires new programs. Sometimes, by just inserting a disc into a 'slot' or 'drive': the computer recognizes and downloads the new program *(code)* and applications. On the other hand, life evolves only when the cells adapt and reprogram, which is called 'mutation'. During mutation, living cells acquire, install and activate new genetic programs. The origin of new genetic software, its installation and activation is no less than pure magic!

- Like a living cell, a computer may also get infected with 'viruses' and may cause everything to crash. Both need protective *('anti-virus')* mechanisms to stay away from invading 'bugs' and for removing corrupted patches. A computer even has a metabolism: it consumes energy from an electrical outlet or a battery.

- A multi-cellular organism is like a network of computers. It requires an efficient 'server', especially while operating human systems with billions or trillions of cells. The nervous system and the hormonal system are two important network hubs.

- Finally, the single-cell organisms *(eg. bacteria)* and multi-cellular life forms *(eg. mammals)* can be compared with handheld calculators and desktop personal computers *(PCs)*, respectively. Like eukaryotes, PCs have huge memory capacity, intricate structure and elaborate networking capability.

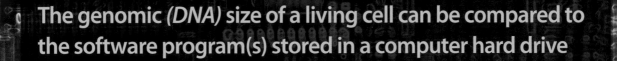

The genomic *(DNA)* size of a living cell can be compared to the software program(s) stored in a computer hard drive

Applying the Equation: 4 Nucleotides (DNA) = 8 bits = 1 byte

CELL TYPE	Corresponding Program Storage Capacity
E.coli **bacterium**	a handheld calculator with about 200 kilobytes
Yeast cell	a personal computer with 12 megabytes
Human cell	a personal computer with 1.5 gigabytes

Thus, a human body would correspond to a computer network of about 100x trillion PCs or more such units (each 1.5 G-bytes)

1.3 | What is **Aging?**

AGING is the biological deterioration of a human or animal over the sequential passage of time. Aging increases susceptibility to disease and vulnerability to toxic environmental conditions. It also leads to deterioration in mobility and flexibility. Aging, in and of itself is not a disease; but a natural process that is characterized by a decline in the resilience of the body's organs, that some scientists refer to this process as "biological entropy".

The signs and symptoms of aging do not surface overnight; this process is gradual, hardly noticeable and no two people experience this phenomenon in quite the same way. Body changes at a cellular level during an aging process, with deterioration of DNA, protein, and lipid molecules; all of which predispose to age-related diseases. Though it is not an implicit part of aging, the probability of a disease condition increases with age. In the continuing struggle between chemistry and biology, chemistry is always the short-term, tactical winner – death of the individual is inevitable. However, barring the extinction of species, biology is the long-term, strategic victor – life survives, and the struggle continues to adapt to adversity and evolve!

Aging theories cover the *genetic, biochemical,* and *physiological* properties of a typical organism, and the way these properties change with time. 1) *Genetic theories* deal with speculations regarding the identity of aging genes, accumulation of errors in the genetic machinery, programmed senescence, and telomeres. 2) *Biochemical theories* are concerned with energy metabolism, generation of free radicals, the rate of living, and the health of mitochondria. 3) *Physical theories* deal almost entirely with the endocrine system and the role of hormones in regulating the rate of cellular senescence. In the end, aging is a complex interaction of genetics, chemistry, physiology and behavior.

1) Genetic Theories of Aging

Genetic theory of aging is limited to the chromosomes in sperm and egg cells. The genes in the chromosome are passed down from generation to generation. However, certain changes may occur to these genes after inheritance, which cannot be passed down to the offspring. No matter what genes have been inherited, the body continuously undergoes complex biochemical reactions. Some of these reactions cause damage and ultimately age the body.

Genetic inheritance plays a significant role in aging. Each individual is born with a unique genetic code that predetermines the qualities of our physical and mental function. Genes also influence on how fast we age and how long we live. As if, each of us has a biological clock ticking away and set to go off with a pre-program to self-destruct the body, first to age and then to die. However, as with all aspects of the genetic inheritance the timing of this genetic clock is subject to enormous variation, depending on what happens during growth and on the actual lifestyle (the old *'nature versus nurture'* debate).

i) Programmed Theory: Dr August Weismann (1834–1914 AD) proposed the first programmed theory of aging. This theory postulates that aging and death are necessary parts of evolution. If a species is devoid of the genetic capacity for aging and death, then it would not be forced to replicate to survive. Individuals in the species would just keep on living until a climate or other changes wipe them all out. The key point here is that if biological individuals live forever, there would be no evolution. The purpose of this programmed elimination of old is to clean up the living space and to free up resources for younger generations.

Are we programmed to get old? If we are, is it like the program that guides our development from a single fertilized egg to a multi-cellular organism? Or is aging the unfortunate side effect of adaptations that make it possible for an organism to have and protect its offspring? Many scientists believe that aging is a matter of evolutionary neglect, rather than design.

ii) Hayflick Limit: In early 1960s, Dr Leonard Hayflick made one of the greatest contributions to the history of cellular biology by demonstrating the senescence of cultured human cells. Hayflick theorized that the aging process was controlled by a biological clock contained within each living cell. The 1961 studies concluded that human fibroblast cells (lung, skin, muscle, heart) have a limited life span. They divided approximately 50 times over a period of years and then suddenly stopped. Nutrition seemed to have an effect on the rate of cell division: overfed cells made up to 50 divisions in a year, while underfed cells took up to times as long as normal cells to make divisions. Alterations and degenerations occurred within some cells before they reached their growth limit. The most evident changes took place in the cell organelles, membranes and genetic material. This improper functioning of cells and loss of cells in organs and tissues may be responsible for the effects of aging.

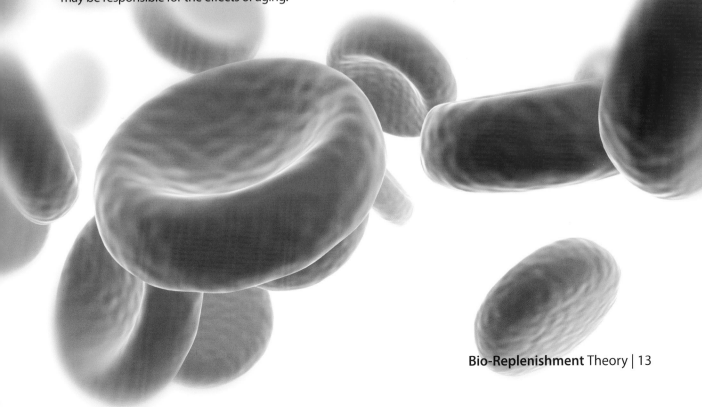

iii) Cellular Senescence: Human body is an amazing, open and a dynamic organism formed by the assembly of 12 organ systems. Each organ contains tissues designed for specific functions such as absorption and secretion. Tissues are made of cells that are formed together to perform those special functions. Each cell is made of smaller components called organelles, one of which is called the nucleus.

Cellular aging, or senescence, is analogus to a wind up clock. If the clock stays wound, a cell becomes immortal and constantly produces new cells. If the clock winds down, the cell stops forming new cells and dies.

The nucleus contains structures called chromosomes that are actually "packages" of all the genetic information that is passed from parents to their children. The genetic information or "genes" are a series of base pairs called Adenine *(A)*, Guanine *(G)*, Cytosine *(C)*, and Thymine *(T)*. These base pairs make up our cellular alphabet and create the sequences, or instructions needed to form our bodies. In order to grow and age, our bodies must duplicate their cells. This process is called mitosis. Mitosis is a process that allows one "parent" cell to divide into two new "daughter" cells. During mitosis, cells make copies of their genetic material. Half of the genetic material goes to each new daughter cell. To make sure that information is successfully passed from one generation to the next, each chromosome has a special protective cap called a *telomere* located at the end of its "arms". Telomeres are controlled by the presence of the enzyme telomerase.

2) Biochemical Theories of Aging

Error-based theories blame environmental insults to living organisms that induce cumulative damage at various levels as the cause of aging. One potential cause of senescence is the accumulation of mutations in DNA, eventually leading to the progressive loss of key genes.

The cells of our body continuously multiply from the time of conception. With each cell division, there is a possible risk that some of the genes are copied incorrectly – a phenomenon called *'mutation'*. Such mutations could also occur with exposure to toxins, radiation or ultraviolet light. The body can correct or eliminate most of these mutations, but not all of them. Eventually mutant cells could copy themselves and accumulate to cause problems to the bodily functions related to aging.

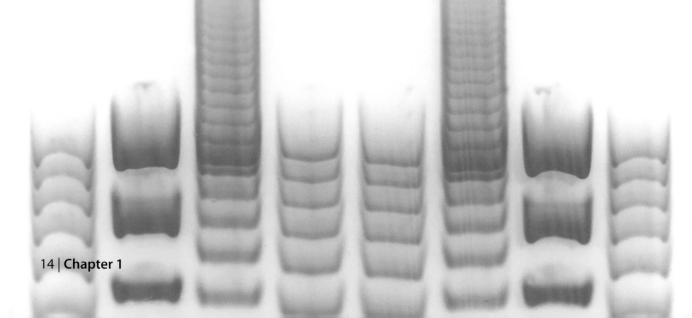

iv) Rate of Living Theory

In 1908, German physiologist Max Rubner found a link between metabolic rate, body size and longevity. Accordingly, he theorized that humans (or animals) are born with a limited amount of energy reserve. Utilization of energy at a slower pace decelerates the rate of aging process. On the other hand, any faster consumption of energy leads to an accelerated aging.

Other rate-of-living theories focus on limiting factors such as amount of oxygen inhaled or number of heartbeats spent. There is some evidence, when comparing species, that organism with faster oxygen metabolism die younger. Tiny mammals with rapid heartbeats metabolize oxygen quickly and have short lifespan. Tortoises, on the other hand, metabolize oxygen very slowly and have long lifespan.

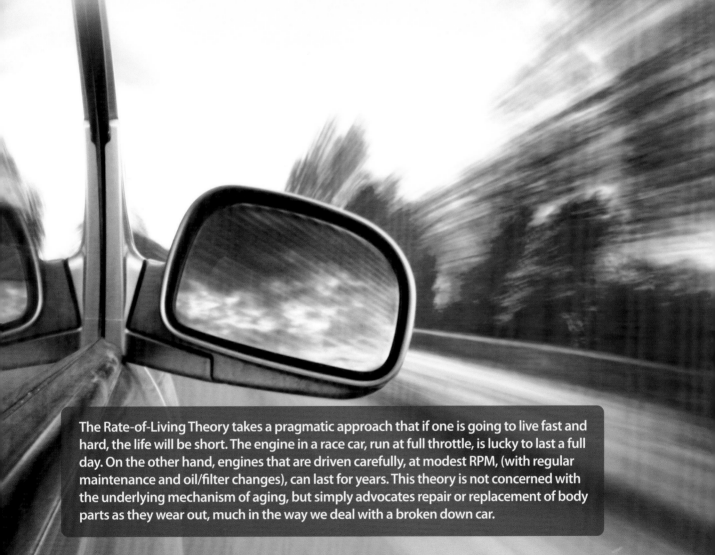

The Rate-of-Living Theory takes a pragmatic approach that if one is going to live fast and hard, the life will be short. The engine in a race car, run at full throttle, is lucky to last a full day. On the other hand, engines that are driven carefully, at modest RPM, (with regular maintenance and oil/filter changes), can last for years. This theory is not concerned with the underlying mechanism of aging, but simply advocates repair or replacement of body parts as they wear out, much in the way we deal with a broken down car.

Death, in general is an organized process, however, like the aging of a car, the rate of living for a human is a uni-directional phenomenon. Death is due to the failure of a specific system (cardiovascular, central nervous, gastro-intestinal, renal, pulmonary, etc). Like cars, our lifespan depends on genetics (make and model), nutrition (fuel), lifestyle (use), environment (exposure) and maintenance.

> *Human organs and tissues do not age at the same rate.* Irrespective of the chronological age, a human body is many years younger. In fact, though a person is middle aged, most of the individual's body could be just 10 years old or less! This amazing biological revelation is due to the fact that human body continuously replaces its cells; renews and repairs its tissue. Every seven years, 90 percent of the cells in the human body are brand new!

Recently, Dr Jonas Frisen (from the Karolinska Insitute, Sweden) postulated that the average age of all the cells in an adult human body could be as young as 7 to 15 years. Laboratory studies showed that cells from the rib muscles have an average age of 15.1 years. Though it may appear that the human body is fairly a permanent structure, most of it is in a continuous state of reorganization. In the process, old cells die and disappear (discarded), while new ones appear (generated) to take over the emptied sites in the body. Each type of tissue is programmed with a specific (pre-determined) turnover time, based on its workload and endurance. Cells that form the stomach lining last only 5 days. The red blood cells bruised and battered after roving nearly 1,000 miles through the maze of the body's circulatory system, max out their survival chances in about 120 days before being dispatched to their graveyard in the spleen. The epidermis, or surface layer of the skin, is replaced every 2 weeks. The rapid turnover of the epidermis is due to the fact that the skin layer works like a 'saran wrap' for the body, which can be easily damaged by scratching, solvents, wear and tear. Liver, the detoxifier of the body, confronts all the chemical poisons and drugs that enter the body through the digestive process. Due to the continuous chemical warfare, the lifespan of a liver is cut short for about 10 to 15 months.

Finally, other tissues have expiry dates measured in years, but are still far from immortal. Though bones have endured with evolutionary existence past the Jurassic era to fascinate the paleontologists; they undergo a non-stop makeover. The entire human skeleton is replaced in about every 7 years in adults, as two opposite cellular crews of 'bone-demolition' (dissolving) and bone-construction (rebuilding) work on a regular basis to remodel and shape the skeletal frame.

Brain cells from the visual cortex are truly exceptional; since they maintain exactly the same chronological age of an individual. *This cellular phenomenon is of galactic importance in order to make our memories last!* However, cells of the cerebellum are slightly younger than those of the cortex, which fits with the idea that this part of the brain does not cease its development after birth. The only parts that last a lifetime seem to be the neurons of the cerebral cortex, cells of the eye inner lens and the muscle cells of the heart.

Aging (Rate of Living) of an Automobile

In theory, the human aging can be compared with the wearing away of an automobile, which is also made of complex, multi-component systems. With time, it's major operating systems (engine, transmission, cooling, electrical, etc.) and sub-systems (fuel injector, driveshaft, radiator, battery, wheel bearings, etc.) gradually deteriorate as a result of chemical and physical damage, eventually leading to a critical failure. Barring serious accidents, most new cars last for 10–15 years, then disappear from the road. Despite the manufacturer's warranty, a new car may still fail in performance due to defective parts (like human congenital disorders). An extended manufacturer's warranty (like the *human health insurance policy*) and a comprehensive automobile insurance *(life insurance)* are precautious efforts. The death rate of a car reaches maximum at its mean lifespan, and the probability for the car to survive an extra year decreases with increasing usage and age.

Similar to that of humans, the aging *(rate of living)* of an automobile depends on numerous factors, including its make, model, design and manufacture *(genetics)*; maintenance, fuel *(nutrition)* and exposure *(environment)*. Like the humans, cars require increasing maintenance with age and stop working as a result of cumulative deterioration. Eventually, a critical component or system fails due to external challenges – overheating in the summer or difficulty in starting during the winter. Neither all of the components age (wear and tear) at the same rate, nor do they all fail simultaneously. The failure of any one component may be the decisive factor in the fate of the car.

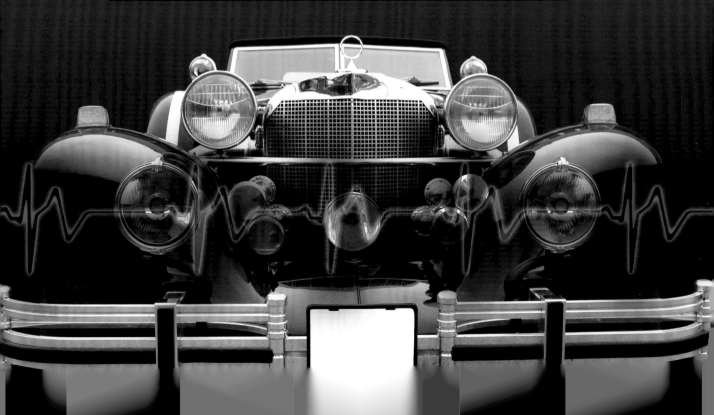

v) Free Radical Theory: Introduced by Dr Rebecca Gerschman in 1954, and developed by Dr. Denham Harman, this theory asserts that many of the changes that our bodies experience as we age are caused by free radicals. Damage to DNA, proteins and other biochemicals has been attributed to free radicals.

Free radicals are molecules that have an unpaired electron, which makes them highly reactive. One of the most important, the oxygen free radical, is a toxic exhaust produced by mitochondria during metabolic process called – *oxidative phosphorylation*. This process produces the ATP that cells need to survive. The oxygen free radical can remove an electron from virtually any molecule in the cell, including DNA, RNA, proteins and the lipids. When it does so, it triggers a chain reaction of destabilized molecules reacting with other molecules to form new free radicals and a variety of potentially dangerous compounds (similar to the nuclear chain reaction with a bomb). It has been postulated that free radicals are directly responsible for cellular senescence and the aging process.

Free radical damage to DNA is implicated in the causation of cancer and its effect on LDL cholesterol is very likely responsible for heart disease.

Free-radical damage begins at birth and continues until death. The extent of free radical damage is relatively low during youth, since the body has extensive repair and replenishment mechanisms to keep cells and organs in working order. However, with the progression of aging, the accumulated effect of free-radical damage consequently takes its toll. Free-radical activity can be compared to that of biochemical electricity, without which the body can not produce energy. The body's electricity enables the movement of muscles and transmission of nerve impulses.

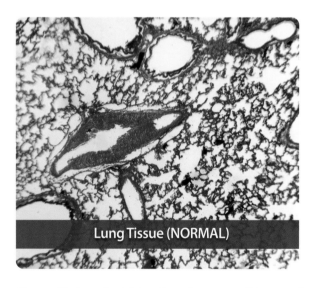

Lung Tissue (NORMAL)

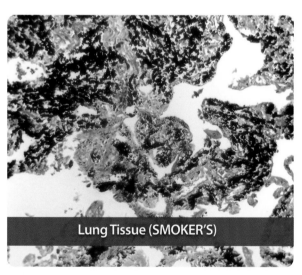

Lung Tissue (SMOKER'S)

One puff of smoke (cigarettes, cigars, marijuana, opium or crack) introduces about 375,000 free radicals into the lungs. One free radical in the wrong place at the wrong time – that all it can take to get lung cancer!

vi) Waste Accumulation Theory: During their lifespan, cells produce a lot of waste that needs proper elimination. This waste includes free radicals and various toxins, which when accumulated to a certain level, can interfere with normal cellular function and ultimately kill the cell. Evidence supporting this theory is the presence of a waste product called lipofuscin. Lipofuscin is formed by a complex reaction that binds the cellular proteins with fat. This waste accumulates in the cells as small granules and increases in size as a person ages. Excess of lipofuscins in the body cause darkening of the skin, known as the "aging spots." Lipofuscins interfere with the ability of cells to repair and multiply, disturb DNA and RNA synthesis, interfere with protein synthesis, lower energy levels, prevent the body from building muscle mass and destroy cellular enzymes that are needed for vital body functions. Cells that generally contain lipofuscin are nerve and heart muscle cells, both critical to life.

Lipofuscin slowly builds up with the aging process; therefore, it has been described as "the ashes of our dwindling metabolic fires"

vii) Mitochondria - the powerhouses in each human cell, have the crucial job of generating energy for use throughout the body. With the advancing age and cumulative free radical attack; however, mitochondria can become less efficient, leading to degenerative changes associated with aging.

Spread throughout the jelly-like cytoplasm within the cells, the mitochondrial count range from hundreds to thousands per cell. They generate energy in the form of ATP, an essential molecule for our survival. *They do so, however, at a price.* According to the mitochondrial theory of aging, free radicals are generated as a byproduct of aerobic respiration. Mitochondria are also one of the easiest targets of free-radical injury because they lack most of the defenses found in other parts of the cell. Progressive respiratory chain dysfunction follows; mitochondrial damage accumulates slowly, eventually this leads to degenerative changes associated with the aging.

Mitochondrion

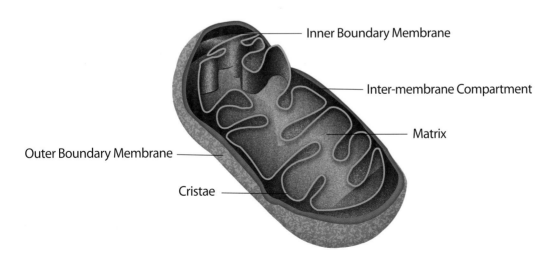

Inner Boundary Membrane

Inter-membrane Compartment

Matrix

Outer Boundary Membrane

Cristae

viii) Cross-linking Theory: Developmental aging and cross-linking were first proposed in 1942 by Johan Björksten. This theory has been applied to aging diseases such as sclerosis, a declining immune system and the most obvious example of cross-linking, is the loss of elasticity in the skin.

The cross-linking theory of aging is based on the observation that with age, proteins, DNA and other structural molecules develop inappropriate attachments or cross-links with one another. These unnecessary links or bonds decrease the mobility or elasticity of proteins and other molecules.

Cross-linking of the skin protein collagen has been shown to be at least partly responsible for wrinkles and other age-related changes to the skin. Cross-linking of proteins in the lens of the eye plays a role in age-related cataract formation. Researchers speculate that cross-linking of proteins in the walls of arteries or the filtering systems of the kidney account for at least some of the atherosclerosis (once called hardening of the arteries) and age-related decline in kidney function observed in older adults.

ix) Death Hormone Theory: Unlike other cells, neurons (brain cells) do not replicate. Humans are born with roughly 12 billion neurons and over a life time about 10 percent perish. Donner Denckle, an endocrinologist formerly at the Harvard University, was convinced that the "death hormone" or DECO (decreasing oxygen consumption hormone) released by the pituitary glands can revitalize the immune system, reduce the rate of cross-linking in cells, and restore the cardiovascular functions. Denckle suggested that with human aging the pituitary begins to release DECO and inhibits cellular ability to use thyroxine hormone. Thyroxine is critical in metabolic regulation; the rate at which cells convert food to energy. Thus, low metabolic rate triggers and accelerates the process of aging.

Skin - Cross Section

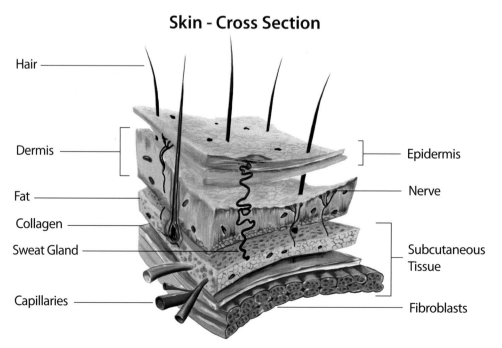

Hair

Dermis

Fat

Collagen

Sweat Gland

Capillaries

Epidermis

Nerve

Subcutaneous Tissue

Fibroblasts

x) Caloric Restriction (CR) Theory: CR or energy restriction is a theory proposed by gerontologist, Dr Roy Walford. After years of animal experiments and research on longevity, Walford suggested that under-nutrition with malnutrition could dramatically hamper the functional, if not the chronological aging process. He emphasized the importance of low calorie diet with moderate vitamin and mineral supplements coupled with regular exercise.

A starvation diet appears to increase the mean life span of an animal. CR is important from a theoretical point of view, but it is never likely to form a practical therapy. Industrialized nations in general find it difficult to maintain even modest shifts in eating habits. The typical CR diet that can reduce caloric intake to one-third of normal levels is not likely to attract a large following. However, CR experiments do highlight the importance of diet on the rate of aging, and this could at least encourage healthier, low-caloric eating habits.

An individual on the CR diet would lose weight gradually until a point where metabolic efficiency reaches its maximum health and life span.

3) Physical Theories of Aging

It is almost as though Mother Nature is saying, *"I will do what I can to get you up to your reproductive years, so you can have offspring, but after that you are on your own."* Being on our own has meant that our bodies begin to break down soon after the peak reproductive years have finished. The elderly can not run far, think as fast, or fight off infectious diseases nearly as well as they did when they were young. Physical appearances change dramatically with age. The hair turns gray, muscle mass declines, the ears get bigger, and the skin becomes thin and wrinkled. At a more subtle level, men and women approaching their 80s converge on a common physical appearance, men become more feminine and women become more masculine. In men, this trend becomes more apparent as the shoulders get narrower, hips broader, beard thinner, and the voice develops a higher pitch. In women, the shoulders become broader, the voice huskier, and hair begins to grow on the chin and upper lip.

Given its broad-spectrum of influence, it is no wonder the endocrine system has captured the attention of gerontologists, many of whom believe that aging of an organism as a whole begins with the senescence of the *hypothalamus*. In this sense, the hypothalamus is like a clock that regulates the rate at which the individual grows older. With the age-related failure of the command center, hormonal levels of the body begin to change, and this in turn produces the physical symptoms of age.

xi) Hormone or Endocrine Theory: Developed by Vladimir Dilman, this theory proposes that endocrine system is responsible for the aging process. Endocrine system controls the hormones that regulate many body processes. During the aging process, endocrine system becomes less efficient, leading to changes in the body such as menopause in women and andropause in men.

Hormone theory explains that endocrine changes eventually lead to several effects on aging. When hormone production decline with aging, it also slows down the body's ability to repair and regulate other internal systems. Hormone production is highly interactive; therefore, any drop in one hormone is likely to have a feedback effect on the entire endocrine system. Accordingly, other organs release lower levels of hormones with disastrous effects on body functions.

Hormone levels tend to be high among young individuals, accounting for among other things, menstruation in women and high libido in both sexes. *Growth hormones* that help in the formation of muscle mass, for example, drop dramatically with aging. As a result, an elderly person though has not gained weight; he or she is prone to an increase in the fat-to-muscle ratio. Hormonal changes are an integral part of aging. Whether they control the pace at which aging happens or are a consequence of other changes in the body is unknown.

xii) Thymic-Stimulation Theory: "Thymus is the master gland of the immune systems," says Alan Goldstein, at the George Washington University. The size of this gland reduces from about 250 grams at birth and then shrinks to around 3 grams by age 60. Scientists are investigating whether the disappearance of the thymus contributes to the aging process by weakening the body's immune system.

Studies have shown that thymic factors are helpful in restoring the immune system of children born without them as well as rejuvenating the poorly functioning immune systems of the elderly. Thymic hormones may also play a role in stimulating and controlling the production of neurotransmitters and brain and endocrine system hormones which means they may be the pacemakers of aging itself, as well as key regulators responsible for immunity.

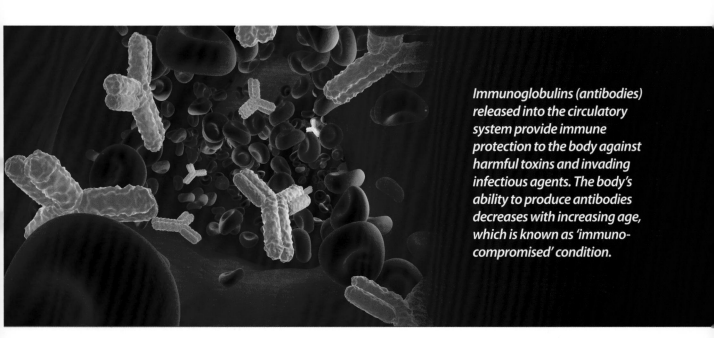

Immunoglobulins (antibodies) released into the circulatory system provide immune protection to the body against harmful toxins and invading infectious agents. The body's ability to produce antibodies decreases with increasing age, which is known as 'immuno-compromised' condition.

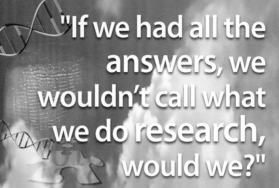

"If we had all the answers, we wouldn't call what we do research, would we?"

– Albert Einstein

A World without Aging

Imagine! If all age-related illnesses are eliminated and the vitality of the body is maintained indefinitely! Such an age-less world will face several issues of over population. Another problem with an unlimited lifespan is the compatibility of a 200-year-old to absorb new ideas. If not, we would have age differences in the mind instead of the body, which could lead to cultural stagnation. As German physicist Max Planck once put it, "A new scientific truth does not triumph by convincing its opponents and making them see the light, but rather because its opponents die, and a new generation grows up that is familiar with it."

Furthermore, there is a danger that dictators will remain in power much longer. Convicted criminals would eventually get released; since, they keep young bodies, could continue to pose a threat to the society. The 'Fountain of Youth' probably will trigger huge social reforms, and perhaps some bizarre situations: your children dating your grandparents' friends, for example; or your children looking younger than your great-grandchildren!

1.4 | What are **Building Blocks** of **Life?**

CELL is the basic unit of life. Every cell is enclosed by its own outer membrane and contains an array of instructions necessary for its operation, maintenance and reproduction. Every living cell uses an exclusive operating system, in which the *DNA makes RNA makes Protein*. DNA is a long complex nucleic acid that carries all vital instructions to operate the cell. During the cellular operation, DNA is transcribed into RNA – another long complex molecule similar to DNA; finally, the RNA transcript is translated into protein. There are hundreds of billions of different proteins used by living organisms – all of them are made from the same 20 amino acids, the *'building blocks of life'*.

Amino acids *(AAs)* play a central role both as building blocks of proteins and as intermediates in metabolism. Chemical properties of the AA determine the specific biological activity of a protein. Proteins not only catalyze all (or most) of the cellular reactions, they virtually regulate all vital processes in a living organism. Proteins make up the muscles, tendons, organs, glands, nails and hair. Growth, repair and maintenance of all cells are dependent upon them. Next to water, protein makes up the greatest portion of our body weight. There are two types of AA's.

i) Essential AAs are so called not because they are more important to life than the others, but because the body is unable to synthesize them, and so must be obtained from the diet. There are 8 AAs generally considered essential for humans: *phenylalanine, valine, threonine, tryptophan, isoleucine, methionine, leucine* and *lysine*. Tryptophan is essential for the body to create neurotransmitters *serotonin* and *melatonin*. Unlike fat and starch, the human body does not store excess AAs for later use; therefore, these amino acids must be provided through food every day. Failure to obtain enough, even 1 of the 8 essential AAs has serious health implications and can result in degradation of the body's proteins. Muscle and other protein structures may be dismantled (degraded) to obtain the one amino acid that is needed.

Plants can make all 20 amino acids. Humans do not have the necessary processes to make 8 of the 20 amino acids. Therefore, human life has an obligate dependence on plants.

ii) Non-essential AAs are the remaining 12 AAs humans can produce: *alanine, arginine, asparagine, aspartic acid, cysteine, glutamic acid, glutamine, glycine, histidine, proline, serine* and *tyrosine*. Tyrosine is produced from phenylalanine (essential AA), so if the diet is deficient in phenylalanine, tyrosine needs to be supplemented through the diet. Cysteine (or sulfur-containing amino acids), tyrosine (or aromatic amino acids), histidine and arginine are additionally required by infants and growing children. In addition, the amino acids arginine, cysteine, glycine, glutamine, histidine, proline, serine and tyrosine are considered 'conditionally essential', meaning they are not normally required in the diet, but must be supplied exogenously to specific populations that do not synthesize it in adequate amounts.

TABLE : *Recommended Daily Allowance (RDA = mg/kg body weight) for essential AAs (highlighted in light blue rows) in adult humans according to the World Health Organization (WHO) guidelines*

Amino Acid	Symbol	Abbr.	RDA*	Works with	Augments
Alanine	A	Ala			
Arginine	R	Arg		Zinc	Immunity, Healing, Muscles
Aspargine	N	Asn			Central nervous system
Aspartic acid	D	Asp			Central nervous system, Brain
Cysteine	C	Cys		B6, Vitamin - E	Skin, Hair
Glutamic acid	E	Glu		Vitamin - B6	Brain
Glutamine	Q	Gln			Brain
Glycine	G	Gly		GABA, taurine	Body protein
Histidine	H	His			Blood, Allergy, Sex
Isoleucine	I	Ile	20		Muscles
Leucine	L	Leu	39		Blood, Muscles, Hormone
Lysine	K	Lys	30	Calcium	Triglycerides
Methionine	M	Met	15	Selenium, Zinc	Hair, Skin, Chelator
Phenylalanine	F	Phe	25	Vitamin - B6	Depression
Proline	P	Pro		Vitamin - C	Collagen, Elastin
Serine	S	Ser		Choline	Blood sugar
Threonine	T	Thr	15		Collagen, Tooth enamel
Tryptophan	W	Trp	4		Depression
Tyrosine	Y	Tyr		Vitamin - B6	Thyroid
Valine	V	Val	26		Muscles

* RDA for children aged 3 years and older is 10% to 20% higher than adult levels and those for infants can be as much as 150% higher in the first year of life

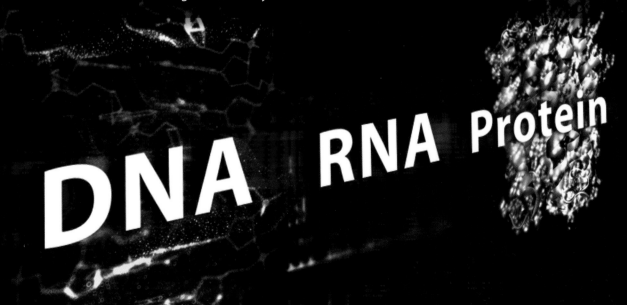

1.5 | What is **Bio-Replenishment?**

LIFE is a member of the class of phenomena that are open or continuous systems able to decrease its internal *entropy* at the expense of substances or *free energy* obtained from the environment and subsequently rejected in a degraded form. Specific chemical reactions result in biological transformation and adaption of life with its environment. These biological processes collectively refer to as 'metabolism'. **The innate ability of a living organism to continuously refill its expended (depleted) chemicals that are vital to maintain homeostasis and negative entropy, while aging is 'Bio-Replenishment'.** Any breakdown in bio-replenishment process can lead to cellular dysfunction, system failure and in severe cases even death.

Living organisms are not perfect. Through internal breakdowns, errors, insufficient skill or strength, or sheer bad luck; eventually their vital processes crash, leading to disease or death.

Therefore, life is based on chemical systems that respond to environmental changes, in order to promote its own survival, growth and multiplication. Aging provides an interesting perspective about living systems. All the apparent regularities in the growth of an organism fluctuate around average normal values. During human growth, concentration(s) of vital organic matter progressively change over time as the body passes from infancy into adulthood and decays during old age.

Survival

Survival of an organism is threatened by various external factors; however, such threat do not always remain inside the body. Disease causing agents, such as bacteria or viruses often infect the system. In higher organisms (eg. humans), the immune system battles such invaders to defend the body. At times, the immune system also attacks the body's own cells if they become cancerous. Besides handling such external threats, the

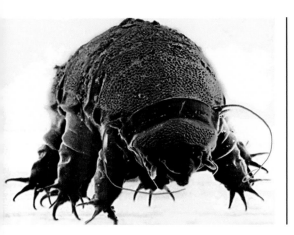

MYSTERIES OF SURVIVAL: The tiny creatures, known as tardigrades or water bears, are certainly strange-looking with their eight chubby legs, little claws and probing heads. They are the toughest life forms that exist in nearly all ecosystems on the planet. Water bears are virtually indestructible even if they are boiled, frozen, squeezed under pressure or desiccated. When dehydrated, they enter into a dormant state in which the body contracts and metabolism ceases. In this death-like dormant state, water bears manage to retain the structures in their cells until water is available to 'reactivate'. In fact, they can be completely dried out for years - and then spring back to life as if nothing had happened.

body must also coordinate with many internal processes during the course of its day-to-day functions.

Several human activities have no obvious bearing on survival. Humans eat because of hunger, not with any intent of biological necessity to survive. However, the instinct to eat when hungry is one of many behaviors that promote survival. Intellectual understanding of nutrition, physiology and health does not necessarily change human behavior to improve chances of survival. For instance, individuals tend to eat more and exercise less; a human behavior that is totally against good health. Presumably, in the old times food supply was irregular and the necessity to perform physical activity was compulsory, therefore, the survival instincts were high among our ancestors.

According to Schrödinger, the energy content of food that we eat does matter. Energy is essential to replace not only the mechanical energy of the bodily exertions; but also the heat that continually releases into the environment. Release of heat energy by the body is not accidental, but essential. Accordingly, in a precise manner, the body disposes surplus entropy that is continuously generated during physical life processes. Burning calories is an essential thermodynamic phenomenon in a biological system.

Food is not simply a source of energy (calories); it is also a source of chemicals for the body to build tissues and perform repairs. However, from a thermodynamic standpoint, food needs to be destroyed before a body can process and assimilate its chemical components. In general, humans eat something only after it is dead (eating anything that is *live,* such as a harmful bacteria or parasite is otherwise called 'infection'). Sequentially, the food is chopped into pieces, cooked, and chewed into a mashed pulp before being swallowed. The digestive process then breaks down several complex organic chemicals (eg. *proteins, carbohydrates and lipids*) into simpler forms (eg. *amino acids, sugars and fatty acids*) to allow assimilation by the body. All proteins are broken down into amino acids and reassembled into proteins of an assimilating body. Thus, the body consumes matter (mostly other life forms) from its environment; destroys most of the order in this matter to produce building blocks that are then absorbed and rearranged into the body's preexisting chemicals (order).

Eating is so common that we tend to forget what a magical process digestion is. We eat chicken, and yet, we do not become chicken. The chicken is transformed into us!

A clear distinction can be drawn between body's exchange of organic matter (chemical nutrients) from its environment and the *bio-replenishment*. Food undergoes a breakdown and transformation through body's assimilation process. *On the other hand, bio-replenishments are body's own chemicals that regulate the essential steps of an assimilation process and maintain the internal order ('homeostasis and negative entropy').*

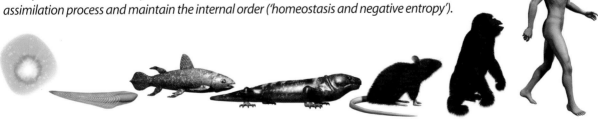

Growth

Growth is an integral part of the living process, during which the body transforms on a continuous basis, also known as 'aging'. On a microscopic level, chemical composition of the body constantly changes during growth. On a macroscopic level, the physical body renovates with each voluntary or involuntary action (*eg.* walking, breathing, and eating). Body alterations are often in response to lifestyle practices, nutritional and environmental conditions; however, the cumulative effect of these external factors on the final structural transformation of a body is unpredictable.

But how a living organism can sustain growth when there is an ongoing decay due to chemical disintegration? The assimilation process (eating, drinking, breathing, digestion, etc.) can only exchange chemical nutrients from its environment; for which the technical term is *metabolism* (the Greek word means 'change' or 'exchange') is used. However, the mere bio-availability of nutrient chemicals (or building blocks) could neither prevent life from decay nor support growth without several innate reactions. Several innate biochemicals are expended through a cascade of internal pathways for the integration of building blocks into the specific blue print of an organism. Calcium metabolism, for example, will strengthen the internal skeleton when accessed by a human blue print; while the same elemental calcium is exchanged differently to form an outer shell in a snail's blue print. The regulation of a physiological blue print is accomplished with molecules specific for each individual species; and these molecules are continuously expended in renovating the biological parts such as the human bone or shell of a snail. Adequate reserves and continuous supply of these regulatory molecules are essential for the growth and survival of a living organism.
Bio-replenishment of these regulatory molecules gradually decreases with growth and aging. Failure to supply adequate amounts of a bio-replenishment to meet the growing biological demand could result in bodily dysfunction disease or death.

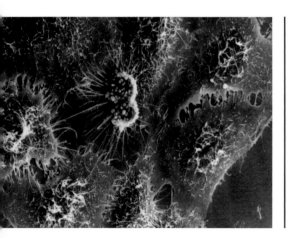

MYSTERIES OF MULTIPLICATION: 'HeLa' cells (from the cervix of Henrietta Lacks, a woman who lived in Washington, D.C.) continue to be grown in several laboratories around the world, despite Lane's death from cervical cancer in the 1950's. In scientific terms, HeLa cells are still alive, but Henrietta Lane is not. This is an interesting example of an individual who is not alive, but her constituent parts are continuing to reproduce, for over half a century! In fact, dead bodies in general should be considered living, at least until decay destroys the internal structures of the cells. Tissue culture is a well developed technology, frequently used in skin grafting and hair transplant procedures.

Humans do not have any characteristics that are perfectly regular; therefore, any signs of growth and aging are highly variable. For instance, body temperature fluctuates around an average, body height varies on a daily basis, due to compression of the vertebral column; ears and nose continue to grow randomly during adulthood, and eyes may be bloodshot one day and clear the next.

Human DNA can develop frequent genetic errors; although various correction mechanisms in the cell take care of this problem. Uncontrollable cell growth with inadequate bio-replenishment could also lead to life-threatening condition known as 'cancer'.

Multiplication

Multiplication is a cellular mechanism; while *autopoiesis* is fundamental for survival and growth of an organism. 'Autopoiesis' refers to continuous process of self synthesis, without which, life can not self-sustain – it will die. *Bio-replenishment is a critical part of 'autopoiesis'.*

Sexual reproduction (multiplication) is a costly process. Cellular energy must be expended to construct special reproductive cells and structures (sperm, egg, fallopian tubes, uterus, etc.). Courtship behavior, hormones, colors, scents must be developed. Reproductive timing, finding and recognizing mates, sperm and egg availbility at the same time must occur. The developing embryo and young must be cared for, often for years or decades!

In humans, the process of gastrulation takes place very early during the development of the embryo. This process reorganizes the embryonic cells into 3 layers: ectoderm, endoderm, and mesoderm. The ectoderm forms the skin and the central nervous system; the mesoderm gives rise to the cells from which blood, bone, and muscle are derived; and the endoderm forms the respiratory and digestive tracts

Human body is made of numerous living cells – each capable of self-replication. Many human cells can multiply both in the body as well as in a laboratory *(see figure on pg. 28)*. Cell multiplication endows the body with a power to repair and heal the damaged tissues. The ability to self-repair is essential for overall health. For example, the human body gets a new stomach lining every 5 days, a new liver every 10 to 15 months, and the skin substitutes itself every 2 weeks. This non-stop cellular replacement is accomplished with 'multiplication'. The human body demands a continuous input of chemical energy and nutrients (food) to fulfill several vital processes.

One of life's great dramas: the development of an offspring in the image of its parents

Cellular multiplication involves feedback mechanisms. In other words, internal processes of growth are regulated according to the necessity. Negative feedback is a key component by which the organism coordinates its internal systems and promotes homeostasis. Any failure in these vital process manifest as visible effects of aging, such as wrinkles, and invisible ones, such as deterioration of the heart and eyes, are due to inadequate revitalizing chemicals (bio-replenishment). Aging and cumulative damage to the body is, therefore, the result of a balance between the rates of cellular multiplication, exposure and turnover of regulatory molecules (bio-replenishments). **The half-life or lifespan of a bio-replenishment is an important determinant of the extent of chemical aging and over all life expectancy of a living organism.**

Naidu
Bio-Replenishment
Theory

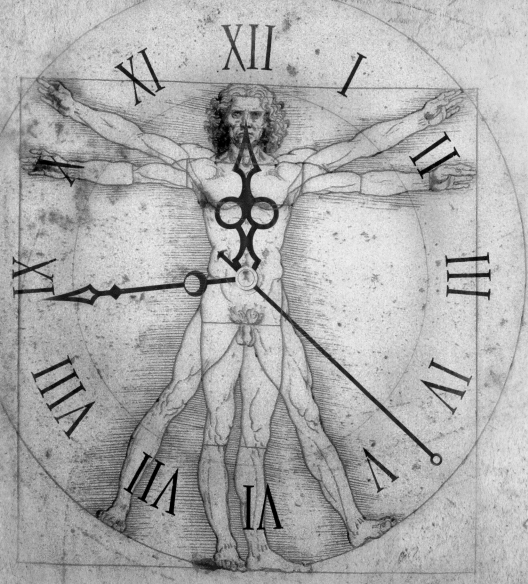

Genotype is the inheritable data and *phenotype* is the physical and functional design of a species. Living organisms reproduce and transfer data about their designs to their descendents. The descendents are enabled to construct themselves in a similar design as their parents. Bio-Replenishment supports the construction, repair and maintenance of a species following the genetic blue print.

LIFE is an organized chemical system founded on three gases that are abundant in the universe, namely, hydrogen *(H)*, oxygen *(O)* and nitrogen *(N)*; and a fourth element that replicates life with precision using an organic 'carbon *(C)*' copy process. The H, O, N, and C are distinguished from all other elements essential for life in several ways: they make up the bulk of organic matter, they are common to all proteins, and their entry, exit, or both is in gaseous state in most organisms. Specific interaction of H, O, N, and C with other minerals (i.e. iron, phosphorus, sulfur, calcium) results into a 'mass-energy transformer' called cell – the fundamental unit of life.

Mortality isn't just ashes to ashes, dust to dust; from a biochemical perspective it is also gas to gaseous.

Energy is at the root of all life forms and the driving force underlying each single biochemical reaction. Every cell needs energy for its survival, growth and multiplication. Most of the energy is used for the synthesis ('anabolism') of new molecules such as proteins and for the breakdown ('catabolism') of large compounds such as carbohydrates into simple sugars. In order to sustain the threshold of life, cells need to recharge their energy supply on a regular basis by using oxygen for fuel oxidation ('metabolism').

Energy is captured, contained and expended via covalent bonds. Such covalent (phosphate-phosphate) bonds form high-energy compounds such as adenosine diphosphate *(ADP)* and adenosine triphosphate *(ATP)*. *ATP has therefore been known as the energy currency for cellular metabolism.* The amount of bio-available energy from ATP is related to the difference in energy levels between the end-product and substrate of the reaction is called the *change in Gibbs free energy (ΔG)*. In cells, the ΔG for ATP production from fuel oxidation must be greater than the ΔG of the energy-requiring processes, such as protein synthesis or muscle contraction, for life to continue.

The 'life motor' keeps running until the internal batteries (ΔG) of its recalibrated cells are good enough to sustain metabolism in auto-mode.

Cellular metabolism is a continuous process and its maintenance requires higher entropy due to increased energy demand. *For example: A new house requires less maintenance while an inhabited house requires more recycling and up keeping.* Cell, like a lithium battery, could recharge only for limited cycles until its functional and organizational abilities dwindle down or discharge – it simply dies. The rate at which a cell dies (or lives) is dependant on the functionality of its internal parts, its inter-cellular communication skills to regulate patterns of growth and differentiation, and the cumulative damage (wear and tear) that occurred during its functional performance over a period of time. Recalibration of cellular metabolism of old cells through internal repair and regeneration of new cells to replace old ones is highly critical for the survival of a living organism.

Sensation of hunger and thirst are homeostatic mechanisms that help maintain optimum levels of energy, nutrients, and water.

Bio-Replenishment Theory elucidates the intricate relationship between cellular homeostasis and entropy as a function of time (aging). Aging and natural death probably arose with the development of multi-cellular life. Treatment for aging could result in delaying or relieving age-related diseases that now kill more than 80 percent of the people who die in the developed world and substantially extend the length and quality of countless lives.

Bio-Replenishment and Homeostasis

Life systems can function only within a narrow range of milieu conditions as temperature, pH , ion concentrations, and nutrient availability. Yet, organisms tend to survive the adversities of an unpredictable environment. *Homeostasis is the maintenance of equilibrium, or steady-state conditions, in a living system with automatic (self-regulating) mechanisms that counteract influences driving toward imbalance.*

Homeostatic mechanisms in living systems operate at molecular, cellular, tissue and organ/system levels. In humans, homeostasis involves constant monitoring and regulation of numerous factors, including the gases oxygen and carbon dioxide, nutrients, hormones, and organic and inorganic substances. The concentrations of these substances in body fluid remain unchanged, within limits, despite changes in the external environment.

Several environmental pollutants and life style factors can trigger homeostatic imbalance

Homeostasis is maintained by the endocrine system with the help of hormones, which are often produced in opposing pairs, for example, *insulin* and *glucagon*. Both are produced by the pancreas. *Insulin* is released in response to high blood sugar, and it signals cells (especially in the liver and in skeletal muscle) to take up glucose (thus reducing blood sugar). *Glucagon* is released in response to low blood sugar, and it signals cells (especially in the liver) to release glucose to the blood (thus increasing blood sugar). If homeostasis is not maintained, the sugar metabolism becomes disordered, which can lead to illness of the entire body (diabetes). Any endocrine failure to maintain homeostasis may lead to death or a disease, a condition known as *homeostatic imbalance.*

Introduction of over 100,000 synthetic chemicals during the past century alone, profoundly impacted every organism on the Blue Planet, including the human race. The occurrence of endocrine disrupting chemicals *(EDC)* in food and water supplies has sparked off global emergence of *Sex Hormonal Dysfunctions*, including disorders of sex development or intersex disorders *(eg. hermaphroditism)*, hypogonadism *(eg. ovarian or testicular failures)*, gender identity dysfunction, disorders of the puberty *(delayed or precocious puberty)*, menstrual or fertility dysfunction, etc. The dietary and lifestyle practices have turned into major etiological factors for obesity, diabetes, cardiovascular diseases, thyroid disorders *(eg. goiter, hypothyroidism)*, respiratory *(eg. asthma)* and gastrointestinal *(eg. celiac, inflammatory bowel diseases)* illnesses, various types of tumors and a myriad of metabolic bone diseases *(eg. osteoporosis, rickets, osteomalacia, and Paget's disease)*.

Based on the laws of entropy everything goes from an ordered to a less ordered state with passage of time. Aging is an example of entropy, therefore, a fundamental property of life.

Homeostasis is an integral part of the bio-replenishment process, which helps the body to achieve: i) proper amounts of gases, ions, nutrients and water; ii) maintain the optimal internal temperature and; iii) sustain optimal fluid volume for the health of cells. However, the functional scope of bio-replenishment is more than homeostasis. Biological systems need repair, replacement and refurbishing of the worn out organelles on a regular-basis to sustain life. There are many obvious examples for such phenomenon. For example, fingernails, hair and claws grow to refurbish the worn body parts. Teeth are replaced in many animals. Damaged tissue heals (to certain extent, the repair process varies from species to species). Some life forms can totally replace a lost limb. Cells that are subject to rapid damage and degradation such as the erythrocytes in the blood, epithelial cells in the skin, mucosal cells in the stomach lining, osteocytes in the bone are continuously replaced. Bio-replenishment is an intricately designed "biological maintenance program" that operates beyond diet and nutritional supplementation. If indeed an animal needed significant resources to self-regulate, perform maintenance and repair functions why would it not simply eat more to provide those resources? Therefore, the bio-replenishment is obvious.

Basal metabolic rate *(BMR)* is the amount of energy used by a human body under normal resting conditions. In this resting state, the oxygen consumption is about 200-250 mL per minute, which could fuel an average 70 kg (154 lbs) adult body to burn nearly 60-72 calories of energy per hour. In effect, this is essentially the minimum amount of energy needed to sustain human life. BMR (energy) is critical for the maintenance of body temperature, powering the heartbeat, breathing, and performing other organ functions. An average person's BMR accounts for about two-thirds of the energy expended in the body. Heredity, height, body composition, and age determine the BMR of an individual. About 70% of total energy spent in the human body is due to vital processes within the organs (i.e. liver 27%, brain 19%, skeletal muscle 18%, kidneys 10%, heart 7%, and other organs 19%); about 20% of energy is used for physical activity and the remaining 10% for thermogenesis, or digestion of food. All of these processes require an intake of oxygen along with coenzymes to provide energy for survival (usually from macronutrients like carbohydrates, fats, and proteins) and expel carbon dioxide. **On average, the human body reduces its energy expenditure by about 12 calories every year after the age of 30; a decline of about120 calories every decade. This is mainly due to changes in body composition that occur with aging.**

Bio-Replenishment and Entropy

DNA and protein, the indispensable components of every cell, are exclusively made by and for living organisms. Both types of molecules are much more energy and information rich than their chemical precursors. Thus, the *Gibbs free energy (ΔG)* of living systems is quite high relative to the simple compounds from which they are formed. In humans, the ΔG is derived from eating high energy biomass ("food"), either plant or animal source. Digested food provides a renewable source of energy and raw materials ("biological blocks"). In order to handle biomass from other species as raw materials for its own biological blueprint, life would require more than just a continuous flow of ΔG. It also needs specific innate factors to regulate a highly complex bio-engineering (construction and demolition) process – influenced by genetics, age and environment.

Bio-Replenishment Theory elucidates the nature of regulatory molecules in reversible and irreversible mode of metabolic activities. The reversible pathways in living organisms operate by feed-back mechanism(s) to maintain a steady-state metabolism as a function of optimal 'survival' mass (or concentration), the homeostasis. This biological phenomenon is in line with Schrödinger's postulate that *life is a result of 'negative entropy'.* On the other hand, irreversible pathways force a living system to move forward as a function of optimal 'reproductive' time (or aging), the *senescence*. This aspect of biology conforms to the 2nd law of thermodynamics that *the entropy of an isolated system will tend to increase over time, approaching a maximum value at equilibrium* (in metabolic term – cellular death). Therefore, Bio-Replenishment plays a conservative role in renewable use of ΔG by pushing back negative entropy to keep an organism alive by maintaining homeostasis; simultaneously, Bio-Replenishment takes an assurance role to keep the *basal metabolic rate (BMR)* at optimum while aging.

All organisms on Earth have extensive common chemistry and biology. However, the differences between species are the result of genetic evolution.

Bio-Replenishment and Aging

Aging is considered as a progressive failure of – *homeostasis* involving genes for the maintenance and repair, stochastic events leading to molecular damage and molecular heterogeneity, and involuntary events determining the probability of death.

Human aging is manifested in changes to the body, reduced sexual vigor and reproductive capacity. Some age-related human diseases involve processes that are plausibly a simple function of chronology with time-sequential deterioration of the body. For instance, certain heart diseases involve buildup of deposits in blood vessels, which gradually increase with passage of time. Since maintenance and repair of physiological systems comprise homeostasis, aging can be considered as a progressive decrease in homeodynamic space mainly due to increased molecular heterogeneity.

Diseases that kill large numbers of people such as heart disease, cancer, and stroke all have incidences that are very highly related to age. Global surge in synthetic chemicals, environmental toxicity and stressed lifestyle could induce rapid aging. Reversal of rapid aging symptoms with bio-replenishments could be a possible solution.

Bio-Replenishment and Cellular Program

DNA is the common denominator to all cellular forms. Human DNA is packed with 23 pairs of chromosomes, holding approx. 100,000 genes (around 3 billion base pairs), encoding instructions to make amino acids (the biological 'building' blocks essential for life). Living organisms are unique; they reproduce and transfer information about their designs to their descendents. The descendents are enabled to self-construct in such a way that they have the same or similar design as their parents. Genetic program theories view aging as a biological clock that ticks from early stages of development through growth and puberty. Life span is the result of both genetic and lifestyle factors.

Genotype is the inheritable data of an organism; and phenotype is the physical and functional design of a species.

When cells (for example RBC count in the blood) drop to a certain low ('threshold'), the living system regenerates new cells, which is called *autopoiesis*. The minimum time required to signal autopoiesis is the *threshold time* (T_t). The Bio-Replenishment Theory postulates that during an aging process, the cells of *younger population* can withhold autopoiesis; which means, the T_t for signaling cellular regeneration can be postponed in response to slow cellular death. This is due to adequate bio-replenishment that facilitates repair and maintenance of homeostasis in cellular systems. However, cellular senescence with prolonged toxic insults and accumulated damage, *older population* is forced to respond quickly to its dwindling cell numbers, this eventually shortens the T_t for autopoiesis. Incidence of cancer in aging population is a striking example to this cell signaling phenomenon.

The kinetics of *Bio-Replenishment* (K_{BR}) is dependent on several intrinsic (i.e. genetic program, rate of living) and external (i.e. food and environment) factors of an organism. In general, K_{BR} is equal or higher than the *threshold time* ($K_{BR} > T_t$) in a young normal living system. The, K_{BR} value is expected to decrease gradually with increase in chronological age, as opposed to the T_t values (which rise with senescence). The, K_{BR} value can not be augmented against 'normal aging', which is a function of intrinsic (i.e. genetic program and rate of living) factors. However, the, K_{BR} value can be amplified with *exogenous bio-replenishment* to reverse 'rapid aging' that can be triggered by external (i.e. food and environment) factors. In conclusion, when the kinetics of bio-replenishment regression against threshold time (i.e. $K_{BR} < T_t$); dysfunction, disease or death may result depending on the extent of decline in the Bio-Replenishment value.

> **Bio-Replenishment Theory** elucidates the function of regulatory molecules in reversible and irreversible mode of metabolic activities, while maintaining homeostasis and negative entropy. Bio-Replenishment is an intricately designed "biological maintenance program" that keeps the human basal metabolic rate (BMR) at optimum, while aging.

1.1 | WHAT IS A **THEORY?**

1. Avery J (2003). *Information Theory and Evolution*. World Scientific. ISBN 9812383999.
2. Bengston VL, Schaie KW, Editors (1999) *Handbook of Theories of Aging*. New York: Springer Publishing. ISBN 082611234X.
3. Coveney PV, Fowler PW (2005) Modelling biological complexity: A physical scientist's perspective. *Journal of the Royal Society Interface*. 2 (4):267–280.
4. Groves CP (2008) *A Theory of Human and Primate Evolution*. Oxford: Clarendon Press. ISBN 0198576293

1.2 | WHAT IS **LIFE?**

1. Capra F (1997) *The Web of Life*. New York: Anchor Books. ISBN 0-385-47676-0
2. Haldane JBS (1949) *What Is Life?* London: Lindsay Drummond. ASIN: B0006DINBE
3. Korzeniewski B (2001) Cybernetic formulation of the definition of life. *Journal of Theoretical Biology*. 209 (3):275–286.
4. Lovelock J (2000). Gaia: *A New Look at Life on Earth*. Oxford: Oxford University Press. ISBN 0-19-286218-9.
5. Margulis L, Sagan D (1995) *What is Life?* Berkeley: University of California Press. ISBN 0-520-22021-8.
6. Orgel LE (1973) *The Origins of Life: Molecules and Natural Selection*, John Wiley and Sons, Inc. ISBN 978-0471656920
7. Panno J (2007) *The Science of Aging*. New York: Checkmark Books. ISBN 0-8160-6930-1
8. Schrödinger E (1944) *What is Life? The Physical Aspect of the Living Cell*. Cambridge University Press. ISBN 0-521-42708-8.
9. Whittaker RH (1969). New concepts of kingdoms of organisms. *Science* 163:150–160.

1.3 | WHAT IS **AGING?**

1. Baynes JW (2000) From life to death – the struggle between chemistry and biology during aging: the Maillard reaction as an amplifier of genomic damage. *Biogerontology* 1:235-246.
2. Beckman KB, Ames BN (1998) The free radical theory of aging matures. *Physiological Reviews* 78:547–581.
3. Cutler RG, Rodriquez H, Editors (2002) *Critical Reviews of Oxidative Stress and Aging*. (Vol. 2). ISBN 978-981-02-4636-5 & 6
4. de Grey ADNJ (2003) *The Mitochondrial Free Radical Theory of Aging*. Landes Bioscience ISBN 1587061554
5. Gavrilov LA, Gavrilova NS (2001) The reliability theory of aging and longevity. *Journal of Theoretical Biology* 213:527-545.
6. Gershon D (1999) The mitochondrial theory of aging: is the culprit a faulty disposal system rather than indigenous mitochondrial alterations? *Experimental Gerontology*.34:613-619.
7. Kowald A (2001) Mitochondrial theory of aging. *Biological Signals and Receptors*10:162-175.
8. Le Bourg É (1998) Evolutionary theories of aging: handle with care. *Gerontology* 44:345-348.
9. Mattson MP, Editor (2001) *Telomerase, Aging and Disease*. Elsevier.ISBN 0-444-50690-X.
10. Morley AA (1995) The somatic mutation theory of aging. *Mutation Research* 338:19-23.
11. Perry HM (1999) The endocrinology of aging. *Clinical Chemistry* 45:1369-1376.

12. Ricklefs RE (1998) Evolutionary theories of aging: confirmation of a fundamental prediction, with implications for the genetic basis and evolution of life span. *The American Naturalist* 152:24-44.
13. Skulachev VP (2001) The programmed death phenomena, aging, and the Samurai law of biology. *Experimental Gerontology* 36:995-1024.
14. Terman A (2001) Garbage catastrophe theory of aging: imperfect removal of oxidative damage? *Redox Report* 6:15-26.
15. von Zglinicki T (2003) *Aging at the Molecular Level*. New York: Springer. ISBN 1402017383
16. Westendorp RGJ, Kirkwood TBL (1998) Human longevity at the cost of reproductive success. *Nature* 396:743-746.

1.4 | WHAT ARE **BUILDING BLOCKS** OF **LIFE?**

1. Berg J, Tymoczko J, Stryer L (2002) *Biochemistry*. New York: WH Freeman. ISBN 0-71674-955-6
2. Da Silva JJRF, Williams RJP (1991) *The Biological Chemistry of the Elements: The Inorganic Chemistry of Life*. Oxford: Clarendon Press. ISBN 0-19855-598-9
3. Heymsfield S, Waki M, Kehayias J, Lichtman S, Dilmanian F, Kamen Y, Wang J, Pierson R (1991). Chemical and elemental analysis of humans in vivo using improved body composition models. *American Journal of Physiology* 261:190-198.
4. Lehninger A (1993) *Principles of Biochemistry*, 2nd Ed. New York: Worth Publishers. ISBN 0-87901-711-2.
5. Mitchell P (1979). The Ninth Sir Hans Krebs Lecture. Compartmentation and communication in living systems. Ligand conduction: a general catalytic principle in chemical, osmotic and chemiosmotic reaction systems. *European Journal of Biochemistry* 95:1-20.
6. Price N, Stevens L (1999) *Fundamentals of Enzymology: Cell and Molecular Biology of Catalytic Proteins*. Oxford: Oxford University Press. ISBN 0-19850-229-X
7. Rudolph F (1994). The biochemistry and physiology of nucleotides. *Journal of Nutrition* 124:124S-127S.

1.5 | WHAT IS **BIO-REPLENISHMENT?**

1. Lane N (2004) *Oxygen: The Molecule that Made the World*. Oxford: Oxford University Press. ISBN 0-19860-783-0
2. Rose S, Mileusnic R (1999) *The Chemistry of Life*. New York: Penguin Press Science. ISBN 0-14027-273-9
3. Schneider ED, Sagan D (2005), *Into the Cool: Energy Flow, Thermodynamics, and Life*. Chicago: University of Chicago Press. ISBN 0-22673-936-8
4. Nicholls DG, Ferguson SJ (2002) *Bioenergetics*. New York: Academic Press ISBN 0-12518-121-3
5. Ouzounis C, Kyrpides N (1996). The emergence of major cellular processes in evolution. *FEBS Letters* 390:119–123.
6. Barrett M, Walmsley A, Gould G (1999). Structure and function of facilitative sugar transporters. *Current Opinion in Cell Biology* 11:496-502.
7. Lienhard G, Slot J, James D, Mueckler M (1992). How cells absorb glucose? *Scientific American* 266:86-91.
8. Souba W, Pacitti A (1992). How amino acids get into cells? Mechanisms, models, menus, and mediators. *Journal of Parenteral and Enteral Nutrition* 16:569-578.
9. Ebenhöh O, Heinrich R (2001). Evolutionary optimization of metabolic pathways. Theoretical reconstruction of the stoichiometry of ATP and NADH producing systems. *Bulletin of Mathematical Biology* 63 (1):21-55.
10. Vertuani S, Angusti A, Manfredini S (2004). The antioxidants and pro-antioxidants network: an overview. *Current Pharmaceutical Design* 10:1677-1694.

1.6 | BIO-REPLENISHMENT THEORY: **PREAMBLE**

1. Darwin C (1859) *On the Origin of Species by Means of Natural Selection, or, The Preservation of Favoured Races in the Struggle for Life*. London: J. Murray.
2. Demirel Y, Sandler S (2002). Thermodynamics and bioenergetics. *Biophysical Chemistry* 97:87-111.
3. Dennett DC (1995) *Darwin's Dangerous Idea: Evolution and the Meanings of Life*. New York: Simon & Schuster, Inc. ISBN 978-0684824710.
4. Gavrilov LA, Gavrilova NS (2001) The reliability theory of ageing and longevity. *Journal of Theoretical Biology* 213(4):527-545.
5. Kirkwood TBL, Austad SN (2000) Why do we age? *Nature* 408:233-238.
6. Margulis L (1998) *Symbiotic Planet: A New Look at Evolution*. New York: Basic Books. ISBN 0-465-07271-2.
7. Margulis L, Sagan D (1986) Origins of *Sex : Three Billion Years of Genetic Recombination*. New Haven: Yale University Press, ISBN 0-300-03340-0.
8. Margulis L, Sagan D (2002) *Acquiring Genomes: A Theory of the Origins of Species*. Cambridge: Perseus Books Group. ISBN 0-465-04391-7.
9. Medawar PB (1952) *An Unsolved Problem of Biology*. London: H K Lewis.
10. *Pearl R* (1928) The Rate of Living, Being an Account of Some Experimental Studies on the Biology of Life Duration. *New York: Alfred A. Knopf*.
11. Poundstone W (1985) *The Recursive Universe*. New York: William Morrow & Co. ISBN 0-688-03975-8.
12. Suzuki D, Dressel H (2005) *Naked Ape to Superspecies – Humanity and the Global Eco-crisis*. Vancouver: Greystone Books. ISBN 1-55365-031-X.
13. Varela, FJ, Maturana HR, Uribe R (1974) Autopoiesis: the organization of living systems, its characterization and a model. *Biosystems* 5:187-196.
14. Wickens AP (1998) *The Causes of Aging*. Harwood Academic Publishers. ISBN 90-5702-313-X.
15. Williams GC (1957) Pleiotropy, natural selection and the evolution of senescence. *Evolution* 11:398-411.
16. Wilson EO (2002) *The Future of Life*. London: Time Warner. ISBN 0-316-648531.

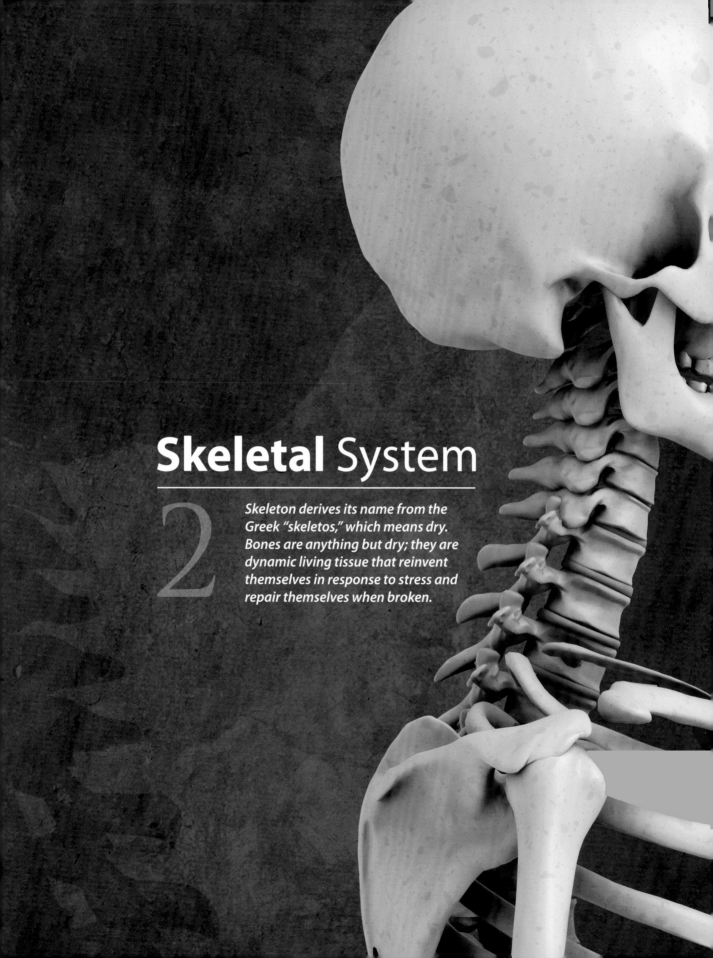

Skeletal System

2

Skeleton derives its name from the Greek "skeletos," which means dry. Bones are anything but dry; they are dynamic living tissue that reinvent themselves in response to stress and repair themselves when broken.

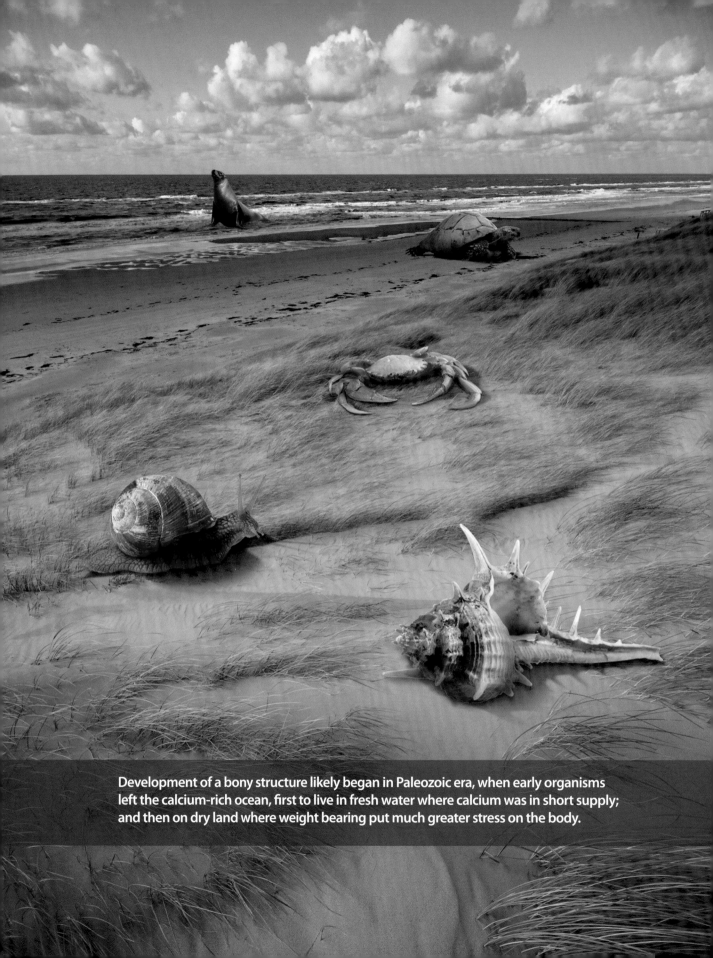

Development of a bony structure likely began in Paleozoic era, when early organisms left the calcium-rich ocean, first to live in fresh water where calcium was in short supply; and then on dry land where weight bearing put much greater stress on the body.

2

2.1 | Skeletal **Evolution**

Bone is a biological marvel from the Mother Nature; it makes vertebrates distinct from other life forms. Bone has the same strength as cast iron, but achieves this remarkable feat while remaining as light as wood. The front leg of a horse can withstand mechanical stress from heavy loads while this 1500 lb animal gallops at 40 miles per hour. The wing bone is able to keep birds aloft through entire migrations, sometimes over 10,000 miles without landing. The antlers of deer, used as weapons in territorial clashes with other deer, undergo tremendous impacts without a fracture – ready to fight another day. Undoubtedly, bone is the ultimate biomaterial. It is light, strong, can adapt to functional demands, and repair by itself.

Fossil records date the evolution of bone to the Paleozoic era some 300 million years ago. When the early life forms emerged from the ocean and evolved into terrestrials, a serious problem became apparent on how to satisfy the calcium needs of these land animals, since calcium absorption from seawater was no longer an option. Humans and other animals evolved an ingenious solution to meet the calcium challenge; building their own skeletal "bone bank", where 99 percent of the bioavailable calcium is deposited for use in times of biological need.

Bone acquired an evolutionary prominence with its terrestrial connections, an extraordinary ability to support a heavy body on land against gravity.

Different types of skeletal systems have evolved to support the calcium and othe mineral needs of various terrestrial organisms. *Exo (outer)-skeleton* in life forms including shells, carapaces (consisting of calcium compounds or silica) and chitinous compounds, offer support, protection and levers for movement. On the other hand, organisms such as sponges (*Porifera* spp.) possess simple *endo (inner)-skeletons* that consist of calcium- or silicon-based spikes and a spongin fiber network. There are other kinds of bone structures that penetrate the skin and exposed to the outside can be formed by a natural process in some animals or due to injury; examples include the horn of a rhino, antlers of a deer, and tusk of an elephant.

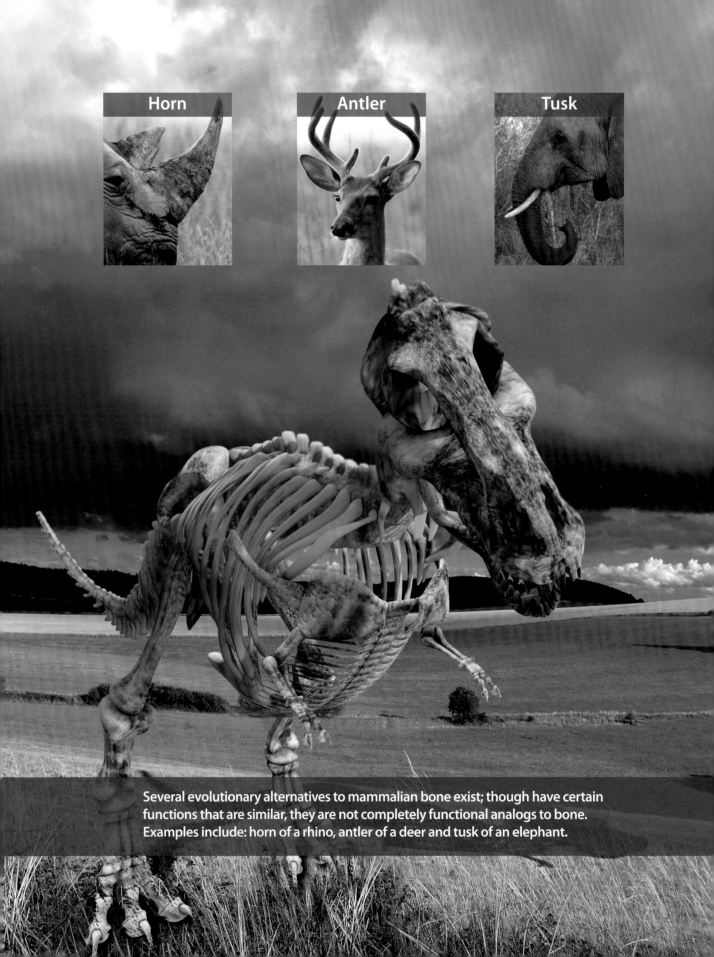

Horn

Antler

Tusk

Several evolutionary alternatives to mammalian bone exist; though have certain functions that are similar, they are not completely functional analogs to bone. Examples include: horn of a rhino, antler of a deer and tusk of an elephant.

The extinct predatory fish "Dunkleosteus", instead of teeth, had sharp edges of hard exposed bone along its jaws. A bird's beak is primarily a bone, covered in a layer of keratin. In the early vertebrates, the skeleton was made of cartilage; however, during growth and development the flexible cartilage gradually changed to a robust bone structure. Interestingly, the skeleton of sharks is entirely made of cartilage, except for the dentin layer in the teeth. The absence of true bone is considered to be a primitive feature, therefore, sharks are considered as ancestors of the bony vertebrates. As an evolutionary remnant, the skeleton of a human embryo is initially composed with soft cartilage; subsequently, this flexible framework transforms into a tough bony skeleton.

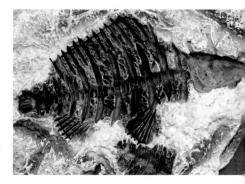

Fossil fish from Devonian period

Humans are vertebrates (animals with spine or backbone). They rely on a sturdy internal frame centered on a prominent spine. They make a perfect combination of form and function: the S-shaped spine keeps the body upright and supports the head, while the pelvis balances the upper body over the feet. Like the framework of a house, skeletons form the internal structure that provides resistance to the force of gravity, move through space, and carry the physical body with grace and dignity.

The male and female skeletons are similar in nature. However, the female frame is usually lighter and smaller than the male, and includes a wider pelvis for childbirth. Bones are rigid organs that form part of the endoskeleton of vertebrates. They come in many shapes with complex internal and external structures.

During the social evolution, human populations have switched from hunting and gathering to a more sedentary lifestyle of farming; accordingly, the strength of their leg bones decreased. Anthropological investigations have elucidated the effects of lifestyle, environment, and diseases on skeletal structures from the historical past. Bone diseases such as osteoporosis, osteomalacia, rickets, and scoliosis were observed in skeletal remains from ancient civilizations excavated from all 6 continents. Bone defects in the skeleton can cause severe dysfunction and aesthetic deformities. In Mayan times "nacre or mother of pearl" was used to reconstruct bone defects and as implants into the tooth bearing areas of the jaws. The first recorded use of an alloplast to restore a skull defect was by Fallopius in 1600, by using a gold plate to reconstruct a skull cap defect.

Bone is one of the hardest structures in the human body; it got certain degree of toughness and elasticity. It is a remarkable organ that serves structural function; provides mobility, support, and protection for the body; and a reservoir function, to store essential minerals. Though delicate in appearance, the bones in our skeletal system are ounce for ounce, stronger than "mild" steel. Human skeleton consists of bones, cartilage, ligaments and tendons that accounts for about 20 percent of the total body weight.

Mummy of Egyptian Queen Hatsheput (1500 B.C.)

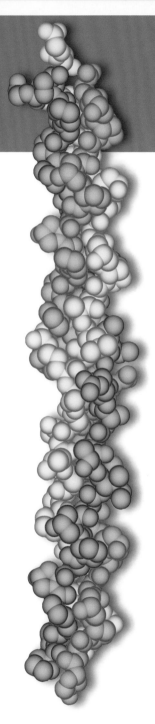

Bone is not a uniform solid material; has some gaps between its regular elements. The primary tissue of bone, "osseous tissue", is a relatively hard and lightweight composite material; made mostly of calcium phosphate in the form of *hydroxyapatite* that gives bone its rigidity. Other types of tissue found in bones include marrow, cartilage, nerves, and blood vessels. While bone is essentially brittle, it also demonstrates a significant degree of elasticity mainly due to the presence of collagen. All bones consist of several living cells embedded in the mineralized organic matrix.

Bone Matrix, the major constituent of the bone, is surrounded by cells. Bone is formed by hardening of the matrix by the entrapped cells. Matrix is composed of two chemical materials – *i) inorganic, and ii) organic.*

i) Inorganic matter is mainly crystalline mineral salts and calcium, which is present in the form of hydroxyapatite *(HA)*. Matrix is initially laid down as unmineralized *osteoid*. Mineralization involves secretion of alkaline phosphatase enzyme containing vesicles by the *osteoblasts* (the bone forming cells). This enzyme cleaves phosphate groups and facilitates calcium and phosphate deposition. These vesicles rupture to act as a centre for crystals to grow on.

ii) Organic matter of the matrix is mainly type-I collagen, made inside the cells and exported outside to form fibrils. The organic part of matrix also includes various growth factors, the functions of which are not fully known.

Other composite materials in the bone matrix include *glycosaminoglycans (GAG), osteocalcin, osteonectin, bone sialo-protein* and *cell attachment factor*. One of the main factors that distinguish the bone from any other biological matrix, is its hardness and rigidity.

i) Woven bone is weak, with a small number of randomly oriented collagen fibers. These fibers are formed rapidly without any pre-existing structure during bone repair or growth.

ii) Lamellar bone is strong, with numerous stacked layers filled with several collagen fibers. These fibers run in opposite directions in alternate layers to enhance ability of the bone to resist torsion forces. After a fracture, woven bone quickly forms and is gradually replaced by slow-growing lamellar bone on pre-existing calcified hyaline cartilage through a process known as *'bony substitution'*.

FIGURE: Collagen Helix

Bone Tissue: Based on packaging form and matrix density, bone tissue is classified in two types – *i) Cortical, and ii) Trabecular*.

i) Cortical (or) compact (or) dense bone is a hard material that gives smooth, white, and solid appearance. It makes up the shaft of long bones and the outer surface of other bones. Compact bone consists of cylindrical units called *osteons* (or *Haversian systems*) that provide canals for blood vessels and nerve fibers pass through the hard matrix. These canals also support exchange of nutrients and wastes within the bone matrix.

ii) Trabecular (or) cancellous (or) spongy bone fills the interior of the cortex shell with porous tissue. The inner trabecular network has two important functions: i) to provide large bone surface for mineral exchange, and ii) to maintain skeletal strength and integrity, particularly, in the spine and at the distal ends of long bones, that are under continuous stress from motion and weight-bearing. Fractures are common at these sites, when bone is weakened. The rods and plates of trabecular bone are aligned in a pattern to provide maximum strength without adding extra bulk, much in the way that architects and engineers design buildings and bridges.

Bone has high compressive strength but poor tensile strength, meaning it resists pushing forces well, but not pulling forces.

Bones are hollow, in order to provide the body with a frame that is both light and strong. Cortical bone, the outer dense shell, makes up about 75% of the total skeletal mass. Though, the trabecular bone accounts for the remaining 25% of total bone mass, it has nearly 10 times the surface area compared to the compact bone. Cortical and trabecular bone respond to stress during physical activity. In most individuals, cortex of their dominant arm is larger than the non-dominant arm. Such difference in cortex size is more prominent among tennis players.

FIGURE: *Cortical and trabecular bone tissue in T-bone steak at a regular grocery.*

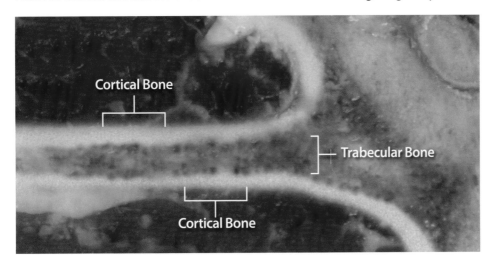

2.3 | Skeletal **Framework**

Skeletal bone framework is adapted to provide adequate strength and mobility to resist factures upon substantial impact, or during vigorous physical activity. Shape and structure of the bone are equally important as its mass in providing such strength.

Bone is a composite material, with mineral crystals bound to protein. This provides both strength and resilience so that the skeleton can absorb impact without fracture. A structure made only of mineral would be more brittle and break more easily, while a structure made only of protein would be soft and bend too easily. The mineral phase of bone consists of small crystals containing calcium and phosphate, called *hydroxyapatite (HA)*. This mineral is bound in an orderly manner to a matrix that is made up largely of a single protein, *collagen*. Collagen is made by bone cells and assembled as long thin rods containing 3 intertwined protein chains. These chains gather into larger fibers that are strengthened by various chemical bonds *(see figure on pg. 44)*. Other proteins in bone can help to strengthen the collagen matrix even more and regulate its ability to bind mineral. Small changes to the bone shape can affect the cells inside bone (the *osteocytes*) to produce chemical signals. This phenomenon allows the skeleton to respond to changes during mechanical loading.

Bone Shapes

Both the amount of bone and its architecture or shape is determined by the mechanical forces on the skeleton. Genetics of each species, including humans, also has a critical role in the structural outcome of a skeleton to suit its function. Significant skeletal variations could occur within a species due to genetic trait, therefore, some might have strong bones, while others with weak bones.

Most bones are hollow structures in which the outer cortical shell defines shape. Cortical shell provides strength, sites for firm attachment of the tendons and muscles.

Bone mass and architecture continuously change throughout life in response to mechanical stress and function. Bones will weaken if they are not subjected to adequate weight bearing function for sufficient periods of time. Therefore, weightless condition such as space travel could cause rapid bone loss. The functional philosophy of *'use it or lose it'* aptly applies to bones.

The bones of the human body come in a variety of sizes and shapes. Accordingly, there are 5 different types of bones: *long, short, flat, irregular and sesamoid.*

Long bones are longer than they are wide, consisting of a lengthy shaft with two bulky ends or extremities. They are primarily made of compact bone but may have a large amount of spongy bone at the ends. Most bones of the limbs (including thigh, leg, arm, forearm and the three bones of the fingers) are long bones.

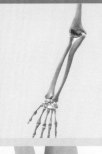

Long

Short bones are roughly cube-shaped, with vertical and horizontal dimensions. They consist primarily of spongy bone covered by a thin layer of compact bone. Short bones break more easily than long bones due to lack of support and extensive bone marrow. Short bones include the bones of the wrist and ankle.

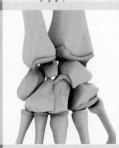

Short

Flat bones are at sites that need extensive protection or provision of broad surfaces for muscle attachment. Flat bones are thin and generally curved, with two parallel layers of compact bones that sandwich a layer of spongy bone. Most of the bones of the skull (cranium), pelvis, sternum, and rib cage are flat bones.

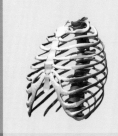

Flat

Irregular bones serve some unique functions. They protection the nervous tissue (eg. vertebrae protect the spinal cord), provide multiple anchor points for skeletal muscle attachment (as with the sacrum), and maintain pharynx and trachea support, and tongue attachment (such as the hyoid bone).

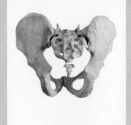

Irregular

Sesamoid bones are embedded in tendons. Since they hold the tendon further away from the joint, the angle of the tendon is increased and thus the force of the muscle is increased. Examples of sesamoid bones are the 'patella (knee cap)' and the 'pisiform'.

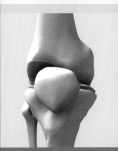

Sesamoid

Body Language - *terms that refer to features and components of the bone*

Bone feature	The 'term' means
articulation	The region where adjacent bones contact each other—a joint.
canal	A tunnel-like foramen; a passage for nerves or blood vessels.
condyle	A large, rounded articular process.
crest	A prominent ridge.
diaphysis	A relatively straight main body of a long bone; the site of primary ossification. Also known as the shaft,
eminence	A relatively small projection or bump.
epicondyle	A projection near to a condyle but not part of the joint.
epiphysis	End regions of a long bone; the sites of secondary ossification.
facet	A small, flattened articular surface.
foramen	An opening through a bone.
fossa	A broad, shallow depressed area.
fovea	A small pit on the head of a bone.
labyrinth	A cavity within a bone.
line	A thin projection with a rough surface. Also known as a ridge.
malleolus	One of two specific protuberances of bones in the ankle.
meatus	A short canal.
metaphysis	The region of a long bone between the epiphysis and diaphysis
process	A relatively large projection or prominent bump.
ramus	An arm-like branch off the body of a bone.
sinus	A cavity within a cranial bone.
spine	A relatively long, thin projection or bump.
suture	Articulation between cranial bones.
trochanter	One of two specific tuberosities located on the femur.
tubercle	A projection or bump with a roughened surface

Surface markings and other characteristics make each bone unique. There are holes, depressions, smooth facets, lines, projections and other markings. These usually represent passageways for vessels and nerves, points of articulation with other bones or points of attachment for tendons and ligaments. Several bone components assemble to form an organ *(eg. skull, vertebra, trunk, limbs, etc.)* to accomplish a specific bodily function.

The Skull

Skull shapes the head and face, protects the fragile brain, and houses and shields special sense organs for taste, smell, hearing, vision, and balance. It is constructed from 22 bones, of which 21 are locked together by immovable joints, to form a strong framework. **Cranial bones** *(n=8)* support, surround and protect the brain within the cranial cavity. They form the roof, sides, and back of the cranium, as well as the cranial floor on which the brain rests. **Facial bones** *(n=14)* form the framework of the face; provide cavities for the sense organs of smell, taste and vision; anchor the teeth; form openings for the passage of food, water, and air; and provide attachment points for the muscles that produce facial expressions. **Maxilla**, the upper jaw bone, contains sockets for the 16 upper teeth, and links all other facial bones apart from the lower jaw bone or mandible. **Mandible** is the only skull bone that is able to move allowing the mouth to open and close, and provides anchorage for the 16 lower teeth.

The smallest bone, stirrup, in the ear has the size of half a grain of rice; the biggest is the femur or thighbone; and the strongest is the jawbone

Skull has several openings *(foramina)* that allow blood vessels and nerves to pass into and out of the cranial cavity. The largest of these openings, the *foramen magnum*, is the point at which the spinal cord connects with the brain. Skull has one of the smallest bones in

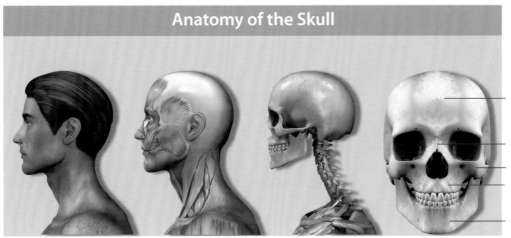

Anatomy of the Skull

Frontal Bone

Nasal Bone

Zygomatic Bone

Maxilla

Mandible

Even the smallest vibration of the eardrum results in a significant resonance. This allows us to hear even the faintest of whispers. our body called the **Auditory Ossicles** ('hearing bones'). Connected by the smallest movable joints in the body, these bones transfer sound vibration from the surface of the ear drum to the delicate oval window of the inner ear. Because the ear drum is much larger than the oval window.

The Vertebra

The vertebral column, or spine, typically consists of 33 vertebrae, which support and stabilize the upper body while forming a strong and flexible housing for the spinal cord. In addition, the spine has three natural curves that help it distribute weight uniformly and absorb shock effectively.

Vertebrae increase in size as they progress down the spine. The vertebrae that make up the spine include:

Vertebral Regions

Brain

Cervical

Thoracic

Lumbar

Sacral

Coccygeal

Cervical Vertebrae, the least robust of the vertebrae, yet strong enough to support the neck and allow a wide range of motion. The first 2 cervical vertebrae the atlas and axis, facilitate complex rotational movements of the head.

Thoracic Vertebrae (n=12) are slightly larger than the cervical vertebrae. Each has a facet, which connects with the head of each of the twelve pairs of the ribs.

Lumbar Vertebrae (n=5) are the largest and strongest of all the flexible vertebrae. They bear the large amount of weight and provide the greatest amount of support.

Sacrum is composed of 5, fused vertebrae. These vertebrae help form the bony pelvis and articulate with an additional 3 to 5 fused vertebrae called the *Coccyx or Tailbone.*

Vertebræ in the upper 3 regions remain distinct throughout life, and are known as true or movable vertebræ; those of the sacral and coccygeal regions, on the other hand, are termed false or fixed vertebræ, since they unite with one another to form 2 bones.

The Trunk

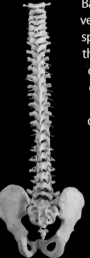

Backbone, also known as the vertebral column, spinal column, or spine, together with the ribs, forms the skeleton of the trunk. Backbone consists of a chain of irregular bones called *vertebrae* that meet at slightly movable joints. Each of the joints permit only limited movement, but collectively the joints give the backbone good flexibility that enables rotation, bending forward, backward and sideways. It also supports the skull; encloses and protects the delicate spinal cord; and provides an attachment point for the ribs, and other muscles and ligaments of the body.

Spinal Cord *(Section)*

It is a long, thin, tubular bundle of nerve fibers and cells; an extension of the central nervous system from the brain, enclosed and protected by the vertebral column. Spinal cord is much shorter than the length of the vertebral column. It is about 45 cm long in men and 43 cm long in women.

There are 12 pairs of curved, flat bones called "ribs", a form of cage that protects the heart, lungs, major blood vessels stomach, liver, etc. Ribs 8 through 10 attach directly to the sternum (breast bone) by cartilage. Ribs 11 and 12 are called "floating ribs" because they do not attach to the sternum. Instead, their floating position allows the sideways bend to provide protection for the kidneys.

The average backbone makes up about 40 percent of the body height. Soft cartilage that covers between adjacent vertebrae are called "discs". Each disc forms a strong, slightly movable joint and cushions the vertebrae against vertical shocks.

The Limbs

Over half the bones in the skeleton are found in the hands and feet. The hand alone has 27 bones - in each one

The appendicular skeleton consists of upper and lower limbs. It is made up of 126 bones, 64 in the shoulders and upper limbs and 62 in the pelvis and lower limbs.

The upper arm bone *(humerus)* is attached at the collar *(clavicle)* and shoulder *(scapula)* bones. The shoulder bone is attached to the rib cage only by muscles. The elbow joint unites the upper arm bone with 2 lower arm bones - the *ulna* and *radius*. Three sets of joints connect the lower arm bones to the bones of the palm *(metacarpals)*, via 8 small wrist *carpals*. Further, the knuckles connect the palm to the proximal *phalanx* of the fingers. Each finger has 3 phalanges except the thumb which has only 2.

The Pelvis transmits the upper body weight to the legs. It begins as 3 hip bones *(ilium, ischium,* and *pubis)* which fuse together when growth is completed. The hip joint unites the pelvis to the thigh bone *(femur)*; the knee joint, which includes the knee cap *(patella)*, links the femur to the lower leg bones - the *tibia* and *fibula*. The body weight transmits to the heel *(calcaneous)* and to the balls of the feet via the *tarsal* and *metatarsal* foot bones. The toes have a phalangeal structure like the fingers.

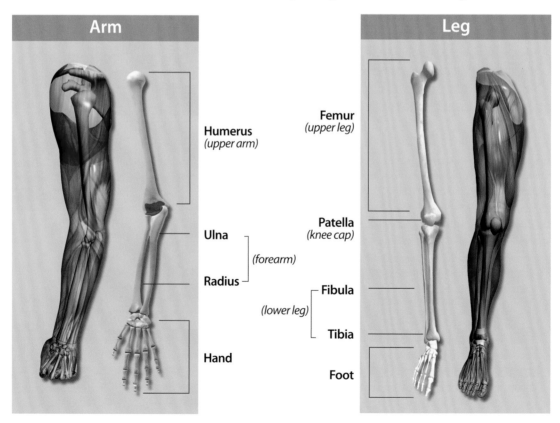

Arm

Humerus
(upper arm)

Ulna

(forearm)

Radius

Hand

Leg

Femur
(upper leg)

Patella
(knee cap)

Fibula

(lower leg)

Tibia

Foot

Bones of the Foot and Hand

Our feet and hands share similar design. The foot has 26 bones, 1 less than in the hand. The bones of the hands and feet are flexible; share similar names. The bones at the back of the foot are comparable to the bones of the wrist. However, bones in the toes are short and thick compared to that of the fingers. This unique feature provides body the ability to balance on two feet.

Foot bones form a system of arches that allow the foot to support large weight

Foot: The 7 bones in the ankle are called *tarsal* bones. The main part of the foot is made of *metatarsal* bones. *Phalanges* are the bones in the toes. The arch in the foot helps to support the body's weight.

Hand: Each hand has 27 separate bones. These are connected with muscles and tendons. Hand bones are also called the *metacarpals*. Just like the foot, the bones in the fingers are called *phalanges*. The fingers have 3 phalanges and the thumb has 2. These joints allow the finger to flex; due to this, the human hand can make more precise and finer movements than other animals.

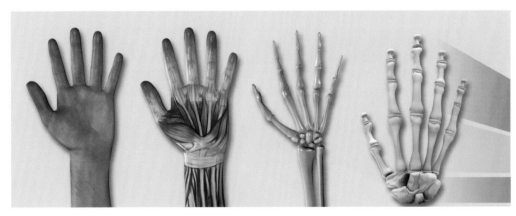

14 Phalanges
(finger bones)

5 Metacarpals
(hand)

8 Carpals
(wrist)

Anatomy of the **Hand and Foot**

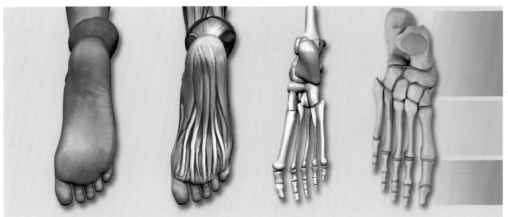

7 Tarsals
(ankle)

5 Metatarsals
(foot)

14 Phalanges
(toe bones)

Oral Cavity

Oral Cavity is the entry to the digestive tract; consisting of the mouth and the structures that are enclosed within it. It's a complex structure with nutritional, respiratory, and communicative functions.

Human dentition began to suffer soon after our early *Homo* ancestors learned to chop and process food with simple tools and, later, to cook it. Subsequently, the particle size and toughness of the food significantly decreased. Molars can be reduced up to 82% smaller in size when eating cooked potato rather than raw. Human dietary habits have been evolved to be *frugivores (eaters of seeds, nuts, tubers, root nodules, leaf shoots and sprouts)*. In comparison, the wild boar has a typical *omnivorous* dental structure. The canines are enlarged to help in tearing and ripping the prey to shreds. The molars are suited for breaking up animal and plant foods. Grass eaters have a front teeth and jaw construction suitable for tearing grass and plant bundles. The lateral rows of teeth are ideal for grating, a good way to break up the plant foods.

It is extraordinary that the normal development of human teeth routinely fails to produce 'ideal' dentition and no one has yet been able to offer an explanation for this phenomenon.

Crooked and disordered teeth may be the result of eating mushy cooked food. The disarray may have developed due to evolutionary pressures. As a result there is often not enough space in the human jaw to accommodate all our teeth. Teeth can also be missing *(wisdom teeth simply do not have enough space to fit into the jaw)* and sometimes do not form at all.

Upper Dentition
(Right and Left)

1 - **Central Incisor**
2 - **Lateral Incisor**
3 - **Canine**
4 - **1st Premolar**
5 - **2nd Premolar**
6 - **1st Molar**
7 - **2nd Molar**
8 - **3rd Molar**
    (**Wisdom Tooth**)

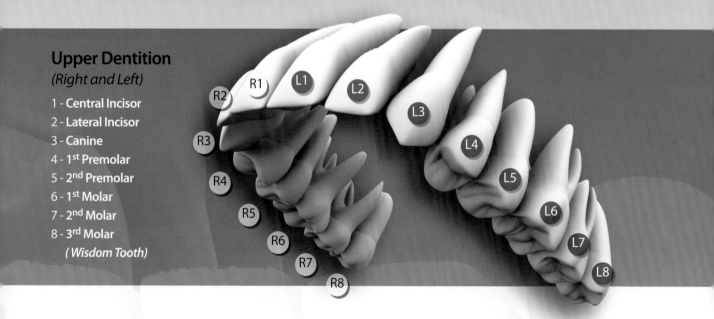

There are three hard materials involved in tooth structure: *enamel, dentin,* and *cementum*. **Enamel** covers the exterior surface of the tooth. It is a thin, brittle coat that easily chips off and almost entirely made of inorganic materials. **Dentin** comprises the bulk of the tooth mass. It is a soft organic matrix, which is located underneath the enamel. **Cementum** is a bone-like substance with embedded *cementocytes*, which covers the root of the tooth, but doesn't project above the gum line.

Teeth are hollow and the space inside is called the *'pulp cavity'*. It contains living cells, and a relatively primitive form of connective tissue. The pulp cavity has blood vessels that run in and out to serve the needs of the connective tissue, and also the nerve fibers.

Teeth are attached to the jaw by a series of very strong, collagenous *periodontal ligament (sometimes called the periodontal membrane)*. It serves as glue for the bony socket, and attaches firmly to the base of the tooth, where the cementum is located. Since the tooth needs blood supply, the *periodontal ligament* serves as the anchoring material and as the conduit through which blood vessels and nerves go to and from the pulp cavity. The gums are also connected to the tooth by a complex series of microscopic fibers; and the gums lay over the tooth-bone attachment like a protective cover. Sometimes teeth get loosened by an impact; when this happens after a while the ligament will repair the damage and the tooth is firmly seated once more.

During the evolution, teeth were derived from bony body scales similar to the placoid scales on the skin of modern sharks. Tooth play an important role in the study of human evolution.

Teeth are made of some of the hardest stuff in organic nature, and many fossil vertebrates are known only from their dental remains.

Try this: grab one of your teeth and push - it will move, just a bit. That's the "give" in the periodontal ligament.

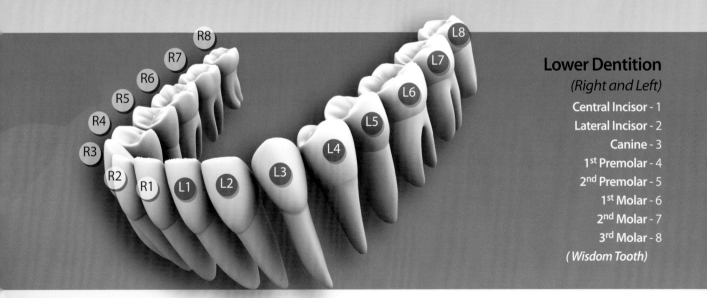

Lower Dentition
(Right and Left)

Central Incisor - 1
Lateral Incisor - 2
Canine - 3
1st Premolar - 4
2nd Premolar - 5
1st Molar - 6
2nd Molar - 7
3rd Molar - 8
(Wisdom Tooth)

Bones, muscles, and joints are integral part of the 'skeleto-muscular system'. Problems with any one part of this system can affect the other components. Thus, weakness of the muscles can lead to loss of bone and joint damage, while degeneration of the joints leads to changes in the underlying bone.

Muscles

Muscles pull on the joints to facilitate movement. Muscles enable the heart to beat, and the chest to rise and fall with each breath. There are tiny muscles that help us smile, blink, twitch or frown. Every kind of movement involves at least one muscle. Human body has three different kinds of muscle: *i) skeletal or voluntary, ii) smooth or involuntary,* and *iii) cardiac,* involved in specific functions.

i) Skeletal or voluntary muscles hold the bones together, give shape and move the body. These muscles work only after a voluntary decision to move them. This muscle is also called *striated*, because when magnified it appears to have stripes or bands. These muscles can contract *(shorten or tighten)* quickly and strongly; but get tired easily, therefore, have to rest between workouts. Skeletal muscles attach to the bone, mostly in the legs, arms, abdomen, chest, neck and face. Most of the muscles in the body are voluntary; involved in regular functions like walking, eating, writing and playing.

ii) Smooth or involuntary muscles are also made of fibers, but this type of muscle looks smooth, not striated. These muscles are under the automatic *(involuntary)* control of the nervous system; and continue to work even during sleep. Smooth muscles take longer to contract than skeletal muscles; however, they are not tired easily and can stay contracted for a long time. Examples of smooth muscles include the walls of stomach and intestines, which help break up food and move it through the digestive system; the walls of blood vessels, which pump the blood and maintain blood pressure.

Bones don't work alone – they need muscles and joints. There are more than 650 muscles that make up 50% of the body weight.

iii) Cardiac muscles are also an involuntary type found in the heart. The walls of the heart chambers are composed almost entirely of muscle fibers. Its rhythmic and powerful contractions pump blood out of the heart as it beats.

Muscles work in pairs of *flexors* and *extensors*. The flexor contracts to bend a limb at a joint. When the movement is completed, the flexor relaxes and the extensor contracts to extend or straighten the limb at the same joint. For example, the *biceps* muscle, in the front of the upper arm, is a flexor; and the *triceps*, at the back of the upper arm, is an extensor.

Skeleto-Muscular Function: Muscle and bone flow seamlessly together and work in tandem at every intersection of the body. The *biceps brachii muscle* helps to flex both the arm and the forearm and also acts to turn the palm upward *("supination")* when the forearm is flexed. The *pronator teres muscle* allows turning the palm downward *("pronation")*. The *intercostal muscles,* located between the ribs, are essential for breathing. Their contractions raise and lower the rib cage, providing room for the lungs as they expand and contract with each breath. The *quadratus lumborum muscles,* wide bands of muscles that connect the lower back to the hip, help to bend the back from side-to-side and to force air out of the lungs. The *biceps femoris,* one of the hamstring muscles, is visible on the back of the thigh. It assists in extending the thigh and in flexing and rotation the leg. Pulled hamstring muscles are common in athletes who perform quick starts and stops.

Human evolution freed upper limbs from the burden of bearing body weight during locomotion; this enabled us to grasp and manipulate objects with precision.

The Olympic is an international multi-sport event. It consists of 35 sports 53 disciplines and more than 400 events. Each of the events is exclusively about the selection of the best "Skeleto-Muscular" performance, for which an athlete receives Gold, Silver or Bronze.

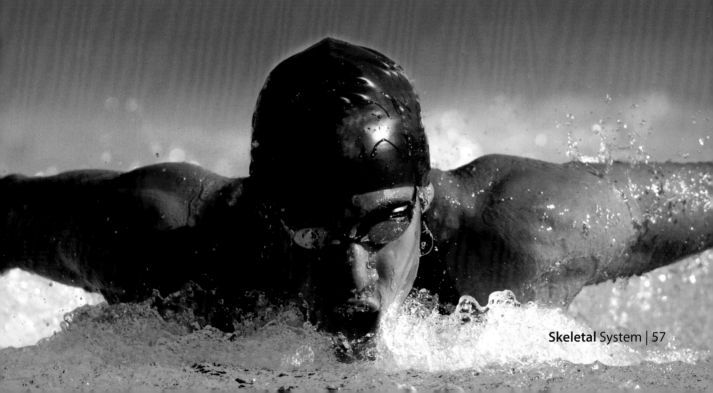

Bone Joints

Many bones in the skeleton are connected by joints, which provide flexibility and movement. These joints are shock absorbers to combat mechanical stress. Bone joints are vulnerable to injury and degeneration with aging.

Joints or Articulations are the areas where bones meet, which are classified by the range of allowable movement. The ends of bone are covered by cartilage, which allows for easy movement of the two bones. The joint capsule is lined with a type of tissue called *synovium*, which produces *synovial fluid*, a clear substance that lubricates and nourishes the cartilage and bones. Joints facilitate different bone movements. For example, hinge joints *(elbows, knees, fingers, and toes)* allow the bones to swing in two directions. Ball and socket joints *(hip and shoulder)* allow some rotation, as well as movement back and forth, and from side-to-side. Pivot joints facilitate a left to right movement similar to the course the head takes as it swivels on the spine.

Knee Joint is the largest and most complex joint in the body – as well as the weakest and most vulnerable to injury. The knee is formed where the rounded end of the *femur (thigh bone)* meets the flattened end of the *tibia (shinbone of the leg)*. The third bone of the knee, the *patella (kneecap)*, is embedded within the tendon of the powerful *quadriceps femoris* muscle of the thigh. The kneecap protects the knee and increase leverage of the quadriceps muscle.

Hip Joint is one of the strongest and most stable joints in the body. The hip joint *(a ball and socket joint)*, is formed where the ball at the head of the femur fits in the socket of the hip bone. This flexible joint structure allows for rotation, as well as movement forward, backward, and from side-to-side. Held in place by 5 ligaments, as well as tough connective tissue deep in the joint, the hip joint is often called upon to withstand 400 lbs *(180 kg)* of force in everyday activities.

Elbow Joint is formed by three bones, three filaments, and fourteen muscles. The elbow joint permits flexion, extension, and rotation of the forearm.

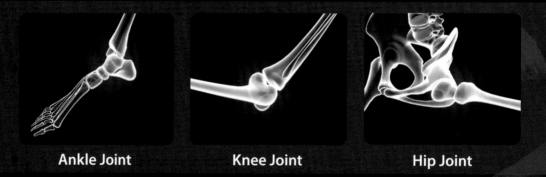

Ankle Joint   **Knee Joint**   **Hip Joint**

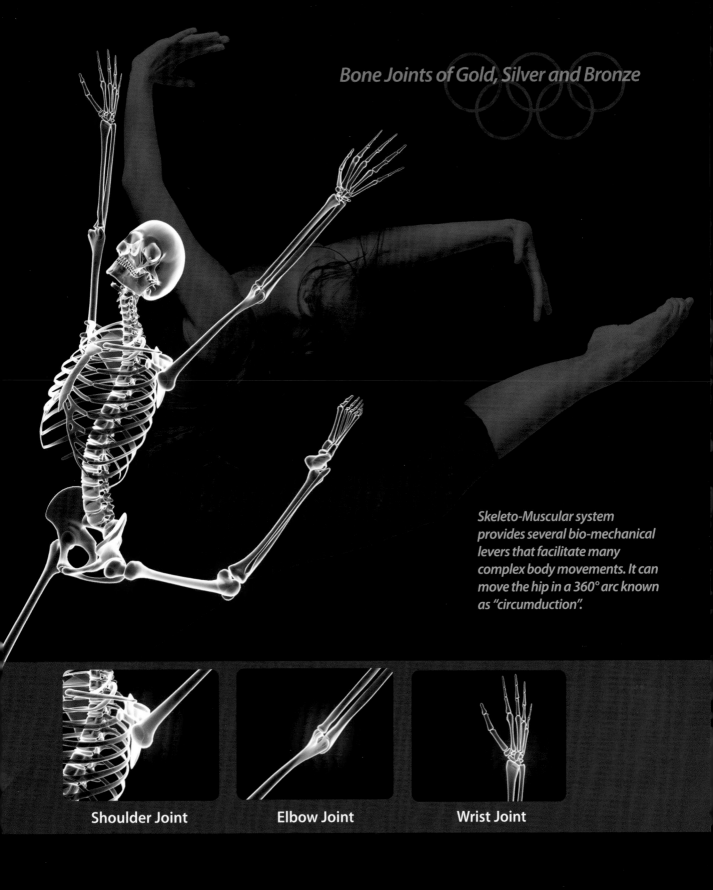

Bone Joints of Gold, Silver and Bronze

Skeleto-Muscular system provides several bio-mechanical levers that facilitate many complex body movements. It can move the hip in a 360° arc known as "circumduction".

Shoulder Joint

Elbow Joint

Wrist Joint

Ligaments connect bone to bone and **tendons** connect muscles to bone; with a purpose to transmit biomechanical forces. The fibers of both ligament and tendon are made of collagen. Normal healthy tendons are composed of parallel arrays of collagen fibers closely packed together. These collagens are held together with other proteins, particularly with *proteoglycan* in compressed regions of the tendon.

Ligaments and tendons play a significant role in the biomechanics of the skeleto-muscular system. The elastic properties have endowed a unique ability for tendons to act as springs. Tendons can passively modulate forces during locomotion, and provide additional stability to bone joints with no active work. It also allows tendons to store and recover energy at high efficiency. For example, during a human stride, the *Achilles* tendon stretches as the ankle joint *dorsi-flexes*. During the last portion of the stride, as the foot *plantar-flexes* (pointing the toes down), the stored elastic energy is released. Furthermore, because the tendon stretches, the muscle is able to function with less or even no change in length, allowing the muscle to generate greater force. Tendons and muscles work together and can only exert a pulling force.

Achilles tendon is a large tendon that connects the heel to the calf muscles. It is named after the mythic hero "Achilles", killed due to an injury to this area.

Mechanical properties of ligaments and tendons increase from early childhood to young adulthood; however, further aging process affects their stiffness. One study found that stiffness of the ligaments decrease by 2-3 folds among the elderly versus younger adult knees. Immobilization of a joint for long periods of time is detrimental for joint structure and function, including decreased range of motion for the joint. The affects of both ligaments and tendons can be severe. Immobilization for 9 weeks can led to a 69% decrease in ultimate load and an 82% decrease in energy to failure. Upon remobilization, the mechanical properties of the ligament are gained back first, followed by the structural properties. Exercise and increased load on tendons and ligaments is believed to alter their structural makeup and lead to increased mechanical properties

Tendon length varies from person to person, and is practically the sensitive factor where muscle size is concerned. For example, should all other relevant biological factors be equal, an individual with a shorter tendon and a longer biceps muscle will have greater potential for muscle mass than a person with a longer tendon and a shorter muscle. Accordingly, successful bodybuilders will generally have shorter tendons. Conversely, athletes from sports such as running or swimming, have longer than average *Achilles* tendon and a shorter calf muscle.

Tendon length is determined by genetic predisposition, and has not been shown to either increase or decrease in response to environment, unlike muscles which can be shortened by trauma, use imbalances and a lack of recovery and stretching.

Cartilage is a dense connective tissue that allows bones to slide over one another at all moveable joints with ease; thereby, reduces friction, and prevents damage. Cartilage is found in many areas in the body including the *articular* surface of the bones, the rib cage, the *bronchial tubes* and the inter-vertebral rdiscs. Its mechanical properties are some what between bone and tendon. Any breakdown of cartilage in the bone joints results in bone damage. Weakened cartilage in the spine can lead to a slipped or crushed vertebral disc. This breakdown of cartilage leads to a severe bone disease – *osteoarthritis (OA)*.

Cartilage is made of specialized bone cells called *chondrocytes* that produce large amounts of extra-cellular matrix composed of *collagen* fibers, *proteoglycan*, and *elastin* fibers. Based on the differences in the relative amounts of these 3 matrix chemicals, cartilage is classified in 3 types, *i) hyaline cartilage, ii) elastic cartilage,* and *iii) fibro-cartilage.*

i) Hyaline cartilage is the most abundant type that covers the end of bone(s) to form a smooth joint surface. Most of the skeleton of a fetus is laid down in cartilage before replaced by the bone. Hyaline cartilage in the adult is found in the nose, parts of the respiratory tract, the larynx and between the ribs and the sternum.

Bend your ear towards the face, it instantly regains the original shape when released. The elasticity of cartilage makes this possible.

ii) Elastic cartilage contains large amounts of elastic fibers *(elastin)* scattered throughout the matrix. It is important to prevent the collapse of tubular structures. Elastic cartilage is found in the *pinna* of the ear, auditory tubes and in the *epiglottis (in the throat).*

iii) Fibro-cartilage is characterized by a dense network of type-I collagen. It is a white, tough material that provides high tensile strength and support; with properties similar to those of tendons. Fibro-cartilage is present in areas most subject to frequent stress like inter-vertebral discs, and the attachments of certain tendons and ligaments.

Cartilage is one of the few tissues in the body that does not have its own blood supply. Therefore, chondrocytes get their nutrients by diffusion. Thus, compared to other connective tissues, cartilage grows and repairs more slowly. Cartilage contains a lot of water, which decreases with age. About 85% of cartilage is water in young people. Cartilage in older people is about 70% water.

TABLE: *Comparison between Bone and Cartilage*

Characteristics	Cartilage	Bone
Mechanical properties	Rigid but flexible	Hard and strong
Cell type	Chondrocytes	Osteocytes
Composition of Matrix	Chondroitin sulfate	Hydroxyapatite
Vascularization	Avascular	Vascular
Covering	Perichondrium	Periosteum

TABLE: *Skeletal system – Number of bones in human body classified by type*

Bone(s)	Number of Bones	Total
Cranial bones 1 Ethmoid bone, 1 Frontal bone, 1 Occipital bone, 2 Parietal bones, 1 Sphenoid bone and 2 Temporal bones.	8	8
Facial bones 2 Inferior Nasal Conchae, 2 Lacrimal bones, 1 Mandible, 2 Maxillae, 2 Nasal bones, 2 Palatine bones, 1 Vomer and 2 Zygomatic bones.	14	14
Ear Ossicles (bones) Malleus *(Hammer)*, Incus *(Anvil)* and Stapes *(Stirrup)*.	3 in each ear	6
Hyoid bone	1	1
Cervical vertebrae	7	7
Thoracic vertebrae	12	12
Lumbar vertebrae	5	5
Sacrum	1	1
Coccyx	1	1
Ribs	12 pairs	24
Sternum	1	1
Clavicle	1 in each shoulder girdle	2
Scapula	1 in each shoulder girdle	2
Humerus	1 in each arm	2
Radius	1 in each arm	2
Ulna	1 in each arm	2
Carpals	8 in each arm	16
Metacarpals	5 in each arm	10
Phalanges	14 in each arm	28
Hip bone	1 in each leg	2
Femur	1 in each leg	2
Patella	1 in each leg	2
Tibia	1 in each leg	2
Fibula	1 in each leg	2
Tarsals	7 in each leg	14
Metatarsals	5 in each leg	10
Phalanges	14 in each leg	28
Total number of bones		**206**

2.1 | SKELETAL **EVOLUTION**

1. Ruben JA, Bennett AA (1987) The evolution of bone. *Evolution* 41(6):1187-1197
2. Volkmann D, Baluska F (2006) Gravity: one of the driving forces for evolution. *Protoplasma* 229:143-148.
3. Donoghue PC, Sansom IJ, Downs JP (2006) Early evolution of vertebrate skeletal tissues and cellular interactions, and the canalization of skeletal development. *Journal of Experimental Zoology (B) Molecular Developments in Evolution* 306(3):278-294.
4. Donoghue PC, Sansom IJ (2002) Origin and early evolution of vertebrate skeletonization. *Microscopic Research and Technology* 59(5):352-372.
5. Eckhardt RB (1989) Evolutionary morphology of human skeletal characteristics. *Anthropologischer Anzeiger (Stuttgart)* 47(3):193-228.
6. Pilbeam D, Gould SJ (1974) Size and scaling in human evolution. *Science* 186:892-901.
7. Graham A (2005) Vertebrate evolution: turning heads. *Current Biology* 15(18):764-766.

2.2 | SKELETAL **CHEMISTRY**

1. Ruff CB (2005) Mechanical determinants of bone form: insights from skeletal remains. *Journal of Musculoskeletal and Neuronal Interactions* 5(3):202-212.
2. Currey JD (2003) How well are bones designed to resist fracture? *Journal of Bone and Mineral Research* 18(4):591-598.
3. Mathews MB (1975) Connective tissue. Macromolecular structure and evolution. *Molecular Biology Biochemistry and Biophysics* 19:13-18.

2.3 | SKELETAL **FRAMEWORK**

1. Sarin VK, Erickson GM, Giori NJ, et al (1999) Coincident development of sesamoid bones and clues to their evolution. *Anatomical Records* 257(5):174-180.
2. Chappard D, Baslé MF, Legrand E, Audran M (2008) Trabecular bone microarchitecture: a review. *Morphologie* 92(299):162-170.

2.4 | SKELETAL **ORGANS**

1. Bruner E (2007) Cranial shape and size variation in human evolution: structural and functional perspectives. *Childs Nervous System* 23(12):1357-1365.
2. de la Fuente L, Helms JA (2005) Head, shoulders, knees and toes. *Developmental Biology* 282(2):294-306.
3. Kumar S (2004) Ergonomics and biology of spinal rotation. *Ergonomics* 47(4):370-415.
4. Hinchliffe JR (2002) Developmental basis of limb evolution. *International Journal of Developmental Biology* 46(7):835-845.
5. Ball KA, Afheldt MJ (2002) Evolution of foot orthotics—part 1: coherent theory or coherent practice? *Journal of Manipulative and Physiological Therapeutics* 25(2):116-124.
6. Ball KA, Afheldt MJ (2002) Evolution of foot orthotics—part 2: research reshapes long-standing theory. *Journal of Manipulative and Physiological Therapeutics* 25(2):125-134.
7. McCollum M, Sharpe PT (2001) Evolution and development of teeth. *Journal of Anatomy* 199:153-159.

8. Russell GV Jr, Stern PJ (1998) The phylogeny of the wrist. *American Journal of Orthopedics* 27(7):494-498.
9. Putz RL, Müller-Gerbl M (1996) The vertebral column—a phylogenetic failure? A theory explaining the function and vulnerability of the human spine. *Clinical Anatomy* 9(3):205-212.
10. Butler PM (1995) Ontogenetic aspects of dental evolution. *International Journal of Developmental Biology* 39(1):25-34.
11. Gans C (1988) Craniofacial growth, evolutionary questions. *Development* 103:3-15.
12. Gracovetsky S, Farfan H (1986) The optimum spine. *Spine* 11(6):543-573.
13. Marshall D (1975) Changes in the skull—past, present and future—because of evolution. *Journal of American Dental Association* 91(5):938-942.
14. Du Brul EL (1974) Origin and evolution of the oral apparatus. *Front Oral Physiology* 1:1-30.

2.5 | SKELETAL **ARTICULATIONS**

1. Blandine C-G (2007) Anatomy of movement. Seattle: Eastland Press, ISBN 978-0-939616-57-2
2. Abrahams P (2008) How the body works. Amber Books Ltd: London, ISBN 978-1-905704-57-6
3. Clarke B (2008) Normal Bone Anatomy and physiology. *Clinical Journal of American Society for Nephrology* 3:S131-S139.
4. Khan IM, Redman SN, Williams R, et al (2007) The development of synovial joints. *Current Topics in Developmental Biology* 79:1-36.
5. Louis DS, Jebson PJ (1998) The evolution of the distal radio-ulnar joint. *Hand Clinic* 14(2):155-159.

Bone Metabolism

3

Bone metabolism is an exclusive mineral management process. It is vital for body functions; such as, bowel movement, heart beat/blood flow, nerve impulse, liver and kidney performance.

Bone Growth and Development

Living bone is a dynamic tissue. During the 1st year of life, almost 100% of the skeleton is replaced. In adults, at any given time, about 5-25% of bone surface undergoes active remodeling at multiple sites.

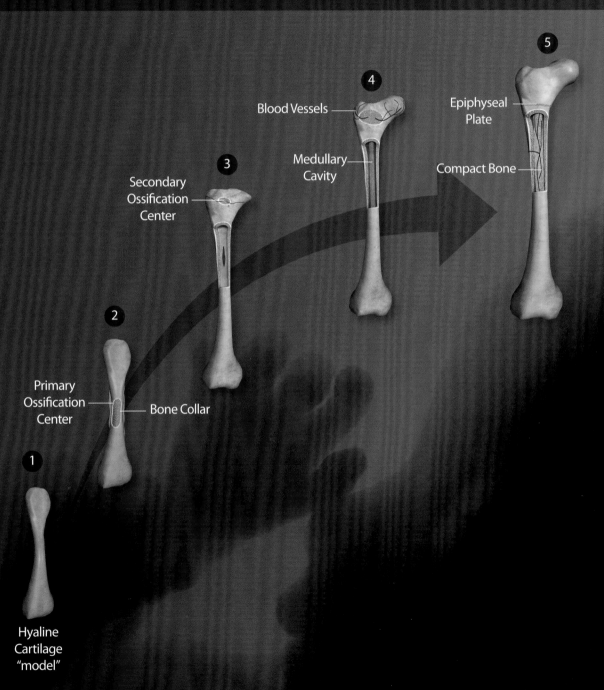

5

4

3

Blood Vessels

Epiphyseal Plate

Secondary Ossification Center

Medullary Cavity

Compact Bone

2

Primary Ossification Center

Bone Collar

1

Hyaline Cartilage "model"

3

3.1 | Osteogenesis

Osteogenesis, the process of bone formation involves three main steps:
i) production of extracellular organic matrix, the *osteoid*; ii) mineralization of the matrix to form bone; and iii) bone remodeling by resorption and reformation processes. The inter-dependent activities of several bone cells are crucial for these processes.

During early stage of human embryonic development, most of the skeletal structure is formed as a soft cartilage. The primitive bone is first laid down in layers as a membrane-bound fiber-like *(soft)* tissue, which subsequently gets replaced by bone tissue through a process called *intra-membranous ossification*. Some bones, such as the flat bones are formed entirely, or in part, by this primary ossification process. In the later stage, the fetal shaft cartilage is replaced by the bone forming cells *(osteoblasts)* and the cartilage matrix is mineralized. This is followed by a resorption process that creates surfaces to facilitate the osteoblasts to lay down woven bone and form primitive bone *(trabeculae).*

This secondary process by which bone tissue replaces cartilage is called endochondral ossification that begins in the femur at about the 9th week of fetal life.

Some of the trabeculae fuse with the new bone; the rest is resorbed to form a cavity to house red bone marrow. In the later months of fetal development, the woven bone is replaced by the *lamellar bone*; and the *bone cortex* becomes thick. The bone structure is once again remodeled to serve mechanical functions; with long canals of the *Haversian systems* containing blood capillaries. Endochondral ossification is repeated to transform bones long in size and large in shape. Linear growth of long bones occurs in the *epiphyseal growth plate*. At age-related intervals, secondary centers of *endochondral ossification* occur at the *articular* side of the growth plate. When skeletal maturity is reached, multiplication of cartilage cells in the growth plate stop, becomes thinner, and replaced by bone fused with the shaft. The structure gradually takes a typical appearance of compact cortical bone as seen in the adult.

3.2 | Bone Modeling and Remodeling

Bones change in size, shape, and position, throughout life. Two processes guide these changes – *modeling and remodeling* of the bone. When a bone is formed at one site and broken down in a different site, its shape and position is changed. This is called "modeling". However, much of the cellular activity in a bone consists of removal and replacement at the same site, by a process called "remodeling".

Modeling and remodeling continue throughout life; and most of the adult skeleton is replaced about every 7 years. While remodeling predominates by early adulthood, modeling can continue throughout life, in response to weakening of the bone. Thus with aging, if excess amount of bone is removed from the inside, some new bone is laid down on the outside, thus preserving the mechanical strength of the bone.

Bone Modeling

During childhood and adolescence bones are sculpted by modeling, which forms new bone at one site and removes old bone from elsewhere within the same bone. This process allows the bone to grow in size and shift in space. During childhood, bones grow because resorption occurs inside the bone while formation of new bone occurs on the outer surface. At puberty, bones get thicker, since formation occurs on both the outer and inner surfaces. As an individual gets older, resorption occurs on inner surface while formation occurs on outer surface. The size and shape of the skeleton follows a genetic program, but can be greatly affected by the loading or impact that occurs with physical activity. Ultimately bones achieve a shape and size that fits best to their function. In other words, *'form follows function'.*

Weight loss with calorie-restricted diets can accelerate bone remodeling and, decrease BMD and increase fragility

Bone Remodeling

Bone remodeling is a life long process that removes old bone from the skeleton where it is not required *(bone resorption)* and adds new bone where needed *(bone formation)*. Remodeling turns into a dominant process by the time a bone reaches its peak mass *(typically by the early age at 20s)*. The remodeling process does not change the bone shape, but it is nevertheless, vital for bone health for several reasons. It regulates calcium homeostasis, repairs micro-damaged bones *(from everyday stress)*, shapes and sculptures the skeleton during growth. It also prevents accumulation of excess old bone, which can lose its resilience and become brittle. Remodeling is critical for skeletal function as a "mineral bank", especially for calcium and phosphorus. Resorption, particularly on the bone surface, can provide calcium and phosphorus when there is a dietary deficiency or in need for the fetus during pregnancy or for an infant during lactation. When calcium and phosphorus supplies are ample, remodeling can deposit these minerals in the bone bank.

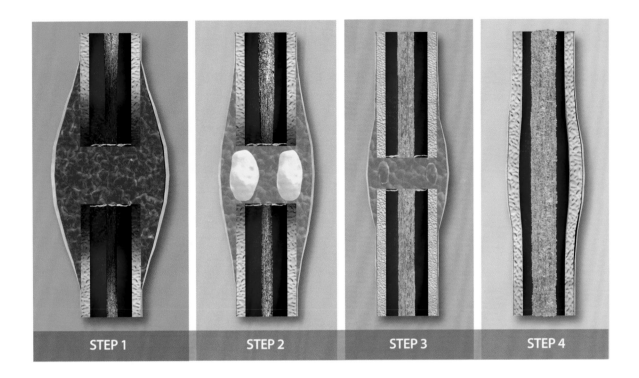

Bone Remodeling and Repair *(Self Healing)*

STEP 1 – Inflammation / Hematoma: When a bone is damaged, either through disease, accident, or surgery, the site of damage will bleed and inflamed. This results in a blood clot around the injured bone, known as *hematoma*.

STEP 2 – Cell Signaling: The body receives a message (via *growth factors*) that a repair is required at the injured bone site and a support is immediately needed from highly specialized cells to rebuild the bone. This internal communication is called *cell signaling*. In response, the bone forming cells *(osteoblasts)* initiate the repair process at the injury site.

STEP 3 – Framework: The osteoblasts need a structure or *framework* to lay down the new bone; which is provided by *hydroxyapatite (HA)*. Bone can not grow in a space where there is no bone at all; but it can grow across a small gap *(e.g. 'bone to bone')* in a minor break or fracture. If the gap is large, the bone needs medical help to heal; for example, *bone graft substitute*, or synthetic bone.

STEP 4 – Remodeling: On a good framework, the osteoblasts start laying down new bone and leave a callous at the site of injury *(similar to a scar after a cut on the skin)*. The final phase of bone repair is *remodeling* of the callous back to as close as possible to the bone's original shape. This task is performed by the osteoclasts.

3.3 | Bone Turnover

Bone is dynamic living tissue under continuous renewal; however, the normal bone maintains equilibrium between old bone being dissolved and new bone being laid down. This process is called – *bone turnover*, which takes place in the adult skeleton at discrete sites. Bone turnover ensures the mechanical integrity of the skeleton throughout life and plays an important role in calcium homeostasis.

Bone Building Process and continuous turnover in response to internal and external signals is carried out by specialized cells that build or break down bone. The cells that form bone are *osteoblasts* and those breaks down the bone are *osteoclasts*. In remodeling, an important local interaction occurs between osteoblasts and osteoclasts. Since remodeling is the main process by which the bone changes in adults; abnormalities during remodeling are the primary cause of bone disease. Therefore, it is critically important to understand the bone turnover process.

Bone Resorption and Osteoclasts

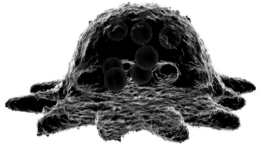

Osteoclast (from the Greek words for *"bone"* and *"broken"*) removes bone tissue by dissolving its mineralized matrix. Osteoclasts are derived from *hematopoietic stem cells (HSC)* that also produce blood and immune cells. HSC are large cells with multiple nuclei and a cytoplasm with typical, "foamy" appearance due to high concentration of vesicles. Osteoclasts are characterized by high expression of two enzymes; *tartrate resistant acid phosphatase (TRAP)* and *cathepsin K*. Osteoclasts remove bone by dissolving minerals and breaking down the matrix by a process called bone resorption. Osteoclast forms a specialized cell membrane, the "ruffled border", which touches the bone tissue surface at the site of active resorption. The ruffled border increases surface area and facilitates the break down of bone matrix, especially, the hydroxyapatite matrix, rich in calcium and phosphate ions. These ions are absorbed into small vesicles, move across the cell and eventually release into the blood.

Osteoclast

Activated osteoclasts move to areas of micro-fracture in the bone; and lie in small cavities or "resorption bays" *(called Howship's lacuna)* that are formed by digestion of the underlying bone. Osteoclasts release hydrogen ions through the ruffled border into the resorption bays; acidify and dissolve the bone mineral matrix into calcium ions (Ca^{2+}), phosphoric acid (H_3PO_4) and carbonic acid (H_2CO_3) and water. Hydrogen ions are driven by proton pumps with the help of a unique enzyme called *ATPase. (This enzyme is an important therapeutic target in the prevention of osteoporosis)*. In addition, several enzymes (eg. *cathepsin and matrix metalloprotease*), are released to digest the organic components of the bone matrix. Several factors regulate osteoclasts, including *parathyroid hormone (PTH)*, *calcitonin (CT)*, and cytokine, *interleukin (IL)*-6.

Bone Formation and Osteoblasts

Osteoblast (from the Greek words for *"bone"* and *"germ"* or embryonic) is responsible for bone formation. Osteoblasts are derived from *mesenchymal stem cells (MSC)* of the bone marrow. MSC possess a single nucleus, and a shape that varies from flat to plump, reflecting their level of activity, and in later stages of maturity line up along bone-forming surface. Osteoblasts synthesize and lay down *Type-I collagen,* which comprises 90-95% of the organic bone matrix. Osteoblasts also produce *osteocalcin,* the most abundant non-collagenous protein in the bone matrix; *proteoglycan,* and *alkaline phosphatase,* an organic phosphate-splitting enzyme. Hormones, growth factors, physical activity, and other stimuli act mainly through osteoblasts to elicit their effects on the bone. Osteoblasts have receptors for PTH and estrogen.

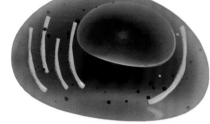

Osteoblast

When the skeleton is subjected to impact, a fluid movement occurs around the *osteocytes (mature cells that make up 90% of the cells in bone).* The long-cell extensions send signals to the bone cells on the surface to initiate an action, either in terms of changes in bone resorption or formation. Osteoblasts produce collagen and deposits this material in a typical pattern, either parallel or concentric layers to form mature *(lamellar)* bone. *Hydroxyapatite,* the calcium- and phosphate-rich mineral is added to the matrix to form a hard, yet resilient tissue – the healthy bone.

However, during rapid bone formation, as in the fetus or certain pathological conditions (e.g. *fracture callus, fibrous dysplasia, hyper-parathyroidism*), collagen is not deposited in a parallel array but in a basket-like weave; which is called woven, immature, or primitive bone. Failure of osteoblasts to make a normal collagen matrix may occur during certain gene disorders (e.g. *osteogenesis imperfecta*). Inadequate bone matrix formation also occurs in *osteoporosis,* particularly in the drug-induced form of *glucocorticoid-induced osteoporosis (GIO).*

Osteoblasts are responsible for mineralization of the osteoid matrix. Osteoblast cell population tends to decrease as individuals become elderly, thus decreasing the natural renovation of the bone tissue.

Osteocytes are mature, non-dividing cells that are housed in small cavities in the bone. These cells contain a nucleus and a thin ring of cytoplasm. Osteocytes are derived from osteoblasts and they represent the final stage of maturation of the bone cell lineage. They are less active than osteoblasts; although not responsible for a net increase in bone matrix, osteocytes are critical for the maintenance of bone structure. These bone cells are involved in the routine turnover of bone matrix, through various mechano-sensory mechanisms.

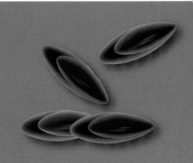

Bone Turnover Mechanisms – **Resorption and Formation**

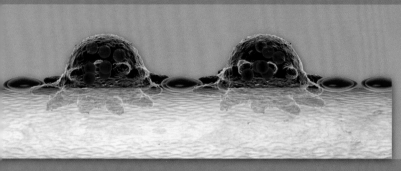

PHASE-I: Bone Resorption

Osteoclasts attach to the trabecular surface and secrete various solvents that erode the bone matrix. First, the acidic milieu dissolves the mineral matrix *(hydroxyapatite)* to release calcium ions, and phosphorus. Osteoclasts also secrete cathepsin, an enzyme that breaks down collagen from the bone matrix.

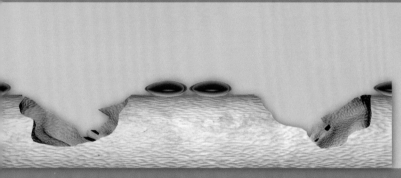

PHASE II: Bone Resorption Complete

In final phase, small cavities or "resorption bays" are created on bone surface; and is prepared for subsequent bone formation. A thin layer of protein, rich in sugars, called the "cement line" is formed that makes a strong bond between the old and newly formed bone. The entire resorption phase is relatively rapid, that lasts about 2 to 3 weeks.

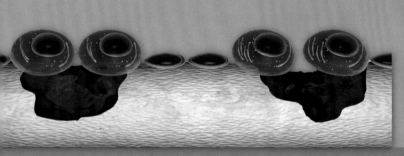

PHASE III: Bone Formation

Osteoblasts repair the bone surface and fill the eroded cavities with new mineralized *(calcified)* matrix. Active osteoblasts lay down successive layers of matrix in an orderly manner that provides added strength. The addition of minerals to the collagenous matrix completes the process of making a strong bone.

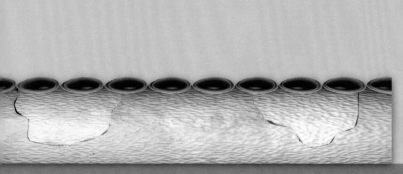

PHASE IV: Bone Formation Complete

In final phase, the bone surface is restored with a layer of protective lining cells. After the new bone is calcified; formation phase is completed. The final phase of bone formation takes longer, lasting up to 3 or 4 months. Active remodeling at many sites can weaken the bone for long periods of time *(even if formation catches up eventually)*.

3.4 | Bone Mineralization

Minerals are the basic elements from the earth and ocean crests, which provide a structural framework for all living organisms on the Blue Planet. All primitive and evolved life forms have specialized built-in systems to acquire, use and dispose minerals via the biological process called 'metabolism'.

Human race has discovered its dependence on minerals and health from ancient times. Perhaps the most extreme example of human eating behavior that may have influenced the mineral intake is called *'geophagy'*. In Ghana, inhabitants continue to this day to mold clay into egg shapes and eat, as an important source of minerals in their diet. Geophagy, *the eating of earth or clay*, is one instance of mineral intake by man, eating a substance that is not food but has an effect on nutrition and health.

Calcium

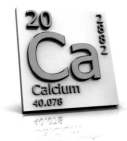

Calcium is one of the abundant minerals in the human body, and perhaps the one with most direct impact on bone health. More than 99% of total body calcium is stored in the bones and teeth, providing vital support to the skeleton. The remaining 1% is distributed throughout the body in blood, muscle, and in the fluid between cells. Calcium levels in most biological systems are about 1 mM, similar to the calcium concentration in the ocean.

Role in Bone Metabolism: A constant level of calcium is required in body fluids and tissues to perform vital body functions. The blood, the heart, the muscular system, the nervous system, the hormonal system, as well as the kidneys, and the gastrointestinal system are all affected by calcium and demand a specific calcium balance. As calcium is transported back and forth between the body fluids and the cells of the various systems, control is maintained in each system. The central nervous system depends on sufficient calcium levels to keep the nerves function properly. If the calcium levels in the body become too low, the nerves become hyper-excited and the muscles go into spasm. Not only does calcium affect the muscles via the nerves, it also has a profound effect on the smooth muscles of the body *(especially the heart)*. Calcium is directly involved in the cardiac muscle tension in the heart walls, which in turn affects the pumping ability of the heart. Calcium levels can be maintained only through diet and supplements, because the human body can not produce calcium by itself.

Deficiency: Thinning bones and onset of osteoporosis are often the first signs of a calcium deficiency. Other symptoms of calcium deficiency include irregular heartbeat, joint problems, nervousness and insomnia. Calcium is lost from the bones during menopause and aging. Characterized by low bone density and bone fragility, osteoporosis affects 1 in 3 women after menopause.

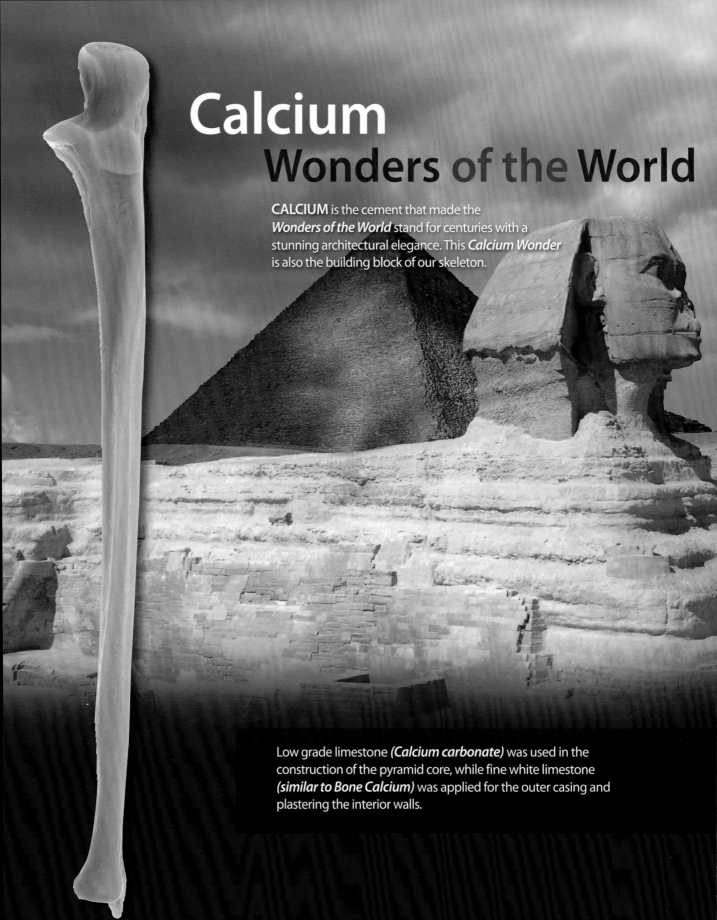

Calcium
Wonders of the World

CALCIUM is the cement that made the *Wonders of the World* stand for centuries with a stunning architectural elegance. This *Calcium Wonder* is also the building block of our skeleton.

Low grade limestone *(Calcium carbonate)* was used in the construction of the pyramid core, while fine white limestone *(similar to Bone Calcium)* was applied for the outer casing and plastering the interior walls.

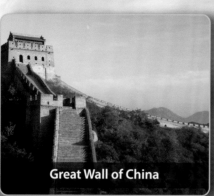

Great Wall of China

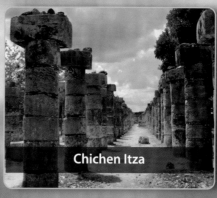

Chichen Itza

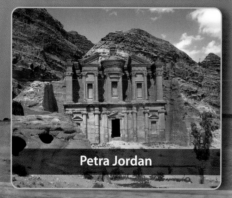

Petra Jordan

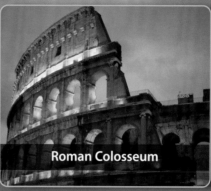

Roman Colosseum

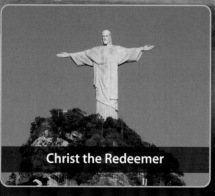

Christ the Redeemer

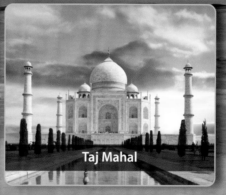

Taj Mahal

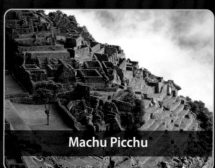

Machu Picchu

Calcium with other minerals such as phosphates has even preserved the bones of dinosaurs and mammoths which are millions of years older than the Pyramids of Giza!

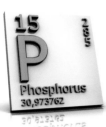

Phosphorus

Phosphorus *(P)* is an essential nutrient present in the body as phosphate; which is required for cellular metabolism and skeletal mineralization. It makes up 1% of total body weight and present in every cell of the body. However, most of the phosphorus in the body is found in the bones and teeth. Bone contains about 85% of the body's phosphate. It is a structural component of nucleic acids as well as of other cellular constituents.

Phosphate concentrations are regulated and range from 3.0 to 4.5 mg/100 mL. Phosphate absorption occurs in the small intestine and is coupled to calcium transfer. However, phosphate absorption is not as tightly controlled as with calcium. Absorbed phosphate is deposited in bone and filtered by the kidneys where most of it is re-absorbed.

Role in Bone Metabolism: The main function of phosphorus is in the formation of bones and teeth. The major structural component of bone is in the form of calcium phosphate salt called hydroxyapatite *(HA)*. It plays an important role in fat and carbohydrate metabolism, protein synthesis and tissue repair. Phosphorus is critical for the making of adenosine triphosphate *(ATP)*, a molecule the body uses for storage and exchange of energy. It also assists in muscle contraction, kidney function, nerve conduction, and for maintaining a regular heartbeat. Phospholipids (e.g., *phosphatidylcholine*) are major structural components of cell membranes. A number of enzymes, hormones, and cell-signaling molecules depend on phosphorylation. Phosphorus also helps to maintain normal acid-base balance *(pH)* by acting as one of the body's most important buffers.

Deficiency: Inadequate phosphorus intake results in low serum phosphate levels *(hypophosphatemia)* which may lead to loss of appetite, anemia, muscle weakness, bone pain, *rickets* (in children), *osteomalacia* (in adults), increased susceptibility to infection, numbness and tingling of the extremities. Since phosphorus is so widespread in food, its deficiency is very rare and is seen only in people who are starving, anorexic, diabetics and those on special diets.

> ***The Power of Phosphorus:*** Nucleic acids (DNA, RNA), which are responsible for genetic code, are long chains of phosphate-containing molecules. Triple phosphate chain in the 'ATP' (nucleotide) molecule stores the cellular energy. Similar to the phosphorus in the head of a match stick that lights up fire upon a strike!

Magnesium

Magnesium *(Mg)* is the fourth most abundant positive ion *(Mg^{2+})* in the body and the second most prevalent mineral within the cells. Magnesium plays an important role in several functions of the human body by participating in more than 300 essential enzymatic reactions. The adult human body contains about 25 grams of Mg^{2+}. Over 60% of all the Mg^{2+} in the body is found in the skeleton, contributing to the structure and strength of the bones and less than 1% is found outside of cells.

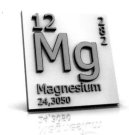

Several enzymes that are involved in the synthesis of carbohydrates and lipids require Mg^{2+}. Glutathione, an important antioxidant, requires Mg^{2+} for its production. Magnesium is required for the active transport of ions like potassium and calcium across cell membranes. Magnesium affects the conduction of nerve impulses, muscle contraction, heart rhythm and the secretion of parathyroid hormone *(PTH)*.

Role in Bone Metabolism: Magnesium has dual role in bone health – it makes bones more flexible and less brittle, and helps regain the bone mineral density *(BMD)*. A positive association exists between Mg^{2+} intake and BMD or bone mineral content *(BMC)* of the lumbar spine and forearm bone in premenopausal women. Similar correlations have been observed for the hip bone density for both men and postmenopausal women. Magnesium intake is also positively correlated with the rate of change in the BMD of *humerus* and *radius*.

Adenosine triphosphate (ATP) that provides energy for all metabolic processes in the body exists primarily as Mg^{2+} complex

Magnesium concentration affect osteoblast function and bone metabolism. The size of mineral crystals in the bone influences its mechanical properties. Magnesium affects the process of bone mineralization. Postmenopausal women with osteoporosis and Mg^{2+} deficiency have larger and more perfect crystals in the *trabecular* bone. When crystals are excessively large, bones become brittle and fail to bear normal loads. Magnesium supplementation can increase the BMD.

Deficiency: Inadequate blood Mg^{2+} levels are known to result in low levels of blood calcium *(hypocalcemia)*, potassium levels *(hypokalemia)*; retention of sodium and resistance to actions of PTH and vitamin-D. Severe Mg^{2+} deficiency has also been associated with hypertension and cardiovascular disease. Mg^{2+} deficiency increases the risk of urinary mineral loss in conditions such as diabetes, gastrointestinal disorders, chronic alcoholism and aging. Magnesium deficiency is prevalent among the elderly due to decreased absorption of magnesium combined with relatively low dietary intake. Magnesium deficiency has been identified as a possible risk factor for osteoporosis.

FIGURE: *Molecular structure of ATP*

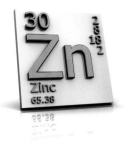

Zinc

Zinc *(Zn)* is an essential trace element for all forms of life. Zinc plays an important role in human growth, development and reproduction; immune and nerve functions. Zinc is essential for protein function, such as the antioxidant enzyme, "superoxide dismutase *(SOD)*". Zinc is necessary for the transport of vitamin-A into the blood and hormone synthesis. Zinc is involved in a critical cellular process called "apoptosis" *(gene-directed cell death)*, which influences growth and development, as well as a number of chronic diseases.

Role in Bone Metabolism: Zinc participates in a broad range of bone metabolic activities. Enzymes like alkaline phosphatase, which is required for deposition of calcium into the bone *(bone calcification)*; and *collagenase* which is required for bone resorption and remodeling, are zinc-dependent "metallo-enzymes". The concentration of zinc in bone is higher than in most other tissues and may have structural role in the bone matrix. Skeleton is a major body store for zinc; about 30% of total body zinc is found in bone. Zinc has a role in slowing down bone resorption and stimulating bone formation. Zinc is bound to fluoride in *hydroxyapatite (HA)*, the major mineral of the bone. Zinc regulates secretion of *calcitonin*, which also influences bone turnover.

Zinc content of the adult human body ranges from 1.4 to 2.5 grams, with the highest concentrations in the bone, liver, kidney, pancreas and muscle tissue.

Deficiency: Zinc deficiency can trigger defects in skeletal development, by causing reduction in osteoblastic activity; collagen and chondroitin sulfate synthesis, and alkaline phosphatase activity. Severe zinc deficiency is caused only in individuals born with genetic disorders and results in impaired uptake and transport of zinc. The major symptoms of severe zinc deficiency include the slowing or cessation of growth and development, delayed sexual maturation and immune system deficiencies.

A milder form of zinc deficiency is caused by malnutrition, malabsorption and with severe or persistent diarrhea. Significant delays in linear growth and weight gain, impaired neuropsychological development and increased susceptibility to life-threatening infections are caused in young children with zinc deficiency. Zinc also affects cell-signaling systems that coordinate the response to the growth-regulating hormone, "insulin-like growth factor-1 *(IGF-1)*". Zinc deficiency is associated with decreased release of vitamin-A (retinol) from the liver, and its conversion to retinal, critical for the night vision. Zinc indirectly contributes to symptoms of night blindness caused by vitamin-A deficiency.

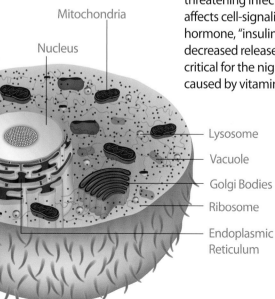

Mitochondria

Nucleus

Lysosome

Vacuole

Golgi Bodies

Ribosome

Endoplasmic Reticulum

> *Zinc is essential for structural stability of the cells. Zinc serves as a cofactor for over 100 enzymes, essential for protein synthesis, integrity of cell membranes, maintenance of DNA and RNA, tissue growth and repair, wound healing, taste acuity, prostaglandin production, bone mineralization, thyroid function, blood clotting and cognitive functions.*

Strontium

Strontium *(Sr)* is a naturally occurring mineral found in food, water and in trace amounts throughout the skeleton. Absorption, bone deposition, intestinal and renal elimination of strontium is similar to that of calcium. Human body contains approximately 320 to 400 mg of strontium; mostly concentrated in the bone, but also found in connective tissue in small quantities.

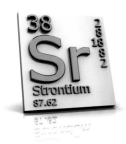

Role in Bone Metabolism: Strontium salts inhibit bone resorption in intact bones and stimulate bone formation in cultured bones. Strontium ranelate is an orally active agent consisting of two atoms of strontium and ranelic acid. Strontium ranelate stimulates formation of new bone tissue, decreases bone resorption without deleterious effects. Strontium has anti-fracture efficacy in the treatment of postmenopausal osteoporosis.

Strontium is currently tested as an investigational drug for lowering the risk of fractures in postmenopausal women.

At the cellular level, strontium enhances the activity of osteoblasts while simultaneously reducing osteoclastic activity. Intestinal absorption of strontium is about 25-30% of which 50-80% is taken up by the bones. In the presence of calcium, strontium absorption is reduced by half. Intestinal absorption is vitamin-D dependent and decreases with aging, food and diets high in other minerals. When unbound by serum proteins, strontium is cleared by urinary and fecal routes. The remaining mineral is retained in soft and mostly calcified tissues.

In a 3-year study on strontium efficacy was evaluated in 1, 442 osteoporotic postmenopausal women with history of at least one vertebral fracture. Those receiving calcium, vitamin-D and strontium ranelate (2-g dosage; 680 mg of elemental strontium), showed an increase in BMD by 12.7% *(lumbar spine)*, 7.2% *(femoral neck)*, and 8.6% (total hip), compared to the placebo. Strontium also increased the bone formation and decreased bone resorption. A hip-fracture prevention and safety study of strontium in 5,091 women with post-menopausal osteoporosis over a 3 year period, showed a 41% reduction in the risk of fracture after a minimum of 18-month treatment. A daily dose of 2-g of strontium ranelate daily was effective with a 44% reduction in the risk of new vertebral fractures after 2 years, compared to placebo.

Strontium Levels: Concentration of strontium in plasma is 29 *mcg*/L. Dietary consumption of strontium is about 1 to 5 mg per day, compared to pharmacological consumption of 1 to 2 grams. Pregnant woman and individuals with decreased renal function should avoid strontium. Both calcium and strontium utilize the same carrier protein for transport and therefore, calcium will impair strontium absorption. High intake of strontium *(1-5 mM)* induce abnormal bone mineral formation other than hydroxyapatite *(HA)*. In a study reported in 1996, onset of *rickets* has been observed in Turkish children who consumed food grown in soil with elevated strontium content.

3.5 | Bone Mineral Absorption

Absorption of minerals in the gastrointestinal tract is highly specific; and regulated by both luminal and tissue factors. Essential dietary cations, such as calcium, magnesium and zinc are generally absorbed 10-100-fold more efficiently than toxic dietary ions – an evolutionary adaption by natural selection.

Metal ions bind and cross the mucus layer with an efficiency highest for *monovalent* (e.g. *Na^+, K^+*); mediocre for *divalent* (e.g. *Mg^{2+}, Ca^{2+}, Zn^{2+}*) and lowest for *trivalent* (eg. *Al^{3+}, As^{3+}, Bi^{3+}*) cations. At the mucosa, the trivalent Fe^{3+} is uniquely reduced to form the divalent Fe^{2+}, for a safe uptake by transport proteins (such as *lactoferrin*) into the blood circulation. The exclusion of trivalent cations minimizes the intestinal absorption of toxic metals such as aluminum *(Al^{3+})*, arsenic *(As^{3+})* and bismuth *(Bi^{3+})*.

Mineral Transport

Ingested minerals are classified in two categories: i) Those soluble throughout the potential pH range of the gastrointestinal lumen, such as Na, K, Mg, and Ca; and ii) Those susceptible to *hydroxy-polymerization*, such as Cu, Fe, Zn, Cr and Al. This latter group termed 'hydrolytic metals' that are acid-soluble, and form insoluble precipitates when pH is raised. Initially, assimilation of metal ions in an available form is facilitated by the intestinal secretions, chiefly soluble mucus *(mucin)* that retards the hydrolysis of ions such as Cu, Fe and Zn. Therefore, intestinal absorption of these mineral categories involves two specific cellular mechanisms: **A)** trans-cellular, metabolically driven active transport and **B)** para-cellular, passive process.

A) Trans-cellular Transport is specific for calcium absorption, which involves three steps: i) *Entry* across the front end of the cell *(facing the intestinal lumen)*, ii) *Diffusion* through the cytoplasm; and iii) *Exit* at the back end of the cell *(release into the blood)*. Calcium crosses the cell membrane through calcium channels, which does not require ATP *(energy)*. However, calcium extrusion from the cell requires energy. The enzyme that facilitates calcium extrusion is *Calcium-ATPase,* which is vitamin-D dependent.

B) Para-cellular Transport is the second major mechanism for calcium and other minerals to mobilize from the intestinal lumen into the blood circulation. The efficacy of para-cellular process is determined by solubility, gut permeability and sojourn time (time spent by the emulsified mineral, *chyme*) in a given intestinal region. Solubility in the chyme is specific for each mineral, influenced by the pH at a given locus and by the nature and quantity of anions (e.g. *chlorides, sulfates, phosphates*). For instance, calcium sulfate is quite insoluble, whereas cadmium sulfate is very soluble. Magnesium citrate is far more soluble than calcium citrate, even though the latter is one of the more soluble calcium salts widely used in dietary supplementation. Based on *in vivo* studies, in a total transit time of about 3-h, chyme passes through the *duodenum* in 2-3 min; stays approximately 45 min in the *jejunum* and the remainder, about 2-h is spent in the *ileum*. The amount of soluble calcium in the intestine is almost similar in all regions at any given time; also the gut permeability is similar in all three major regions of the intestine; therefore, the sojourn time becomes the decisive factor for the bio-availability of calcium and other minerals that follow the para-cellular route.

Calcium Absorption

Calcium absorption varies among individuals; at an average of about 30% of total intake, being more efficient in males than females. Factors that influence calcium absorption include age and health status of the individual, vitamin-D availability, calcium levels in food consumption, type and amount of fiber in the diet. It should be noted that all calcium ingested is not absorbed into the body.

Calcium ion concentration in body fluids is approximately 1.2-1.5 mM. If the calcium ion level in the intestinal lumen is greater than 1.5 mM, calcium will move down without absorption.

Calcium absorption begins in the stomach with its acid (hydrochloric acid), which dissolves, ionizes and facilitates mineral assimilation in the gut. After the acidic, enzymatic and mechanical action of the stomach, calcium (along with other food materials) enters the *duodenum* as a partly digested semi-fluid mass called "chyme". It crosses the intestinal membranes, cell junctions and finally enters the blood circulation. Small intestine secretes several specific chemicals called "ligands" that capture minerals, most notably mucin. Absorption from the mucus layer into the intestinal mucosa may occur either through the mucosal cells called "enterocytes" (trans-cellular) or between enterocyte cell junctions (para-cellular). The para-cellular route is inefficient (usually less than1% absorption) and likely, therefore, only important in the absorption of non-essential polyvalent metals (e.g. Al^{3+} and As^{3+}) that lack a transport system. Efficiency of this route may be increased by the ingestion, or mucosal application of penetration enhancers. Presence of other food materials in the intestinal lumen can also enhance calcium bio-availability. Calcium supplements, in particular calcium carbonate, appear to be absorbed more readily when ingested with food rather on an empty stomach.

Absorbed calcium mixes rapidly with calcium in the circulatory pool. When calcium levels in the blood are normal (2.5 mmol/L), about 50% of its Ca^{2+} ions are deposited into the bone mineral matrix; simultaneously, an equal molar amount of Ca^{2+} ions are withdrawn from the bone, when the blood circulates through the skeleton. A majority of blood calcium is filtered by the renal tube (kidney), and about 70% of the filtered calcium is reabsorbed, when urinal fluid passes through the *nephron*.

Proper level of stomach acid is so important that its shortage in the digestive process can account for as much as 80 percent loss of available calcium absorption.

High intake of calcium not necessarily results in increased BMD or decreased fracture risk. In fact, large doses of calcium may cause an imbalance of other important minerals, for example, high calcium may force magnesium depletion. Therefore, an optimum bio-availability of calcium is important for bone mineral homeostasis.

Calcium Absorption in the Gastrointestinal Tract

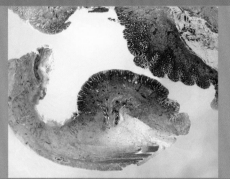

Stomach has a low calcium assimilation capacity due to small surface area and thick layer of pH-buffered mucus, which is impermeable to nutrient absorption. Nonetheless, stomach plays an important role in the 'preparation' of ingested minerals for later absorption. Gastric juice contains soluble mucin (once termed 'gastroferrin'), that helps calcium to remain in solution at neutral pH. This facilitates the calcium-containing 'chyme' to empty into the small bowel in a highly bio-available form.

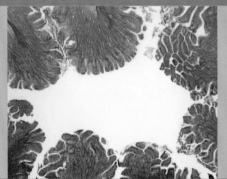

The **small intestine (proximal)** region is where calcium is mostly absorbed by the blood and transported to the bone and other tissues. In the small intestine, calcium transfer occurs by two independent processes: i) a saturable, trans-cellular mechanism, dependent on vitamin-D, which takes place exclusively in the proximal intestine i.e., the duodenum and the upper jejunum; and ii) is a non-saturable para-cellular mechanism, which is independent of vitamin-D.

FIGURE: *Proximal (duodenum) portion of the small intestine (100x).*

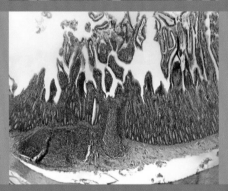

The **small intestine (distal)** part is where the calcium transport occurs between the mucosal cells, predominantly by the non-saturable, para-cellular mechanism, because the trans-cellular process plays only a minor role in the distal jejunum and the ileum. Absorption in this part of the intestine is dependent on adequate supply of calcium in the lumen. Increased absorption via this mechanism becomes possible only when there is an increased dietary intake of the mineral.

FIGURE: *Distal (ileum) portion of the small intestine (100x).*

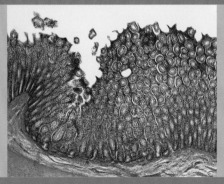

The **large intestine:** In response to high calcium intake, a high proportion of unabsorbed calcium reaches the large bowel. Active calcium transport takes place in the cecum and the ascending colon but not in the transverse colon. The sojourn time in the cecum and ascending colon is about 2½ hours. Assuming that the rate of para-cellular movement is similar for both small and large intestines an estimated 11% of calcium is absorbed in the large intestine.

FIGURE: *Large intestine (villi) showing goblet cells (100x).*

Effectors of Calcium (Mineral) Assimilation

Intestinal Absorption: A marked reduction in gastric hydrochloric acid output *(hypochlorhydria)* can make the dissociation of a mineral ion ineffective from its ingested matrix (e.g. Fe^{3+} in food or Al^{3+} in an antacid), leading to a reduced luminal concentration of solubilized and potentially bio-available metal.

Calcium needs to be ionized and must remain in solution for intestinal absorption. Even if a calcium salt is precipitated due to alkaline conditions that prevail in the small intestine, some Ca^{2+} ions still survive in solution and get absorbed. Calcium present in vegetables or other non-fluid foods fail to go into solution, unless some part of the vegetable (or food) is digested. Foods with high indigestible fiber content are poor sources of calcium than foods that contain less or no fiber but an equivalent amount of calcium (e.g. cereals vs. milk). High fat intake may prevent calcium absorption due to formation of calcium soaps.

To allow for adequate assimilation of calcium into the body, magnesium must co-exist. Also silica eases assimilation of calcium and its easy absorption in the body

Fiber, in particular, cellulose and hemi cellulose, decrease calcium absorption by increasing the bulk of intestinal contents, by minimizing the transit time and also by stimulating microbial proliferation (which can compete with the mineral assimilation). A diet high in *phytic acid*, commonly found in the bran of whole grains, is likely to interfere with calcium absorption. Phytic acid binds to a variety of minerals including calcium and form insoluble salts, called "phytates". Calcium, in its insoluble form is excreted from the body as waste. Also, diets that are high in sodium may interfere with calcium absorption and adversely deplete minerals through urination.

Reduced levels of vitamin-D levels are common in the elderly, especially among women. This vitamin deficiency can affect intestinal calcium absorption. Factors that can influence vitamin-D levels include reduced exposure to sunlight, decreased dietary intake and absorption problems. The ability of vitamin-D to absorb calcium in enhanced in the presence of magnesium and boron. Vitamin-D has been elaborated in different *Sections of Chapters 6 and 7.*

High bioavailability of calcium in milk has been attributed to the co-existence of lactose, peptides and amino acids; the latter derived from hydrolysis of casein in the intestinal lumen. Calcium bioavailability can also be enhanced with compounds such as citric acid, and milk peptides, and by using highly soluble salts such as calcium gluconate or calcium gluconate-glycerophosphate can improve calcium bioavailability.

> *Secretion of stomach acid decreases gradually with age; up to 40% of post-menopausal women are deficient in stomach acid, with a predisposed risk of poor calcium absorption.*

Bone Mineralization. Several hormones affect calcium mineralization in the body. The parathyroid hormone (PTH) transports calcium from the bones into the bloodstream. It also signals the kidneys to conserve calcium and other minerals from the urine. Additionally, PTH signals the kidneys to produce *calcitrol*, which is formed from vitamin-D that signals the small intestine to absorb more calcium. The thyroid gland secretes *calcitonin*, which increases bone mineralization, and decreases the rate of bone breakdown. Any factors that interfere with, or alter the delicate balance maintained by these hormone systems are likely to have a negative impact on bone absorption and mineralization.

The single most powerful cause for low bone mineralization and onset of osteoporosis is lack of hormones. A lack of *estrogen* in post-menopausal women prevents the absorption and utilization of calcium. *Testosterone* is converted to estrogen in the male, therefore, serves the same function as in women. A decrease in testosterone levels with aging contributes to osteoporosis in men as well. For this reason, calcium is generally is given at menopause and andropause as a dietary supplement.

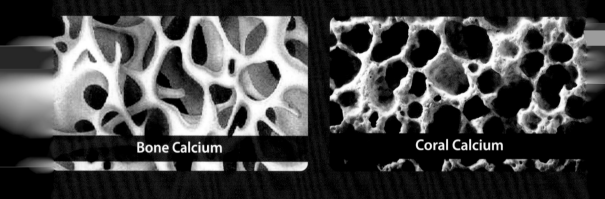

Bone Calcium

Coral Calcium

Microscopic views of different natural forms reflect importance of calcium in the maintenance of structural integrity. Therefore, the source of calcium for human dietary supplementation comes primarily from **ground up rock, clays, sea beds, egg shells, or soils.**

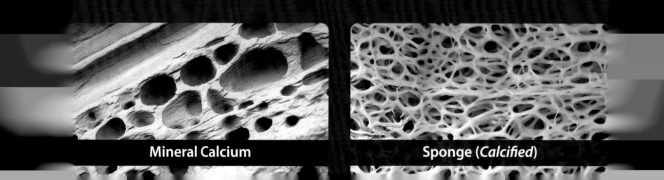

Mineral Calcium

Sponge (*Calcified*)

3.6 | Calcium Homeostasis

Calcium homeostasis is a closely regulated process that maintains the levels of Ca^{2+} ions in the body within a tight normal range. In this process, calcium is removed (resorbed) from the bone and released into the blood circulation to maintain Ca^{2+} at 2.5 mmol/L (normal level).

The typical calcium content of the adult human body is 1 kg, virtually all is found in the skeleton; the amount in body fluids and cells of the soft tissues accounts for the remaining for1% calcium reserve. Accordingly, there are three major pools of calcium in the body: i) *Intracellular pool* refers to calcium inside the cells and stored within the mitochondria, the cellular 'power house'. Intracellular free calcium concentrations fluctuate greatly, from roughly 0.1 to 1.0 *micro-M*. These fluctuations are integral to calcium's role in intracellular signaling, enzyme activation and muscle contractions. ii) *Circulatory pool*, roughly half of the calcium in blood is bound to proteins. The concentration of Ca^{2+} ions in this pool is normally constant at 1 milli-M, or 10,000 times more concentration of free calcium within cells. Also, the concentration of phosphorus in blood is essentially identical to that of calcium. iii) *Skeletal pool* is comprised of the vast majority of body calcium. Within bone, 99% of the calcium is tied up in the mineral phase, but the remaining 1% is in a pool that can rapidly exchange with extracellular calcium.

Calcium homeostasis maintains only with continuous use of energy and depends on the balance flow of several factors including, vitamins, hormones and bone nutrients.

Calcium Fluxes

Calcium in the circulatory pool (constant level: 1 mM) is maintained by frequent adjustments, called as *calcium fluxes* between blood and other body pools. Three organs participate in the supply and removal of calcium from the blood: i) the small intestine is the primary site where dietary calcium is absorbed; ii) the bone serves as a huge reservoir for calcium; and iii) kidney is critical for calcium reclamation. Under normal conditions, most of the calcium that enters the kidney *(glomerular filtrate)* is reabsorbed from the tubular system back into blood, in order to preserve the blood calcium levels. If kidney reabsorption is impaired, then the calcium is lost by urinary excretion.

Variations in body calcium levels, above *(hypercalcemia)* or below *(hypocalcemia)* the normal range can trigger several disorders. *Hypercalcemia* can lead to precipitation of calcium phosphate in tissues, leading to widespread organ dysfunction and damage. *Hypocalcemia* can lead to severe disorders to the neuromuscular system with clinical symptoms such as muscle spasms, tetany and cardiac dysfunction. The above two calcium-based disorders can be prevented by active hormone control systems.

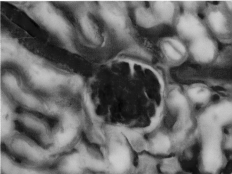

FIGURE: *Microscopic view of kidney glomerulus*

Hormone Control Systems

Sex hormone, estrogen (E) has a positive effect on bone geometric and densitometric development. E suppresses bone turnover during the early pubertal period.

Calcium transfer between the bone 'mineral bank' and circulatory pool is strictly controlled by three hormones, i) the parathyroid hormone *(PTH)*, ii) the calcitonin *(CT)* and, iii) the vitamin-D. Through a combined action, these 3 hormones maintain the normal levels of blood calcium and control the calcium fluxes between blood and cells of various tissues.

Parathyroid hormone *(PTH)* increases calcium levels in the circulatory (blood) pool. This PTH function is achieved by several mechanisms. Primarily, PTH facilitates calcium mobilization from the bone. PTH stimulates formation of active vitamin-D in the kidney, which is necessary for calcium reclamation and minimizing its urinary loss.

Vitamin-D is involved in raising the blood calcium levels. The most important function of vitamin-D is to facilitate calcium absorption from the small intestine. Together with PTH, vitamin-D also enhances calcium fluxes.

Calcitonin *(CT)* activity is exactly opposite to PTH function; it lowers the blood calcium levels. CT is secreted by the thyroid gland, in response to *hypercalcemia*. CT can suppress the kidney (renal tubular)-mediated reabsorption of calcium; in other words, it increases excretion of calcium through urine. CT also inhibits bone resorption, and minimizes calcium fluxes from bone to blood.

The process of calcium homeostasis, the effects of Ca^{2+} deprivation and Ca^{2+} loading and the body responses are summarized in the following **TABLE**.

Measure	Calcium Deprivation	Calcium Loading
PTH	Secretion stimulated	Secretion inhibited
Vitamin-D	Production stimulated by increased PTH secretion	Production inhibited due to low PTH secretion
Calcitonin	Very low level secretion	Secretion stimulated by high blood calcium
Ca^{2+} Absorption *(Intestinal tract)*	Enhanced by vitamin-D	Low basal uptake
Ca^{2+} Release *(from the Bone)*	Stimulated by increased PTH and vitamin-D	Decreased due to low PTH and vitamin-D
Ca^{2+} Excretion *(by the Kidney)*	Decrease due to enhanced tubular reabsorption	Increase due to hampered PTH and low reabsorption
General Response	Long term deprivation leads to osteopenia (bone thinning).	High gut absorption and low urinary excretion leads to hypercalcemia.

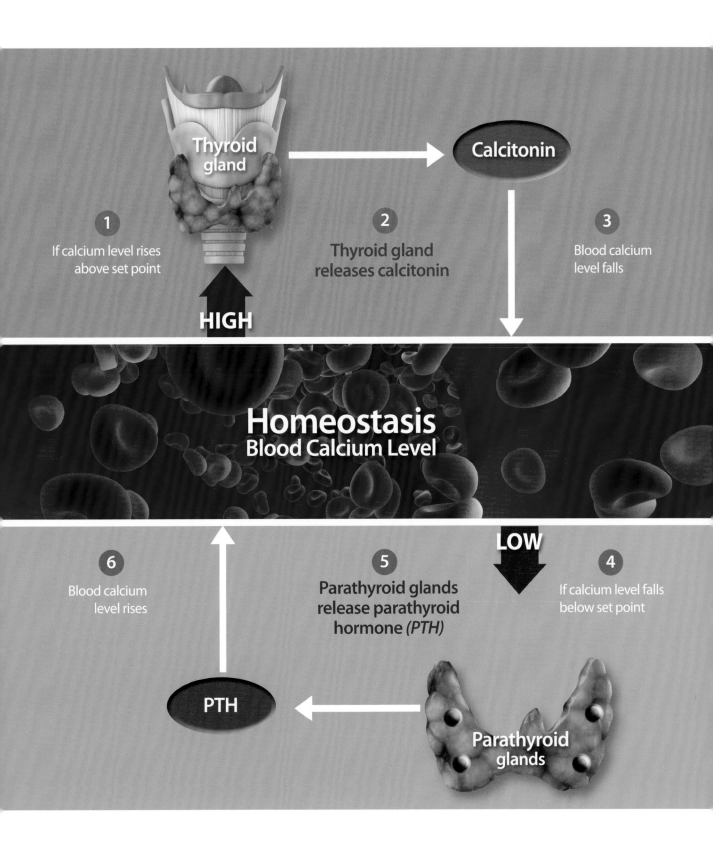

1
If calcium level rises above set point

2
Thyroid gland releases calcitonin

3
Blood calcium level falls

Thyroid gland

Calcitonin

HIGH

Homeostasis
Blood Calcium Level

LOW

6
Blood calcium level rises

5
Parathyroid glands release parathyroid hormone *(PTH)*

4
If calcium level falls below set point

PTH

Parathyroid glands

3.1 | OSTEOGENESIS

1. Deng ZL, Sharff KA, Tang N, et al (2008) Regulation of osteogenic differentiation during skeletal development. *Frontiers in Bioscience* 13:2001-2021.
2. Clarke B (2008) Normal bone anatomy and physiology. *Clinical Journal of American Society for Nephrology* 3:131-139.
3. Wang Y, Wan C, Gilbert SR, Clemens TL (2007) Oxygen sensing and osteogenesis. *Annals of New York Academy of Sciences* 1117:1-11.
4. Weaver CM (2007) Vitamin D, calcium homeostasis and skeleton accretion in children. *Journal of Bone and Mineral Research* 22:45-49.

3.2 | BONE MODELING AND REMODELING

1. Aguila HL, Rowe DW (2005) Skeletal development, bone remodeling and hematopoiesis. *Immunological Reviews* 208:7-18.
2. Hadjidakis DJ, Androulakis II (2006) Bone remodeling. *Annals of New York Academy of Sciences* 1092:385-396.
3. Lemaire V, Tobin L, Greller L, et al (2004) Modeling the interactions between osteoblast and osteoclast activities in bone remodeling. *Journal of Theoretical Biology* 229:293-309.
4. Li Z, Kong K, Qi W (2006) Osteoclast and its roles in calcium metabolism and bone development and remodeling. *Biochemical Biophysical Research Communications* 343(2):345-350.
5. Mackie EJ (2003) Osteoblasts: novel roles in orchestration of skeletal architecture. *International Journal of Biochemistry and Cell Biology* 35(9):1301-1305.
6. Matkovic V (1991) Calcium metabolism and calcium requirements during skeletal remodeling and consolidation of bone mass. *American Journal of Clinical Nutrition* 54:245-260.

3.3 | BONE TURNOVER

1. Caetano-Lopes J, Canhão H, Fonseca JE (2007) Osteoblasts and bone formation. *Acta Reumatologica Portuguesa* 32(2):103-110.
2. Blair HC (1998) How the osteoclast degrades bone. *Bioessays* 20(10):837-846.
3. Phan TC, Xu J, Zheng MH (2004) Interaction between osteoblast and osteoclast: impact in bone disease. *Histology and Histopathology* 19(4):1325-1344.
3. Pogoda P, Priemel M, Rueger JM, Amling M (2005) Bone remodeling: new aspects of a key process that controls skeletal maintenance and repair. *Osteoporosis International* 16:18-24.

3.4 | BONE MINERALIZATION

1. Therapeutic Research Faculty (2003) Natural Medicines: Comprehensive Database. 5th Edition. Therapeutic Research Faculty, Stockton.
2. Lieberman S, Bruning N (2003) The real vitamin and mineral book. New York: Avery. ISBN 1-58333-152-2,
3. Ambard AJ, Mueninghoff L (2006) Calcium phosphate cement: review of mechanical and biological properties. *Journal of Prosthodontology* 15(5):321-328.

4. Bronner F (1997) Calcium. In: Handbook of Nutritionally Essential Mineral Elements (O'Dell, B. L. and Sunde, R. A. eds.), pp. 13–61. New York: Marcel Dekker.

5. Marcus R (1987) Calcium intake and skeletal integrity: Is there a critical relationship? *Journal of Nutrition* 117:631-635.

6. Nordin BE, Need A, Morris H, et al (2004) Effect of age on calcium absorption in postmenopausal women. *American Journal of Clinical Nutrition* 80:998-1002.

7. Baker SB, Worthley LI (2002) The essentials of calcium, magnesium and phosphate metabolism: part I. Physiology. *Critical Care and Resuscitation* 4(4):301-6.

8. Calvo MS, Park YK (1996) Changing phosphorus content of the U.S. diet: potential for adverse effects on bone. *Journal of Nutrition* 126:1168S-1180S.

9. Anderson JJ (1996) Calcium, phosphorus and human bone development. *Journal of Nutrition* 126:1153S-1158S.

10. Renkema KY, Alexander RT, et al (2008) Calcium and phosphate homeostasis: concerted interplay of new regulators. *Annals of Medicine* 40(2):82-91.

11. Takeda E, Taketani Y, Sawada N, et al (2004) The regulation and function of phosphate in the human body. *Biofactors* 21:345-355.

12. Bergman C, Gray-Scott D, Chen JJ, Meacham S (2009) What is next for the Dietary Reference Intakes for bone metabolism related nutrients beyond calcium: phosphorus, magnesium, vitamin D and fluoride? *Critical Reviews in Food Science and Nutrition* 49(2):136-144.

13. Abrams SA, Atkinson SA (2003) Calcium, magnesium, phosphorus and vitamin D fortification of complementary foods. *Journal of Nutrition* 133(9):2994-9299S.

13. Nishi Y (1996) Zinc and growth. *Journal of American College of Nutrition* 15(4):340-344.

14. Yamaguchi M (1992) Role of zinc as an activator of bone formation. *Journal of Nutritional Sciences and Vitaminology* (Tokyo) Spec No:522-525.

15. Vincent JB (2004) Recent advances in the nutritional biochemistry of trivalent chromium. *Proceedings of Nutrition Society* 63(1):41-47.

16. Vincent JB (2000) The biochemistry of chromium. *Journal of Nutrition* 130(4):715-718.

17. Blake GM, Lewiecki EM, Kendler DL, Fogelman I (2007) A review of strontium ranelate and its effect on DXA scans. *Journal of Clinical Densitometry* 10(2):113-119.

18. Marie PJ (2006) Strontium ranelate: a physiological approach for optimizing bone formation and resorption. *Bone* 38:10-14.

3.5 | BONE MINERAL ABSORPTION

1. Bronner F (1996) Cytoplasmic transport of calcium and other inorganic ions. *Comparative Biochemistry and Physiology (Part B)* 115:313-317.

2. Bronner F, Pansu D (1999) Nutritional aspects of calcium absorption. *Journal of Nutrition* 129:9-12.

3. Carter PH, Schipani E (2006) The roles of parathyroid hormone and calcitonin in bone remodeling: prospects for novel therapeutics. *Endocrine Metabolism Immune Disorders and Drug Targets* 6(1):59-76.

4. Duflos C, Bellaton C, Pansu D, Bronner F (1995) Calcium solubility, intestinal sojourn time and paracellular permeability codetermine passive calcium absorption in rats. *Journal of Nutrition* 125:2348-2355

5. Huang CL, Sun L, Moonga BS, Zaidi M (2006) Molecular physiology and pharmacology of calcitonin. *Cellular and Molecular Biology* 52(3):33-43.

6. Khanal RC, Nemere I (2008) Regulation of intestinal calcium transport. *Annual Review of Nutrition* 28:179-196.

7. Powell JJ, Jugdaohsingh R, Thompson RPH (1999) The regulation of mineral absorption in the gastrointestinal tract. *Proceedings of the Nutrition Society* 58:147-153.

8. Recker RR (1985) Calcium absorption and achlorhydria. *The New England Journal of Medicine* 313:70-73.

9. Stein W D (1992) Facilitated diffusion of calcium across the intestinal epithelial cell. *Journal of Nutrition* 122:651S-656S.

10. Hansen M, Sandstrom B, Jensen M, Sorensen SS (1997) Effects of casein phosphopeptides on zinc and calcium absorption from bread meals. *Journal of Trace Elements in Medicine and Biology* 11:143–149.

12. Suzuki Y, Landowski CP, Hediger MA (2008) Mechanisms and regulation of epithelial Ca^{2+} absorption in health and disease. *Annual Review of Physiology* 70:257-271.

13. van de Graaf SF, Bindels RJ, Hoenderop JG (2007) Physiology of epithelial Ca^{2+} and Mg^{2+} transport. *Reviews in Physiology Biochemistry and Pharmacology* 158:77-160.

14. Wasserman RH, Chandler JS, Meyer SA, et al (1992) Intestinal calcium transport and calcium extrusion processes at the basolateral membrane. *Journal of Nutrition* 122:662–671.

15. Cámara-Martos F, Amaro-López MA (2002) Influence of dietary factors on calcium bioavailability: a brief review. Biological Trace Element Research 89(1):43-52.

3.6 | CALCIUM HOMEOSTASIS

1. St-Arnaud R (2008) The direct role of vitamin D on bone homeostasis. *Archives of Biochemistry and Biophysics* 473(2):225-230.

2. Talmage RV, Mobley HT (2007) Calcium homeostasis: reassessment of the actions of parathyroid hormone. *General and Comparative Endocrinology* 156(1):1-8.

3. Talmage RV, Talmage DW (2006) Calcium homeostasis: solving the solubility problem. *Journal of Musculoskeletal and Neuronal Interactions* 6(4):402-407.

4. Doyle ME, Jan de Beur SM (2008) The skeleton: endocrine regulator of phosphate homeostasis. *Current Osteoporosis Reports* 6(4):134-141.

5. Matkovic V, Heaney RP (1992) Calcium balance during human growth: Evidence for threshold behavior. *American Journal of Clinical Nutrition* 55:992-995.

Bone Functions

4

Bone is not just a framework that moves the body; it is a 'Mineral Bank' that runs day-to-day production of blood cells and regulates several internal systems.

Bone Functions

I. Mineral Bank
Bones are storage reserves for calcium phosphorous and other essential minerals.

II. Blood Production
Bone marrow of long bones and inner space of spongy bone, produces blood cells by the *hematopoiesis* process.

III. Protection
Bones protect vital organs. Skull and vertebrae shield the brain and spinal cord. Rib cage is a protective armor for the heart, liver and lungs.

IV. Acid-Base Balance
Bone buffers the blood against excess pH changes by absorbing or releasing alkaline salts.

V. Detoxification
Bone tissues absorb heavy metals and toxins. It removes such compounds from the blood and reduces their toxic effects on the body.

VI. Sound Management
Auditory Ossicles ('hearing bones'), facilitate the physio-mechanical aspect of hearing.

VII. Movement
Bones, skeletal muscles, tendons, ligaments and joints function together to move individual body parts or whole body in 3D space.

VIII. Shape
Bones provide structural frame to stylize the individual appearance of the body .

4

4.1 | The Multi-functional System

Skeleton is a marvelous ensemble of bones designed to perform some extraordinary functions. It resists and balances the body against the pull of gravity. The large bones of the lower limbs not only supported the trunk to stand upright, but also endowed the human race the unique ability to evolve as the only bipedal to walk on this Blue Planet.

Skeleton provides the strongest protective body armor; the fused bones of the cranium enclose the brain and make it less vulnerable to injury; the vertebrae wrap around to protect the spinal cord; and bones of the rib cage efficiently shield the heart and lungs. Bones team up with muscles to develop simple mechanical lever systems to mobilize the body parts. Inner core of the bone is enriched with mineral salts, especially, calcium phosphate. The dynamic process of release and storage of calcium has a multifunctional characteristic, critical for several vital functions, especially for the heart to beat, the nerve cell to flash an electric impulse, the muscle to twitch, the bowel to move and the kidney to filter. Furthermore, the ability to release alkaline salts makes the bone an extraordinary physiological tool for acid-base titration in the body. As a primary site for the formation of blood cells; bone marrow generates red blood cells *(RBC)* that oxygenate the tissues, white blood cells *(WBC)* that provide immune protection against foreign bodies, and platelets that facilitate blood clotting. The 3 tiny 'hearing bones' located in the ear, have bestowed the gift to applaud the sound of music and listen to whispers of the Mother Nature. Finally, bones not only gave us a shape but a face to look into the mirror.

Strength and endurance of the skeletal system is undisputable. Accordingly, bones have served, yet an extraordinary function of documenting the evolution.

Bones have opened a remarkable forensic window to track our ancestry from the 10th century BC, the times of King Solomon from the southern Jordon; or the lost Egyptian kingdom of the Pharaohs. The magnificent skeletons of dinosaurs from the Jurassic era stand with grace and elegance at the National Museum of History to reinforce the power of bones.

4.2 | Bone Function: **Mineral Bank**

Skeleton is body's designated *organ*(ization) that runs a *'Mineral Bank'*, especially the *'checking/saving accounts'* for two minerals, calcium and phosphorus. This mineral bank operates as body's lender in times of need. Maintaining an optimum balance of calcium in the body fluids and an adequate cellular supply of minerals is critical for life.

Bones contain more calcium reserves than any other organ. Calcium is *'withdrawn'* from the bone bank when blood calcium levels drop below normal, to sustain metabolic needs. When blood calcium levels rise, the excess calcium is *'deposited'* in the bone bank. The dynamic transaction of calcium deposits and withdrawals; and process of saving calcium reserves in the *'bone locker'* go on a regular-basis.

A complex group of hormones ensure an adequate supply of bone minerals to support a variety of physiological functions. These hormones not only inspect the bone reserves of calcium, but also transfer calcium and other minerals to support the ongoing functions of various tissue organs, such as the intestine, brain, liver and kidney.

In response to its dual role of deposits-withdrawals of calcium and phosphorus; performing repair services to maintain a functional skeleton, bone is constantly on the run to remodel itself. Old bone breaks down and new bone is formed on a regular basis. In fact, the skeletal tissue is replaced several times during life. This requires a well structured regulatory system, a group of specialized cells and an extensive communication network. This network must respond to several signals, internal and external, mechanical and hormonal, and systemic (affecting the whole skeleton) and local (affecting only a small part of the skeleton). Therefore, it is not surprising, with a plethora of events running concurrently with the bone bank (i.e. growth, maintenance and adaptation), there is always a chance for a pathway in the bone metabolism to go astray. Accordingly, the *"bone mineral overdraft"* sets off the clinical condition – the osteoporosis.

Entire skeleton is replaced every 7 years or so. Balance between bone deposits and withdrawals change with age, which leads to a bone loss over a lifetime of about 15% in men and 30% in women.

Maximum bone deposit, defined as the 'peak bone mass', largely depends on genetics and environmental factors, including adequate nutrition. True strength of a bone bank is defined during the childhood, the teen years and early adulthood. Peak bone mass is reached between 18 and 25 years of age. In youth and young adulthood, daily consumption of enough calcium, regular exercise and a healthy lifestyle makes bone dense (thick) and strong, thereby reduces any risk of osteoporosis later in life.

Nutrition is one of the important modifiable factors in the development and maintenance of bone mineral bank and the prevention and treatment of osteoporosis. The nutrients of most obvious importance to bone health are calcium and phosphorus, since they compose roughly about 80% to 90% of the bone mineral content

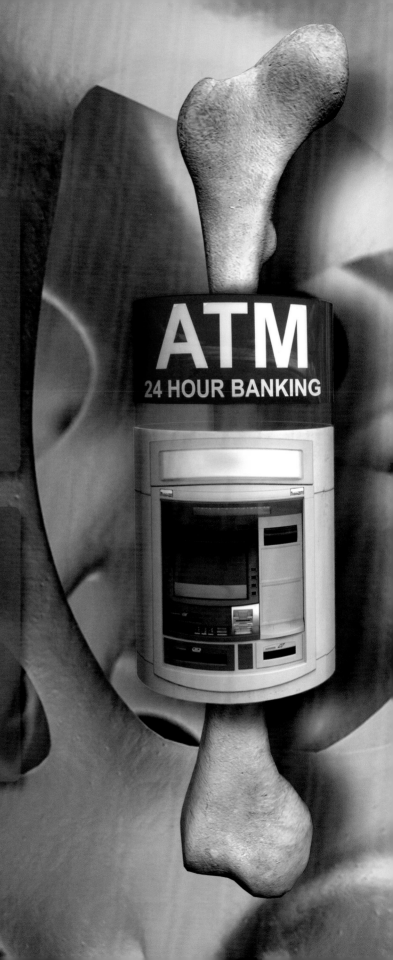

Bone Bank **Withdrawals** is a well articulated mechanism of bone resorption by the osteoclasts; wherein the stored bone minerals, especially calcium, are released into the blood stream. This is an important bone breakdown process to maintain calcium balance in the tissues and extracellular fluids. Too many withdrawals result in mineral depletion, increased porosity and bones become more prone to fractures such as in osteoporosis.

Bone Bank **Deposit** is the skeletal formation process by the osteoblasts; wherein the bone cells actively fish out the circulating calcium in its mineral form, take it from the bloodstream and make a deposit into the bone matrix. This results in an increase of bone mineral density (BMD). Ninety percent of bone mass accumulates by age 20; and 10 percent between age 20 and the early 30s. Peak bone mass is about 30% higher in men than in women.

4.3 | Bone Function: **Blood Production**

Bone marrow is the body's designated *Blood Cell Factory*. Bone marrow constitutes 4% of total body weight (about 2.6 kg or 5.7 lbs.) in adults. There are two types of bone marrow: RED (mainly *myeloid tissue*) and YELLOW (mainly fat cells). Red blood cells *(RBC)*, most white blood cells *(WBC)*, and platelets are produced in the red marrow; while some WBC are manufactured in the yellow marrow.

At birth, all bone marrow is red. However, with age, a majority is converted to yellow. Red marrow is found mainly in the flat bones (hip bone, breast bone, skull, ribs, vertebrae and shoulder blades), and in the spongy material of the long bones *(femur and humerus)*. Yellow marrow is found in the hollow interior of the long bones.

Hematopoiesis is a remarkable self-regulated system that generates all types of blood cells. Approximately a trillion new blood cells are produced daily.

Blood cells are divided into three lineages: *i) Erythroid cells* are the oxygen carrying RBC; *ii) Lymphoid cells* are the players of the adaptive immune system; and *iii) Myeloid cells* include granulocytes, and macrophages, that are involved in innate immunity and blood clotting. Any interruption of hematopoiesis blocks the production of neutrophils (which have a 6-8 h short life span); followed by the inhibition of platelet (with a 10-day life span) synthesis. Anemia develops more slowly, over a longer span of time (since the lifespan of RBC is about 90-20 days).

During child development (beginning at 4 years) the hematopoietic activity moves to the axial skeleton *(flat bones, skull, ribs, sternum, clavicle, vertebrae, pelvic bones)* and proximal ends of long bones *(humerus and femur)*. Move to the axial site is completed by age 18. The remaining marrow cavities are replaced with fat (yellow bone marrow). By age 40, the marrow in *sternum, ribs, pelvis* and *vertebrae* is composed of equal amounts of hematopoietic tissue and fat.

First blood cells are the RBC that forms within 2 to 8 weeks of embryonic development. Granulocytes appear by the 2nd month; by the 5th month bone marrow takes over as the main facility for blood production, which continues for rest of the life. Blood cells develop from the *hematopoietic stem cells (HSC)* found in the red bone marrow. Stem cells make up 10% of cord blood cells and <1% of all adult blood cells. Stem cells are able to multiply and differentiate into different types of blood cells. The average number of HSC in a leg bone is about 440 billion.

An average 70 litre human body contains only about 5 litres (7% by volume) of blood. Of the average 5-L of blood, only 2.25-L (45%) consists of cells. The rest is plasma, which consists of 93% water (by weight) and 7% solids (mostly protein). Of the 2.25-L of cells, only 0.037-L (1.6%) is WBC. The entire circulating WBC, if isolated, would fit in a bartender's jigger. The total circulating platelet volume is even less — about 0.0065-L — or a little over one teaspoonful.

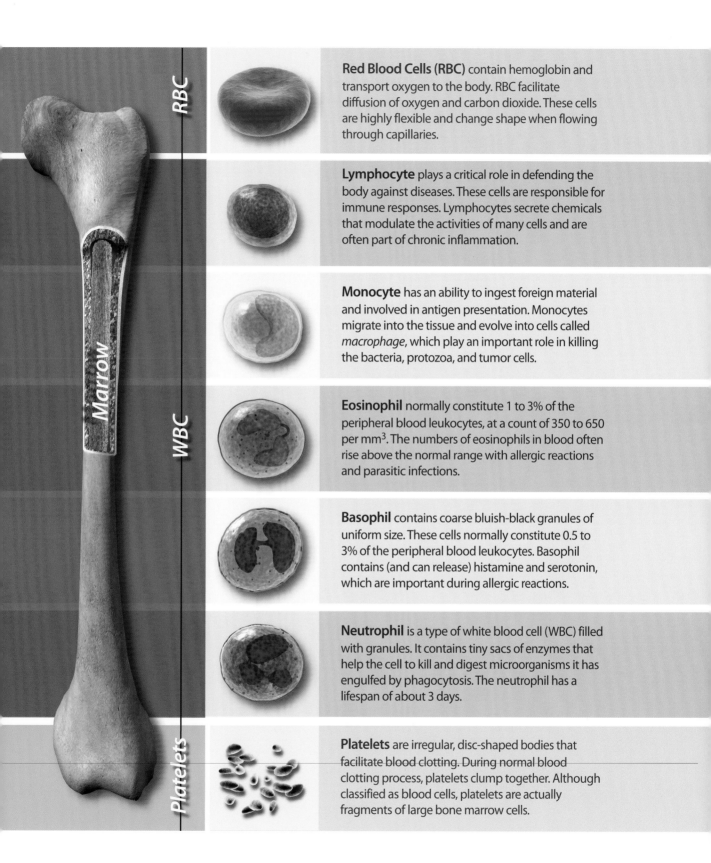

RBC

Red Blood Cells (RBC) contain hemoglobin and transport oxygen to the body. RBC facilitate diffusion of oxygen and carbon dioxide. These cells are highly flexible and change shape when flowing through capillaries.

Lymphocyte plays a critical role in defending the body against diseases. These cells are responsible for immune responses. Lymphocytes secrete chemicals that modulate the activities of many cells and are often part of chronic inflammation.

Monocyte has an ability to ingest foreign material and involved in antigen presentation. Monocytes migrate into the tissue and evolve into cells called *macrophage*, which play an important role in killing the bacteria, protozoa, and tumor cells.

WBC

Eosinophil normally constitute 1 to 3% of the peripheral blood leukocytes, at a count of 350 to 650 per mm³. The numbers of eosinophils in blood often rise above the normal range with allergic reactions and parasitic infections.

Basophil contains coarse bluish-black granules of uniform size. These cells normally constitute 0.5 to 3% of the peripheral blood leukocytes. Basophil contains (and can release) histamine and serotonin, which are important during allergic reactions.

Neutrophil is a type of white blood cell (WBC) filled with granules. It contains tiny sacs of enzymes that help the cell to kill and digest microorganisms it has engulfed by phagocytosis. The neutrophil has a lifespan of about 3 days.

Platelets

Platelets are irregular, disc-shaped bodies that facilitate blood clotting. During normal blood clotting process, platelets clump together. Although classified as blood cells, platelets are actually fragments of large bone marrow cells.

Marrow

Bone Functions | 97

Skeletal system protects the vital body organs. It provides a sturdy *'cage of bones'* designed to house the delicate internal organs and fragile body tissues. The *cranial cage* (skull) encloses the brain; the *rib cage* shields the heart and lungs; and the hollow *vertebral column* (backbone) wraps around the spinal cord.

Skull is composed of 22 bones more or less tightly sutured together to form a *cranial vault* that protects the brain, like a steel helmet. Skull shapes the head and arranges the facial bones; at the same time the sensory organs for taste (tongue), smell (nose), hearing (auditory ossicles), and vision (eye balls).

Ribs are curved, flat bones with a slightly twisted shaft. They are comprised of 24 bones arranged in 12 pairs to form a *ribcage* to fence the upper body and provide the chest its familiar enclosure. Ribs provide an armored cover for the heart and blood vessels to protect from physical injuries and shocks. Lungs are safely housed in the ribcage; where the curved bones support the breathing process. During inhalation, the muscles in between the ribs lift the rib cage up, allowing the lungs to expand. When exhaled, the rib cage shifts down and squeezes air out of the lungs. Ribs also protect parts of the stomach, spleen, liver and kidneys.

Vertebral Column is the major foundation of the skeleton that encircles the spinal cord. The 5 fused *sacral* vertebrae and 4 *coccyx* form part of the *pelvis*, all these units collectively protect the *pelvic viscera*.

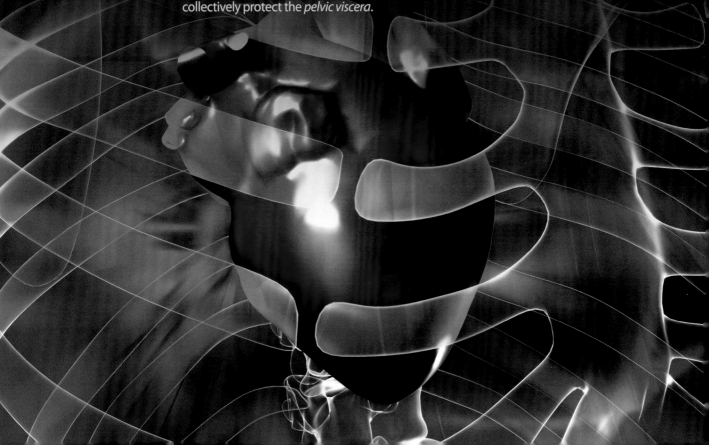

4.5 | Bone Function: **Acid-Base Balance**

Bone contains large stores of buffer, in the form of mineral salts to effectively balance the pH changes that occur in the body. Acid-base balance (or titration) in the body has a significant metabolic outcome on the bone turnover, especially on the rates of bone resorption and calcium mobilization.

Acids are metabolic end products of the body. Digestion of proteins and amino acids from the diet results in production of acids, like sulfuric, hydrochloric, and phosphoric acids. These acids are instantly buffered in the blood and quickly excreted by the kidneys. In the event of inadequate buffering capacity of the blood, the skeletal system provides an acid-alkaline balance by absorbing or releasing alkaline salts into the blood. Bone matrix contains a substantial alkaline reserve of calcium *(Ca^{+2})* and magnesium *(Mg^{+2})*. These cations are released from the bone to titrate an overly acidic milieu. However, repeated borrowing of the bone's alkaline reserves can be potentially detrimental to health. However, if the acid production is increased and its excretion is impaired, a serious clinical condition called *'metabolic acidosis'* will arise. In response, the kidneys react to the circulating calcium in the plasma and increase the excretion of calcium in urine (or *hypercalcinuria*). Metabolic acidosis can onset osteoporosis, muscle wasting and kidney dysfunction (due to increased risk of calcium-based kidney stones).

In adults, the bone buffering capacity is extremely poor due its low water content and highly exchangeable bone mineral surface. Therefore, even a mild acid exposure can trigger the onset of osteoporosis in the elderly. A diet that can neutralize the endogenous acid production may increase calcium and phosphate retention, reduce bone resorption and increase bone formation.

Body Site	pH Range
Blood	7.35-7.45
Muscle	6.1
Liver	6.9
Gastric juice	1.2-3.0
Saliva	6.35-6.85
Urine	4.5-8.0
Pancreatic juice	7.8-8.0

The "potential of hydrogen," or "pH," is based on a logarithmic scale, which is a 10-fold difference between each number going from 1 to 14. The lower numbers (1.0 to 6.99) represent the ACID (or H+ donating) range, and the higher numbers (7.01 to 14.0) represent the ALKALINE (or H+ accepting) range. For the most part, body tissues remain within the neutral pH of 7.0. Some body systems such as the blood (7.35-7.45) are more tightly regulated than others (eg, urine pH ranges from 4.5-8.0). From a physiological perspective, body has compartmental organ systems that operate within a well defined pH range (see TABLE).

4.6 | Bone Function: **Detoxification**

Detoxification is a method of cleansing harmful chemicals by various bodily processes including excretion, neutralization or transformation. This chemical elimination protects the vital body systems from detrimental toxic effects.

Bone, as the elemental storehouse of cations (e.g. Ca^{2+}, Mg^{2+}, Sr^{2+}) and anions (e.g. phosphates, carbonates), can strongly react to various toxic heavy metals that enter the body. Bone minerals form complexes with toxic heavy metals and dispose these artifacts via the circulatory route that runs through the skeletal matrix. Bone-mediated detoxification is a safe containment within its matrix and a controlled excretion from the body.

However, repeated exposure to high doses of heavy metals like cadmium, lead, and mercury can trigger metabolic bone diseases, such as osteoporosis. These heavy metals interact with normal bone minerals and can either destroy or deplete their levels. For example, *lead (Pb)* deposits in the bone through its distal ends or joints and displaces calcium. Lead can also destroy normal cartilage tissue and contribute to arthritis. On the other hand, *cadmium (Cd)* deposits on the bone surface and cause pain. *Berryllium (Be)* can deplete magnesium and disturb calcium and vitamin-D metabolism, leading to the onset of rickets. *Mercury (Hg)* accumulates in tissues such as kidneys, eyes, brain, thyroid, and liver. The function of these five organs can affect bone tissue, and set off osteoporosis.

Bone is also the major disposal sink for *vanadium (V)* that enters the body. The upper respiratory tract is the main target for vanadium exposure. Symptoms include conjunctivitis, asthma, fatigue, cardiac palpitation, gastrointestinal distress, kidney damage, and other neurological disorders. Accumulation of vanadium in bone is useful and efficient biological detoxification process. The high skeletal retention of *vanadate* (vanadium salt) can rapidly exchange with bone phosphate, facilitated by the strong structural similarities between vanadate and phosphate.

Scientific evidence on bone-mediated detoxification of heavy metals can be traced to ancient civilizations. Archeological investigations have detected heavy metals such as copper and lead in human femur samples traced to 10th century BC, around the time when King Solomon is believed to have ruled over the ancient Hebrews – which is the modern day Jordan.

The Human Auditory System is designed to detect several aspects of sounds, including pitch, loudness, and direction. Sound waves are acquired by the external ear and channeled through the ear canal to the eardrum (or *tympanic membrane*).

Auditory ossicles (also known as the *'Hearing Bones'*) are *'3 tiny bones'* that work together as a single unit. The 1st ossicle, the *malleus* (or *hammer*), has a long arm embedded into the eardrum that responds to mechanical vibrations (or oscillations). The 2nd is the *incus* (or *anvil*), a leverage system that amplifies the mechanical vibrations. The 3rd is the *stapes* (or *stirrup*), forms the connection to the inner ear and transmits the vibrations. Bone loss of the auditory ossicles can result in a moderate-to-severe hearing loss.

The ear is organized in three major parts: outer ear, middle ear, and internal (inner) ear. Each part aids in the transmission of the stimulus to the receptor cells.

When sound hits the eardrum, the impact creates vibrations that moves the auditory ossicles. In the inner ear, thousands of microscopic hair cells are bent by the wave-like action of *cochleal fluid*. This *'hair bending'* sets off nerve impulses that pass through the *auditory nerve* to the hearing centre of the brain. The relative length of the hair fibers determine the different sound frequencies - short fibers respond to high frequencies and long fibers respond to lower frequencies. The sensation of sound, of course, occurs only when the vibrations are interpreted by the cerebral cortex of the brain at a conscious level.

The extent of hearing bone vibrations are controlled by contractions of the *auditory muscles*. These muscles become rigid and dampen the response of acoustic stimulation, especially during the transmission of low frequency sound *(frequencies below 1000 Hz)*. It takes about 40 to 80 milliseconds *(1000th fraction of a second)* to cause such contraction. The auditory muscle contraction can reduce a sound transmission by 30 to 40 decibels, which is about the difference between a loud noise and the sound of a whisper

Nerves
(Connects to the Brain)

Semi-Circular Canals

Cochlea

Outer Ear Canal

Stirrup

Hammer

Eustachian Tube
(Connects to the Nose)

Anvil

Ear Drum

Inner Ear	Middle Ear	Outer Ear

4.8 | Bone Function: **Movement**

Movement is a basic function of the *musculo-skeletal system*, which manifests into postures and motions. This function is dependent on several muscles that attach to the bones through tendons, ligaments and cartilage. Muscle contraction flexes the *'biceps'* or tightens the *'abs'*, is the quintessential force that enables mobility.

Humans are the only obligate *bipeds* that walk on this *Blue Planet*. Skeletal adaptations, especially to the lower limbs, have evolved a strong foot-hold to balance and propel the human body in a bipedal motion. Locomotion, whether to walk, skip, jump, swim or run is a voluntary human behavior. Muscles work in opposing pairs and coordinate the body movement. However, from a biological standpoint, locomotion should not be considered a life function because not every organism that is alive is able to move (e.g. plants, barnacles).

Basketball players and long-distance and marathon runners have a high percentage (about 80%) of slow-twitch fibers; sprinters have 60% of fast-twitch fibers; weight lifters and football players have an approximately equal number of fast- and slow-twitch fibers.

Three types of muscle fibers play an integral part in the mechanism of skeleto-muscular motion. These fibers are recognized on the basis of size, speed of reaction, and endurance, accordingly: i) *Red slow-twitch fibers* have endurance capability (or fatigue resistance), however, these fibers can generate only a limited power; ii) *White fast-twitch fibers* are suitable for short-term (but easily fatigued), rapid intense movements, such as jumping; iii) *Intermediate fast-twitch fibers* are rich in blood supply, depend on aerobic metabolism, and somewhat fatigue resistant. The fiber network of a skeletal frame is hereditary; therefore, individuals are made of different muscular types to facilitate specific activities.

Normal human locomotion requires a complex interactive control between multiple limb and body segments to provide shock-absorbing and energy-efficient system. This skeletal function is also dependent on, and is serviced by the cardiovascular, respiratory and nervous systems. Skeletal locomotion is also relevant for excretory and reproductive functions.

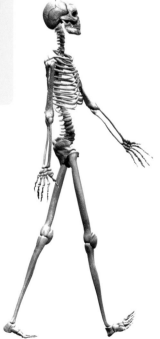

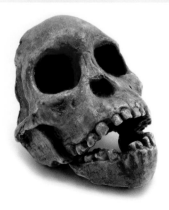

Australopithicus afarensis , nick name "Lucy" was found in 1974 near Hadar in Ethiopia. Her skeleton (traced back to 4 million years) has provided a wealth of information about the ancestral line of human beings, some of it quite surprising. She was only about 3 feet, 8 inches tall; and the way the hip joint and pelvis articulated indicated that "Lucy" walked upright like a human – the first documentation of a bipedal.

4.9 | Bone Function: **Shape**

Shape or figure of a human body is defined exclusively by the structural frame of the skeleton. Skeletal structure (or size of the bone) grows and changes only up to the point at which a human reaches the adulthood and remains essentially same for rest of the life.

Genetics, gender and lifestyle play a cumulative role in the overall development and appearance of the body shape. Males are generally taller with broad shoulders and expanded chest. The shoulder bones widen and the ribcage expands due to the effects of *testosterone* during puberty. The wide shoulders result in a swagger in males as they walk. Due to the testosterone activity, males develop facial-bone features during puberty that comprise a more prominent brow bone, a square jaw, and a large nose bone.

Body shape affects posture, gait, and also implies good bone health and overall fitness of an individual.

Females demonstrate widening of the hip bones and pelvis in response to *estrogen* as a part of sexual differentiation to permit childbirth. The *sacrum* in females is short, wide, and directed more towards the rear that affects their walking style, resulting in hip sway. Also, females generally stand with hips relaxed to one side. Females have a small nose that makes for a fuller upper lip. Hence female faces are generally more close to those of pre-pubertal children.

Body shape usually reaches its optimum between the ages of 13 and 18; by then the *epiphyseal plates* of long bones close, allowing no further growth. Body shape is important for physical attraction between the opposite sexes.

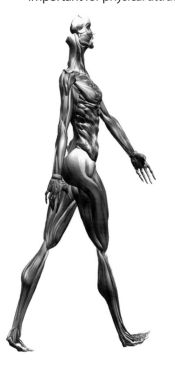 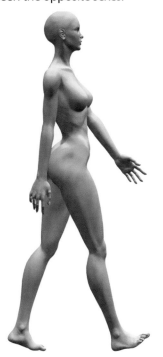 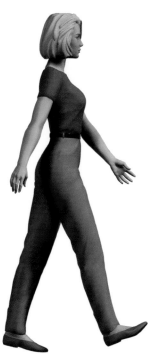

4.1 | MULTIFUNCTIONAL SYSTEM

1. Pyatt FB, Barker GW, Birch P, et al (1999) King Solomon's miners—starvation and bioaccumulation? An environmental archaeological investigation in southern Jordan. *Ecotoxicology and Environmental Safety* 43:305–308.

4.2 | MINERAL BANK

1. Kerstetter J, O'Brien KO, Insogna KL (2003) Low protein intake: The impact on calcium and bone homeostasis in humans. *Journal of Nutrition* 133(3):855S-61S.
2. Marcus R (1987) Calcium intake and skeletal integrity: Is there a critical relationship *Journal of Nutrition* 117:631-635.
3. Matkovic V, Heaney RP (1992) Calcium balance during human growth: Evidence for threshold behavior. *American Journal of Clinical Nutrition* 55:992-995.
4. Mundy GR, Guise TA (1999) Hormonal control of calcium homeostasis. *Clinical Chemistry* 45:1347-1352.

4.3 | BLOOD PRODUCTION

1. Weiss L (1976) The hematopoietic microenvironment of the bone marrow: An ultra structural study of the stroma in rats. *Anatomical Record* 186 (2):161-184.
2. Travlos GS (2006) Normal structure, function, and histology of the bone marrow. *Toxicology and Pathology* 34(5):548-565.
3. Yin T, Li L (2006) The stem cell niches in bone. *Journal of Clinical Investigation* 116(5):1195-1201.
4. Aguila HL, Rowe DW (2005) Skeletal development, bone remodeling, and hematopoiesis. *Immunological Review* 208:7-18.
5. McGrath K, Palis J (2008) Ontogeny of erythropoiesis in the mammalian embryo. *Current Topics in Developmental Biology* 82:1-22.

4.4 | PROTECTION

1. Ross FP, Christiano AM (2006) Nothing but skin and bone. *Journal of Clinical Investigation*116(5):1140-1149.
2. Johnson RB (1998) The bearable lightness of being: bones, muscles, and spaceflight. *Anatomy Records* 253:24-27.
3. Martin B (1993) Aging and strength of bone as a structural material. *Calcified Tissue International* 53:S34-S39;
4. Meghji S (1992) Bone remodelling. *British Dental Journal* 172(6):235-242.
5. Gordan GS, Genant HK (1985) The aging skeleton. *Clinical Geriatric Medicin* 1:95-118.

4.5 | ACID-BASE BALANCE

1. Barzel US (1995) The skeleton as an ion exchange system: Implications for the role of acid-base imbalance in the genesis of osteoporosis. *Journal of Bone and Mineral Research* 10(10):1431-1436.
2. Brenner RJ, Spring DB, Sebastian A, et al. (1982) Incidence of radiographically evident bone

disease, nephrocalcinosis and nephrolithiasis in various types of renal tubular acidosis. *The New England Journal of Medicine* 307(4):217-221.

3. Bushinsky DA (2001) Acid-base imbalance and the skeleton. *European Journal of Nutrition* 40(5):238-244.
4. Bushinsky DA, Frick KK (2000) The effects of acid on bone. *Current Opinion in Nephrology and Hypertension* 9(4):369-379.
5. Green J, Kleeman CR (1991) Role of bone in regulation of systemic acid-base balance. *Kidney International* 39:9-26.
6. Tucker KL, Hannan MT, Kiel DP (2001) The acid-base hypothesis: diet and bone in the Framingham Osteoporosis Study. *European Journal of Nutrition* 40(5):231-237.

4.6 | DETOXIFICATION

1. Baran EJ (2008) Vanadium detoxification: chemical and biochemical aspects. *Chemistry and Biodiveristy* 5:1475-1484.
2. Etcheverry SB, Apella MC, Baran EJ (1984) A model study of the incorporation of vanadium in bone. *Journal of Inorganic Biochemistry* 20:269-274.
3. Minich DM, Bland JS (2007) Acid-alkaline balance: Role in chronic disease and detoxification. *Alternative Therapies* 13(4):62-65.
4. Oniki T, Doi K (1983) ESR spectra of VO^{2+} ions adsorbed on calcium phosphates. *Calcified Tissue International* 35:538-541.

4.7 | SOUND TRANSDUCTION

1. Stenfelt S, Goode RL (2005) Bone-conducted sound: physiological and clinical aspects. *Otology and Neurotology* 26(6):1245-1261.
2. Mallo M (2003) Formation of the outer and middle ear, molecular mechanisms. *Current Topics in Developmental Biology* 57:85-113.
3. Austin DF (1994) Acoustic mechanisms in middle ear sound transfer. *Otolaryngologic Clinics of North America* 27(4):641-654.
4. Bowden RE (1977) Development of the middle and external ear in man. *Proceeding of the Royal Society of Medicine* 70(11):807-815.

4.8 | MOVEMENT

1. Rose J, Gamble J (1994) Human walking, 2nd ed. Baltimore: Williams and Wilkins.
2. Dugan SA, Bhat KP (2005) Biomechanics and analysis of running gait. *Physical Medicine and Rehabilitation Clinics of North America* 16(3):603-621.
3. Harcourt-Smith WE, Aiello LC (2004) Fossils, feet and the evolution of human bipedal locomotion. *Journal of Anatomy* 204(5):403-416.
4. Andriacchi TP, Alexander EJ (2000) Studies of human locomotion: past, present and future. *Journal of Biomechanics* 33(10):1217-1224.

4.9 | SHAPE

1. Lovejoy CO (2005) The natural history of human gait and posture. Part 1. Spine and pelvis. *Gait Posture* 21:95-112.
2. Lovejoy CO (2005) The natural history of human gait and posture. Part 2. Hip and thigh. *Gait Posture* 21:113-124.
3. Lovejoy CO (2007) The natural history of human gait and posture. Part 3. The knee. *Gait Posture* 25:325-341.

Bone Facts

- A newborn has 350 bones in the body; 144 of these fuse together to form the final 206 bones in the adult.

- Babies are born without knee caps, which do not appear until the child reaches 2-6 years of age

- Bones are 4 times stronger than concrete. Adult human bones account for 20% of the body's total weight.

- The only bone in the human body not connected to another is the hyoid, a V-shaped bone located at the base of the tongue between the mandible and the voice box. Its function is to support the tongue and its muscles.

- When a person weighing 150 lbs jogs three miles, the cumulative impact on each foot is greater than 150 tons.

- The big toe is important for body balance. When walking without it, one would simply fall over.

- A person is taller in the morning than at night. This occurs with vertebral compression due to standing upright at daytime.

Bone Diseases

5 Bone diseases are conditions that impair normal bone functions and make bones weak. Fragile bones should not just be excused as a natural part of aging.

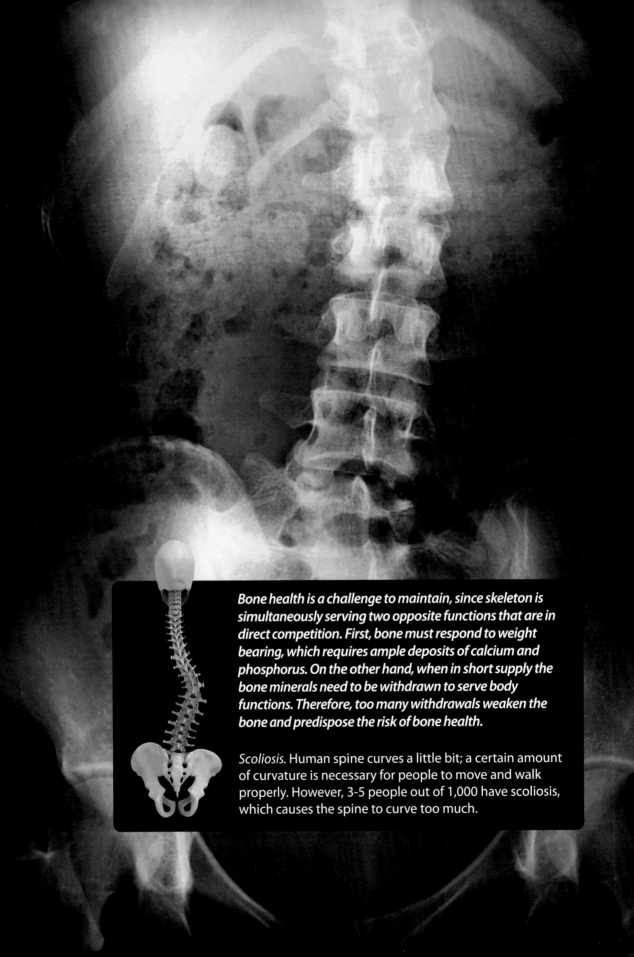

Bone health is a challenge to maintain, since skeleton is simultaneously serving two opposite functions that are in direct competition. First, bone must respond to weight bearing, which requires ample deposits of calcium and phosphorus. On the other hand, when in short supply the bone minerals need to be withdrawn to serve body functions. Therefore, too many withdrawals weaken the bone and predispose the risk of bone health.

Scoliosis. Human spine curves a little bit; a certain amount of curvature is necessary for people to move and walk properly. However, 3-5 people out of 1,000 have scoliosis, which causes the spine to curve too much.

5

5.1 | Metabolic Bone Diseases

Maintenance of strong healthy skeleton is complex and involves a cascade of metabolic pathways. Several factors such as genetics, diet, environment and lifestyle influence the outcome of bone structure and its function. Deficiency or dysfunctions of .any of the above factors lead to *Metabolic Bone Disease*.

Genetic abnormalities can result in weak, thin or overly dense bones. The hereditary disease, *osteogenesis imperfecta* is due to abnormalities in the collagen protein, which weakens the bone matrix and predisposes multiple fractures. Another congenital (hereditary) disorder, *osteopetrosis*, tends to make highly dense bone. This malfunction leads to a defective bone marrow with a failure to produce normal blood cells. There are other genetic abnormalities that affect bone size and shape; causing skeletal deformities.

Nutritional deficiencies, particularly of vitamin-D, calcium and phosphorus, can result in the formation of weak, poorly mineralized bone. In children, vitamin-D deficiency causes rickets, with typical weak bones, bowing of the long bones and a characteristic deformity due to overgrowth of cartilage at distal ends of the bone. In adults, vitamin-D deficiency leads to softening of the bone (a condition known as *osteomalacia*), which can cause fractures and skeletal deformities.

Rickects is deformation of bone due to vitamin-D deficiency

Hormonal disorders can cause serious skeletal problems. Overactive parathyroid glands (or *hyper-parathyroidism*) can cause excess bone breakdown and increase the risk of fractures. In severe cases, large holes appear in the bone, which makes the bone highly fragile. Deficiency of the growth hormone can inhibit skeletal development leading to short body stature. Loss of gonadal function (or *hypogonadism*) in children and young adults can set off severe osteoporosis due to loss of testosterone and estrogen.

In addition, too much cortisol production by the adrenal gland can trigger *Cushing's syndrome*.

Inflammation can lead to bone loss around the affected joints in individuals suffering from arthritis. Bacterial infections, such as gingivitis can initiate bone loss around the teeth, and osteomyelitis can set off bone loss at the site of infection. This type of bone loss is due to direct damaging effect of bacterial toxins and production of bone dissolving factors by the white blood cells.

Blood Sugar Imbalance (e.g. diabetes) could affect bone health in different ways. Type 1 diabetes is associated with modest reductions in bone mineral density *(BMD)*. Type-2 diabetes, the most common form, is often characterized by elevated BMD. However, recent studies indicate that diabetes is associated with increased fracture risk to the hip, *proximal humerus*, and foot. Subjects with type-1 diabetes or juvenile diabetes have lower *tibia trabecular* and femoral neck density. Altered bone mineral acquisition in adolescents with type-1 diabetes may limit peak bone mass acquisition and increase the risk of osteoporosis in later life.

Several factors including obesity, changes in insulin levels, higher concentrations of advanced *glycation end products (AGEs)* in bone collagen, high calcium and glucose excretion in the urine, reduced function of the kidneys and inflammation contribute to bone loss in diabetic adults. Also, diabetes is known to induce complications of capillaries (micro-vasculature) that reduce blood flow to the bone leading to bone loss and fragility. Blood levels of *Insulin-like Growth Factor-1 (IGF-1)* and bone formation marker, *Osteocalcin* are reduced in diabetic individuals, suggesting that the *osteoblasts* are defective. These abnormal osteoblasts can reduce bone formation and increase fracture healing time.

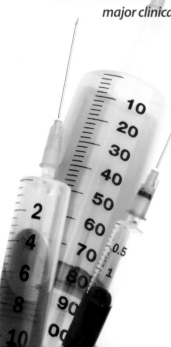

Glucocorticoid-Induced Osteoporosis (GIO) is by far the most common form of osteoporosis produced by drug treatment. This form of bone loss has become a major clinical concern.

Medications can directly cause unusual and massive bone loss; these include inhaled *glucocorticoids* (for asthma), corticosteroids, thyroid hormones, blood thinners *(heparin, warfarin), gonadotropin-releasing hormone agonists* for prostate cancer treatment, contraceptives *(medroxyprogesterone), lithium* (for bipolar disorder treatment), anticonvulsants, aluminum-containing antacids and tetracycline. Other medications like tranquillizers, sedatives, and antidepressants increase the risk of osteoporotic fractures; 11% of all hip fractures are attributed to prescription drugs that leave the elderly sedated or imbalanced.

Glucocorticoids, which are widely used in the treatment of several inflammatory conditions (e.g., *rheumatoid arthritis, asthma, emphysema, chronic lung disease*), can decrease bone formation and increase bone resorption; leading to *trabecular* bone loss at the spine and hip, especially in postmenopausal women and older men. The most rapid bone loss occurs early in the course of treatment, and even small doses increase bone fractures.

5.2 | Osteoporosis

Osteoporosis or *"porous bone"* is a skeletal disorder characterized by compromised bone strength, and increased risk of fracture. This disease manifests due to an imbalance between bone formation and bone resorption. As a result, BMD is reduced, bone architecture is disrupted, and the quality of bone matrix is altered. Osteoporosis is a *metabolic bone disease* (MBD) with characteristic fragile bones that break easily. Osteoporosis may significantly affect life expectancy and quality of life.

Advanced aging is the common underlying cause for the onset and progression of osteoporosis in both men and women. Women, especially with estrogen deficiency after menopause are prone to rapid reduction in BMD; in men a decrease in testosterone levels has a comparable effect.

Malnutrition, parenteral nutrition and malabsorption can lead to osteoporosis. Nutritional and gastrointestinal disorders that can predispose osteoporosis include *Celiac disease, Crohn's disease,* lactose intolerance, surgery (after gastrectomy, intestinal bypass surgery or bowel resection) and severe liver disease. Patients with *bulimia* can also develop osteoporosis. Endocrine disorders (e.g. diabetes) and use of corticosteroids can induce bone loss. During pregnancy and lactation, there can be a reversible bone loss.

After the age of 30, average bone loss is about 0.5% per year. And, for 8-10 years of post-menopause, women lose bone mass at a rate of about 2-5% per year.

Localized osteoporosis can occur after prolonged immobilization of a fractured limb in a cast. Bone loss takes place also in wheelchair-bound or bedridden individuals.

TABLE: *Life style factors that can onset and advance osteoporosis*

Vitamin-D Deficiency	Elevates parathyroid hormone (PTH) level, which in turn increases bone resorption, leading to bone loss.
Excess Alcohol	Chronic heavy drinking (alcohol intake greater than 2 units/day), especially at a younger age, increases the risk.
Tobacco Smoking	Inhibits bone formation. Smoking results in increased estrogen breakdown, lower body weight and early menopause; all contribute to lower BMD.
Malnutrition	Low dietary intake of calcium, proteins, vitamins K and C, negatively affects peak bone mass during adolescence and lowers BMD in the elderly.
Heavy Metals	A strong association exists between cadmium, lead and osteoporosis. Higher cadmium exposure results in osteomalacia (softening of the bone).
High Body Mass Index	Incidentally, overweight protects against osteoporosis, either by increasing load or through the hormone leptin.
Physical Inactivity	In adults, physical activity helps maintain bone mass, and increases the BMD by 1 or 2%. Conversely, physical inactivity can lead to bone loss.
Excess physical Activity	Excessive exercise can lead to constant bone damage. In women, heavy exercise leads to decreased estrogen levels that predispose osteoporosis.
Soft Drinks	Soft drinks (containing phosphoric acid) may interfere with calcium absorption in the gut and negatively affect the BMD.

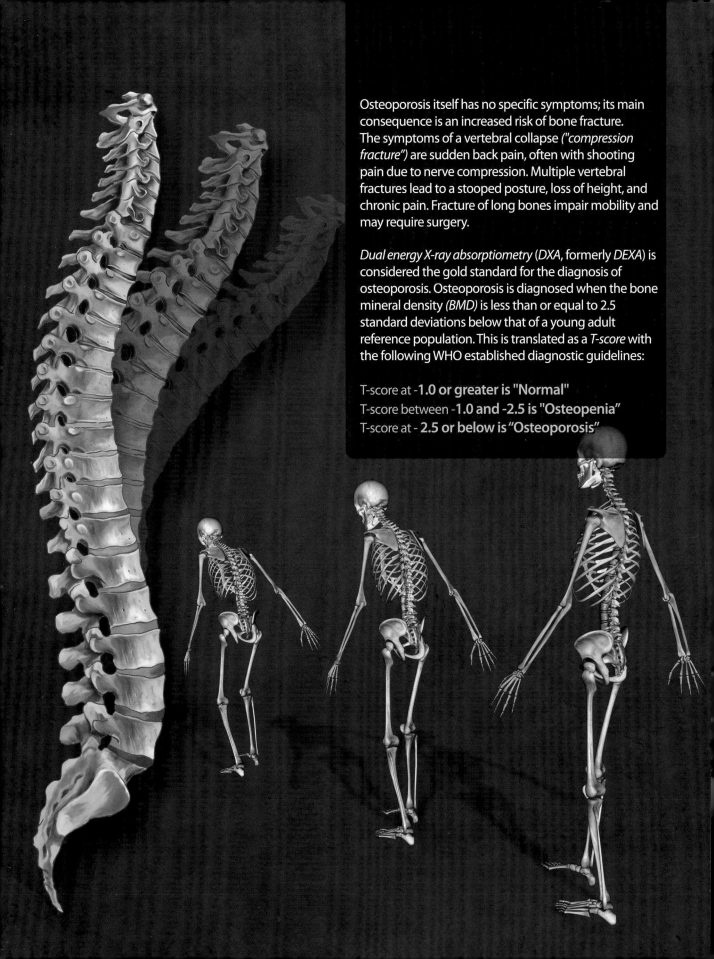

Osteoporosis itself has no specific symptoms; its main consequence is an increased risk of bone fracture. The symptoms of a vertebral collapse *("compression fracture")* are sudden back pain, often with shooting pain due to nerve compression. Multiple vertebral fractures lead to a stooped posture, loss of height, and chronic pain. Fracture of long bones impair mobility and may require surgery.

Dual energy X-ray absorptiometry (DXA, formerly *DEXA)* is considered the gold standard for the diagnosis of osteoporosis. Osteoporosis is diagnosed when the bone mineral density *(BMD)* is less than or equal to 2.5 standard deviations below that of a young adult reference population. This is translated as a *T-score* with the following WHO established diagnostic guidelines:

T-score at **-1.0 or greater is "Normal"**
T-score between **-1.0 and -2.5 is "Osteopenia"**
T-score at **- 2.5 or below is "Osteoporosis"**

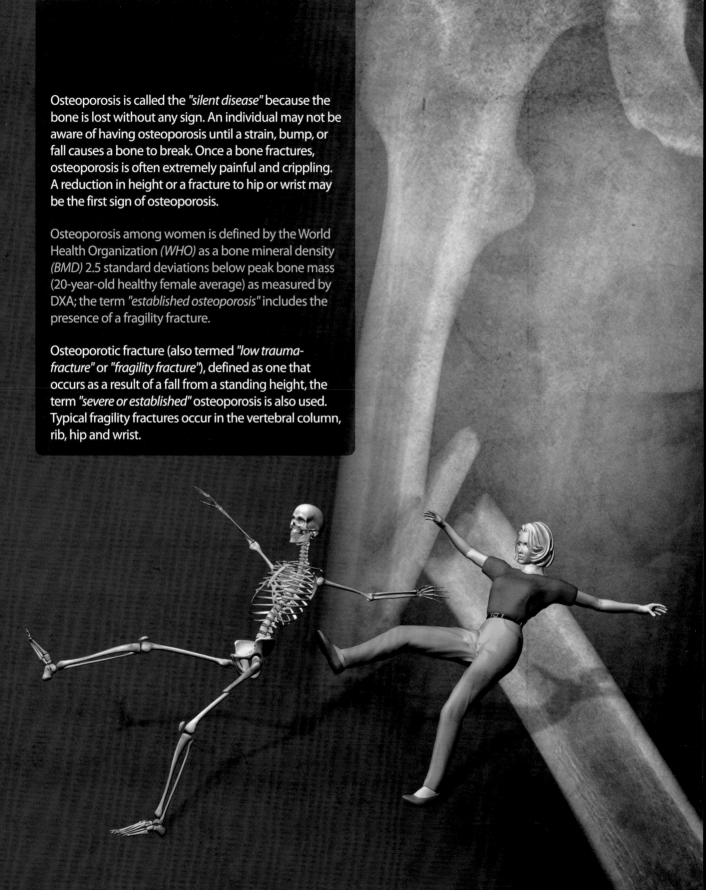

Osteoporosis is called the *"silent disease"* because the bone is lost without any sign. An individual may not be aware of having osteoporosis until a strain, bump, or fall causes a bone to break. Once a bone fractures, osteoporosis is often extremely painful and crippling. A reduction in height or a fracture to hip or wrist may be the first sign of osteoporosis.

Osteoporosis among women is defined by the World Health Organization *(WHO)* as a bone mineral density *(BMD)* 2.5 standard deviations below peak bone mass (20-year-old healthy female average) as measured by DXA; the term *"established osteoporosis"* includes the presence of a fragility fracture.

Osteoporotic fracture (also termed *"low trauma-fracture"* or *"fragility fracture"*), defined as one that occurs as a result of a fall from a standing height, the term *"severe or established"* osteoporosis is also used. Typical fragility fractures occur in the vertebral column, rib, hip and wrist.

5.3 | Osteoarthritis *(OA)*

Osteoarthritis *(OA)* is a degenerative bone disease, caused by the breakdown and eventual loss of the cartilage in one or more joints. Cartilage serves as a "cushion" between the bone joints. In severe OA, complete loss of cartilage cushion causes friction between bones, causing pain during rest or pain with limited joint mobility.

OA occurs more frequently with aging. Before age 45, OA occurs more frequently in males. After age 55 years, it is more common among females. Although OA generally accompanies aging, osteoarthritic cartilage is chemically different from normal cartilage of the same age. As *chondrocytes* (the cells that make up cartilage) age, they lose ability to produce more cartilage. This process plays an important role in the clinical development and progression of OA.

Body's ability to repair cartilage decreases with increasing age. Nearly all vertebrates suffer from OA, including porpoises and whales, as did dinosaurs.

Primary OA is mostly related to aging, wherein the water content of the cartilage increases, and the protein makeup of cartilage degenerates. Eventually, cartilage begins to ware off by flaking or forming tiny cracks. In advanced condition, a total loss of cartilage cushion between the bone joints is evident. Repetitive use of the worn joints over the years can irritate and inflame the cartilage, causing joint pain and swelling. Inflammation of the cartilage can lead to new bone outgrowths (or spurs) around the joints. Several studies have shown a high prevalence of this disease between siblings, especially identical twins, indicating a hereditary (genetic) trait. Up to 60% of OA cases may result from genetic factors.

Repeated trauma to joint tissues can lead to early OA of the knees in soccer players. Interestingly, recent studies did not find any risk of OA in long-distance runners.

Secondary OA is caused by conditions that include obesity, repeated trauma or surgery to the joint structures; abnormal joints at birth (congenital disorders), gout, diabetes and other hormonal dysfunctions. Crystal deposits in the joints, especially uric acid, can degenerate the cartilage and cause arthritis in gout; while calcium pyrophosphate crystals cause arthritis in *pseudogout*. Individuals born with abnormal joints (congenital deformities) are vulnerable to mechanical wear and tear, which leads to early degeneration and loss of joint cartilage. OA of the hip joints is commonly related to congenital abnormalities. Hormonal disorders, such as diabetes and growth hormone malfunction, can trigger early cartilage destruction and secondary OA.

OA commonly affects the hands, feet, spine, and large weight-bearing joints, such as the hips and knees. With the progression of OA, the affected joints appear larger, stiff, painful and usually feel worse, when frequently used over the day; thus distinguishing it from rheumatoid arthritis. Next to aging, obesity is the most common risk factor for OA of the knee, due to increased mechanical stress on the cartilage. The early development of OA of the knees among weight lifters is common.

OA is commonly identified by the following symptoms:

- Pain that worsens during activity and gets better during rest. Pain and stiffness of the joints can also occur after long periods of inactivity, for example, sitting in a theater.

- Pain is generally described as a sharp ache, or a burning sensation in the associated muscles and tendons. There can be swelling, warmth and creaking of the affected joints.

- Pain can increase in humid weather. Occasionally, the joints may also be filled with fluid.

- Some may have muscle spasm and contractions in the tendons.

- Knee may cause a crackling-like noise (called *crepitus*) when moved or touched.

- Weight-bearing joints (like the knee) can develop a limp. Limping can worsen as more cartilage is destroyed.

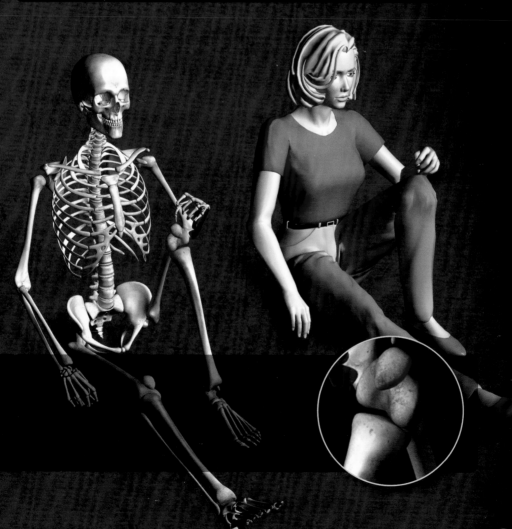

5.4 | Rheumatoid Arthritis *(RA)*

Rheumatoid arthritis *(RA)* is an inflammatory bone disease that causes pain, swelling, stiffness, and loss of joint function. RA is derived from the term *"rheumatic fever"*, an illness that includes joint pain; the Greek word rheumatos ("flowing") and the suffix-oid ("resembling") gives the translation as joint inflammation that resembles rheumatic fever.

RA is an autoimmune condition with several clinical features that make it unique from other types of arthritis. Individuals with RA may experience fatigue, occasional fever and a general sense of not feeling well. Increased stiffness upon waking up from sleep is a prominent feature of this disease, which may last for more than an hour. Although RA is often noticed in middle age and occurs with increased frequency among the elderly, children and young adults are also show symptoms of this disease. RA affects women 3 times more often than men. Risk is high among women between 40 and 50 years of age, and for men somewhat later. RA is 4 times more common in smokers than non-smokers.

Daily activities are impaired in most individuals. After 5 years of disease, about 33% of sufferers will not be working. After 10 years, about half will have substantial functional disability

Rheumatoid arthritis is due to synovitis, which is inflammation of the synovial membrane that lines joints and tendon sheaths. The inflamed *synovium* turns thick and the joints become swollen, tender, warm, reddend and stiff; collectively preventing the joint mobility and function. As the disease progresses, the inflamed synovium destroys the cartilage and bone within the joint. Most commonly, small joints of the hands, feet and cervical spine are affected, but larger joints like the shoulder and knee can also be involved. RA can lead to erosion of the joint surface, causing deformity and loss of function.

The symptoms of RA may vary among individuals, for some, it lasts only for few months or a year and goes away without causing any noticeable damage. Whereas, others may demonstrate mild or moderate forms of the disease, with bouts of worsening symptoms, called flares; and periods of feeling better, called remissions. Still others have a severe form of the disease that is active most of the time, lasts for many years or a lifetime, and leads to serious joint damage and disability. Permanent damage occurs to the joints at an early stage of the disease. Anti-inflammatory agents and analgesics (pain killers) improve stiffness and pain but do not prevent joint damage or slow the disease progression.

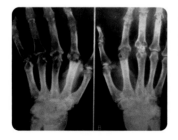

RA generally occurs in a symmetrical pattern, meaning that if a knee or hand is involved, the other one is also affected. The symptoms are often manifested with the wrist and finger joints closest to the hand.

Rheumatoid Arthritis - Joint inflammation of the hand .

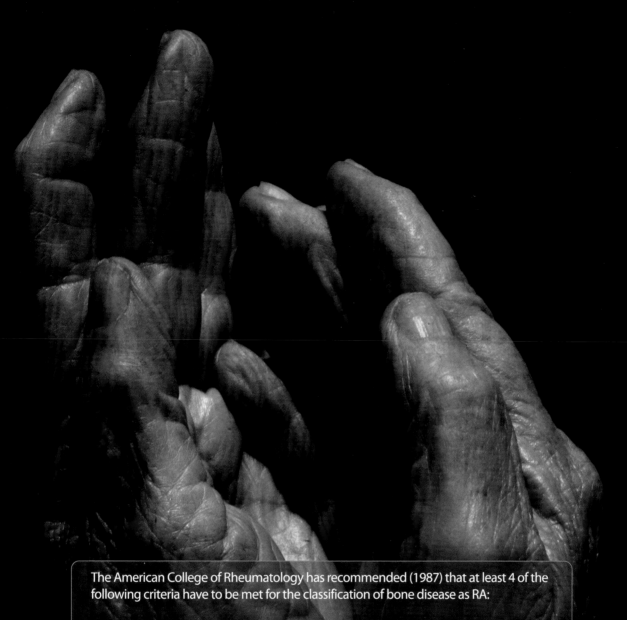

The American College of Rheumatology has recommended (1987) that at least 4 of the following criteria have to be met for the classification of bone disease as RA:

- Morning stiffness of >1 hour, for at least 6 weeks.

- Arthritis and soft-tissue swelling of 3 to 14 joints, for at least 6 weeks.

- Arthritis of hand joints, present for at least 6 weeks.

- Symmetric arthritis, present for at least 6 weeks.

- Subcutaneous nodules in specific places.

- Rheumatoid factor at a level above the 95th percentile.

- Radiological changes suggestive of joint erosion.

5.5 | Bone Disorders

Bone Disorders often result in weak bones that can lead to painful and debilitating fractures. The symptoms of bone disorders manifest into skeletal deformities, in some cases can be *irreversible*, affecting the posture and mobility of the body. Certain affected individuals are seriously handicapped and restricted to wheel chair. Some chronic bone disorders are extremely severe and life-threatening.

Paget's Disease

Paget's disease (also known as *osteitis deformans*), is a chronic disorder of the skeleton in which areas of bone undergo abnormal turnover, resulting in areas of enlarged and softened bone. Excessive breakdown (bone loss) and rapid production of new tissue makes the bone more susceptible to deformity or fracture. Paget's disease can affect any bone; most commonly involves the pelvis, thigh bone *(femur)*, skull, shin (tibia), spine, collarbone *(clavicle)* and upper arm bone *(humerus)*.

Paget's disease is the second most common bone disease after osteoporosis. This disease rarely occurs in people younger than 40. Men are 50% more commonly affected than women.

Symptoms of the disease may include deep, aching and occasionally severe bone pain, which may worsen at night. The enlarged bones may compress nerves and cause shooting pain. Enlarged skull bones may damage the inner ear that can lead to hearing loss, dizziness and headaches. The vertebrae may enlarge, weaken and buckle, resulting in loss of height and a hunched posture. Damaged vertebrae may pinch the nerves of the spinal cord, that may cause pain, numbness, tingling, weakness, or, very rarely, even paralysis of the legs.

Hereditary involvement in the Paget's disease (where more than one family member has the disease) ranges from 10 to 40%. Environmental factors are likely to play a role in certain cases. Involvement of slow virus infection *(e.g. Measles, Canine Distemper virus)* in the incidence of Paget's disease has also been reported.

Rickets and Osteomalacia

Consuming large amounts of antacids (containing aluminum hydroxide) can interfere with the absorption of dietary phosphate, which may lead to osteomalacia.

Rickets is a bone disorder that primarily affects children causing skeletal deformities, especially bowed legs. Deficiency of vitamin-D and lack of adequate calcium in the diet may also lead to rickets with severely softened and weak bones. Rickets is among the most frequent childhood diseases in many developing countries, usually resulting from malnutrition, famine or starvation. Occasionally, rickets may also occur in children with liver dysfunction, or with disability to convert vitamin-D to its active form. This bone disorder can also strike children who are confined to indoors due to chronic illness or frailty.

Osteomalacia is the equivalent of rickets among adults; where the deficiency in bone mineralization does not cause skeletal deformity but can lead to fractures, particularly of the weight-bearing bones such as pelvis, hip, and feet. Certain individuals may experience bone pain and aggravated muscle weakness.

Osteomalacia may also result due to severe loss of phosphorus from the body. This condition may coincide with congenital illness or can develop among individuals with phosphorus transport disorder. Individuals with gastrointestinal tract ailments, such as gastrectomy, malabsorption syndromes and small bowel resection, are at higher risk, since these conditions reduce the absorption of vitamin-D from the diet.

Major symptoms of rickets and osteomalacia include decreased muscle tone (loss of muscle strength); defects in the structure of teeth (holes in the enamel, dental cavities); impaired growth; increased bone fractures; muscle cramps; short stature (adults less than 5 feet tall); skeletal deformities; asymmetrical or odd-shaped skull; bowlegs; bumps in the ribcage *(rachitic rosary)*; breastbone protrusion *(pigeon chest)*; pelvic deformities; spine deformities (abnormal spine curvature, including *scoliosis*).

The cure for OI is yet to be found. Therefore, treatment for the disease focuses on managing the symptoms. Treatments include exercise, pain medicine, physical therapy, wheelchairs, braces and surgery.

Osteogenesis Imperfecta *(OI)*

Osteogenesis Imperfecta (OI), the term means imperfect bone formation. This disease is characterized by unusually fragile bones that break easily, often under loads that normal bones bear or with no apparent cause. Multiple fractures are common, and in severe cases, can occur even before birth. Milder cases may involve only a few fractures over a person's lifetime. OI can also cause weak muscles, brittle teeth, curved spine *(scoliosis)* and hearing loss.

The cause of OI is a faulty gene that impairs the body's ability to make collagen. Collagen is an important protein in the bone matrix and its impairment leads to a clinical outcome of weak or fragile bones. The child of an affected parent will have a 50 percent chance of developing OI.

There are at least eight recognized forms of OI, designated as type I through type VIII. Type I is the mildest form and type II, the most severe; other types of OI have signs and symptoms that fall somewhere between these two categories. The milder forms of OI, including type I, are characterized by bone fractures during childhood and adolescence that often arise from minor trauma. Fractures occur less frequently in adulthood. People with mild forms of the condition typically have a blue or grey tint to the part of the eye, which should normally be white *(the sclera)*; and may also develop hearing loss in adulthood. Other types of OI are more severe; with frequent bone fractures that may begin before birth and result from little or no trauma. Additional features of these conditions can include *blue sclerae*, short stature, hearing loss, respiratory problems, and a defective tooth development called *dentinogenesis imperfecta*. The most severe forms of OI, particularly type II, can include an abnormally small, fragile rib cage and under developed lungs. Infants with such abnormalities may have life-threatening problems with breathing and often die shortly after birth.

5.1 | METABOLIC BONE DISEASES

1. Ahlborg HG, Johnell O, Turner CH, et al (2003) Bone loss and bone size after menopause. *The New England Journal of Medicine* 349(4):327-334.
2. Cizza G, Ravn P, Chrousos GP, Gold PW (2001) Depression: A major, unrecognized risk factor for osteoporosis? *Trends in Endocrinology and Metabolism* 12(5): 98-203.
3. Heap J, Murray MA, Miller SC, et al (2004) Alterations in bone characteristics associated with glycemic control in adolescents with type 1 diabetes mellitus. *Journal of Pediatrics* 144(1):56-62.
4. Jeffcoat MK, Lewis CE, Reddy MS, et al (2000) Post-menopausal bone loss and its relationship to oral bone loss. *Periodontology 2000* 23:94-102.
5. Kanis JA, Johnell O, Oden A, et al (2000) Risk of hip fracture according to the World Health Organization criteria for osteopenia and osteoporosis. *Bone* 27(5):585-590.
6. Michelson D, Stratakis C, Hill L, et al (1996) Bone mineral density in women with depression. *The New England Journal of Medicine* 335(16):1176-1181.
7. Saag K (2003) Glucocorticoid-induced osteoporosis. *Endocrinology Metabolism Clinics of North America* 32(1):135-157.
8. van Staa TP, Leufkens HGM, Cooper C (2002) The epidemiology of corticosteroid-induced osteoporosis: a meta-analysis. *Osteoporosis International* 13(10):777-787.

5.2 | OSTEOPOROSIS

1. Fleming LA (1992) Osteoporosis: Clinical features, prevention, and treatment. *Journal of General Internal Medicine* 7:554-562.
2. Khosla S, Lufkin EG, Hodgson SF, et al (1994) Epidemiology and clinical features of osteoporosis in young individuals. *Bone* 15(5):551-555.
3. Marcus R, Feldman D, Kelsey J (editors) *Osteoporosis*, 2nd Edition. Volume 2. San Diego (CA): Academic Press; pp. 207-27; 2001.
4. Melton LJ, Thamer M, Ray NF, et al (1997) Fractures attributable to osteoporosis: Report from the National Osteoporosis Foundation. *Journal of Bone and Mineral Research* 12:16-23.
5. Morris CA, Cheng H, Cabral D, Solomon DH (2004) Predictors of screening and treatment of osteoporosis: A structured review of the literature. *Endocrinologist* 14(2):70-75.
6. Raisz LG, Rodan GA (2003) Pathogenesis of osteoporosis. *Endocrinology Metabolism Clinics of North America* 32(1):15-24.
7. Riggs BL, Melton LJ (1995) The worldwide problem of osteoporosis: Insights afforded by epidemiology. *Bone* 17(5):505S-511S.
8. Seeman E (2003) Invited Review: Pathogenesis of osteoporosis. *Journal of Applied Physiology* 95(5):2142-2151.
9. Stein E, Shane E (2003) Secondary osteoporosis. *Endocrinology Metabolism Clinics of North America* 32(1):115-134.
10. WHO (1994). Assessment of fracture risk and its application to screening for post-menopausal osteoporosis. Report of a WHO Study Group. *World Health Organization Technical Report Series* 843:1–129.

5.3 | OSTEOARTHRITIS

1. Favus MJ, Editor (2003). Primer on the metabolic bone diseases and disorders of mineral metabolism. 5th Edition. Washington, DC: American Society for Bone andMineral Research.

2. WHO Scientific Group on the Burden of Musculoskeletal Conditions at the Start of the New Millennium. (2003) The burden of musculoskeletal conditions at the start of the new millennium: Report of a scientific group. Geneva, Switzerland: *World Health Organization Technical Report Series* 919; pp. 57.

3. Gregory PJ, Sperry M, Wilson AF (2008) Dietary supplements for osteoarthritis. *American Family Physician* 77(2):177-184.

4. Sun BH, Wu CW, Kalunian KC (2007) New Developments in Osteoarthritis. *Rheumatic Disease Clinics of North America* (33):135-148.

5. Zhang W, Moskowitz RW, Nuki G, et al (2008) OARSI recommendations for the management of hip and knee osteoarthritis, Part II: OARSI evidence-based, expert consensus guidelines. *Osteoarthritis Cartilage* 16:137-162.

6. Poolsup N, Suthisisang C, Channark P, Kittikulsuth W (2005). Glucosamine long-term treatment and the progression of knee osteoarthritis: systematic review of randomized controlled trials. *The Annals of Pharmacotherapy* 39(6):1080-1087.

7. Reichenbach S, Sterchi R, Scherer M, et al (2007). Meta-analysis: chondroitin for osteoarthritis of the knee or hip. *Annals of Internal Medicine* 146(8):580-590.

5.4 | RHEUMATOID ARTHRITIS

1. Alamanos Y, Voulgari PV, Drosos AA (2006). Incidence and prevalence of rheumatoid arthritis; based on the 1987 American College of Rheumatology criteria: a systematic review. *Seminars in Arthritis and Rheumatism* 36:182-188.

2. Arnett F, Edworthy S, Bloch D, et al (1988). The American Rheumatism Association 1987 revised criteria for the classification of rheumatoid arthritis. *Arthritis and Rheumatism* 31:315-324.

3. Haugeberg G, Orstavik RE, Kvien TK (2003) Effects of rheumatoid arthritis on bone. *Current Opinion in Rheumatology* 15(4):469-475.

4. Majithia V, Geraci SA (2007). Rheumatoid arthritis: diagnosis and management. *American Journal of Medicine* 120: 936-939.

5. O'Dell J (2004). Therapeutic strategies for rheumatoid arthritis. *The New England Journal of Medicine* 350:2591-2602.

6. Turesson C, O'Fallon WM, Crowson CS, et al (2003). Extra-articular disease manifestations in rheumatoid arthritis: incidence trends and risk factors over 46 years. *Annals of Rheumatic Diseases* 62(8):722-727.

5.5 | BONE DISORDERS

1. Chesney RW (2001) Vitamin D deficiency and rickets. *Reviews in Endocrine and Metabolic Disorders* 2(2):145-151.

2. Drezner MK (2003) Hypophosphatemic rickets. *Endocrine Reviews* 6:126-155.

3. Morales-Piga AA, Rey-Rey JS, Corres-Gonzalez J, et al (1995) Frequency and characteristics of familial aggregation of Paget's disease of bone. *Journal of Bone and Mineral Research* 10(4):663-670.

4. Nield LS, Mahajan P, Joshi A, Kamat D (2006) Rickets: not a disease of the past. *American Family Physician* 74:619-626

5. Pettifor JM (2002) Rickets. *Calcified Tissue International* 70(5):398-399.

6. Rauch F, Glorieux FH (2004) Osteogenesis imperfecta. *The Lancet* 363:1377-1385.

7. Siris ES, Ottman R, Flaster E, Kelsey JL (1991) Familial aggregation of Paget's disease of bone. *Journal of Bone and Mineral Research* 6(5):495-500.

8. Tiegs RD, Lohse CM, Wollan PC, Melton LJ (2000) Long-term trends in the incidence of Paget's disease of bone. *Bone* 27(3):423-427.

Fractures

When a bone breaks it is called a *"fracture"*. A break can be anything from a hairline fracture *(a thin break in the bone)* to the bone snapped in two pieces like a broken tree branch. A broken bone takes about 12 weeks to heal. Fractures are described in the following ways:

Complete fracture is when bone has broken into two pieces.
Greenstick fracture is when the bone cracks on one side only, not all the way through.
Single fracture is when the bone is broken in one place.
Comminuted fracture is when the bone is broken into more than two pieces or crushed.
Bowing fracture, which only happens in kids, is when the bone bends but doesn't break.
Open fracture is when the bone is sticking through the skin.

Crush fractures of the vertebrae are common in osteoporotic individuals. Many elderly women have fractured spines and go unnoticed because they don't feel or hear the bone crack. When older women lose height, suffer back pain, or develop a protruding abdomen or *Dowager's Hump* on the back – it is a sign of vertebral fracture. About 700,000 women suffer vertebral fractures each year.

Hip fractures are the most devastating type of bone fracture and account for almost 300,000 hospitalizations each year. Of hip fracture patients: 20% die within a year of the fracture and 20% end up in a nursing home within a year.

The Osteoporosis Dilemma

Osteoporosis is believed to be a preventable and treatable bone metabolic disorder that affects an estimated 75 million people in the United States, Europe and Japan. Yet, the medical (diagnostic) definition of this disease still remains as conceptual, with no scientific consensus. Consider the definition offered by the NIH Consensus Development Conference: *"A systemic skeletal disease characterized by low bone mass and micro-architectural deterioration with a consequent increase in bone fragility and susceptibility to fracture."* By contrast, a Working Group of the WHO attempted to assign a numerical value to its definition and proposed that osteoporosis be defined as BMD (T score) that is 2.5 SD below the mean peak value in young adults.

The limitations of this definition include:

- By focusing on BMD, it ignores other important determinants of bone strength;
- It does not specify the methodology for determining BMD;
- It fails to take into account increased vulnerability to fracture of bones of older women; and
- It does not address the important issue of wide variations in mineral densities in different bones of the same individual.

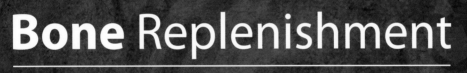

Bone Replenishment

6

Bone Replenishment is to maintain homeostasis of bone turnover (resorption vs. formation) in the skeletal system with relation to age and sex of an individual.

This Chapter elucidates the molecular mechanisms of bone replenishment with an emphasis on the anabolic aspects of skeletal metabolism. New strategies are discussed in view of the latest developments in biomedical technology and ever expanding knowledge on theories of aging, metabolic homeostasis, human genomics and proteomics. A major endeavor is to identify proteins with central role in the anabolic phases of bone metabolism, especially pathways that are regulated by sex hormones. Selective stimulation of anabolic effectors with bone-replenishments, form the basis for maintaining a healthy functional bone.

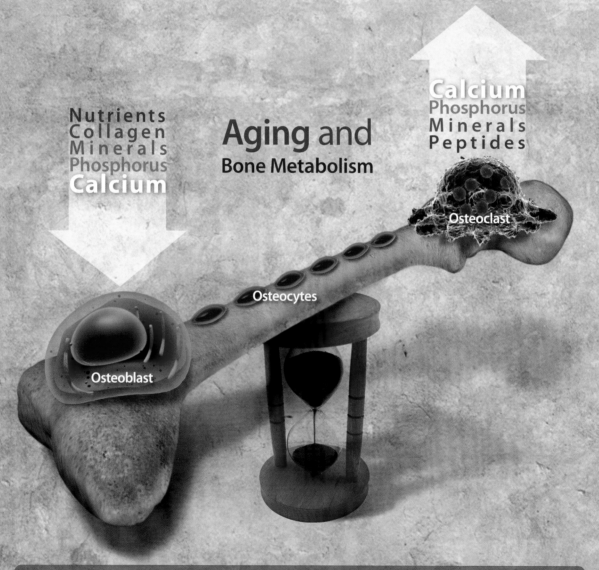

Nutrients
Collagen
Minerals
Phosphorus
Calcium

Aging and
Bone Metabolism

Calcium
Phosphorus
Minerals
Peptides

Osteoclast

Osteocytes

Osteoblast

6

6.1 | Bone Replenishment: **Perspective**

BONE quality (structure) and quantity (mass), at macroscopic and microscopic level, are determined by the genetic blueprint and factors that regulate bone modeling and remodeling. Genetic transcription is responsible for the highly conserved anatomical shape of bones and most likely in restoring a fractured bone to its original shape. Bone replenishment is a steady-state biochemical management that encompasses vital activities of bone turnover, maintenance and repair of the skeletal system.

During bone turnover, the skeleton undergoes continuous destruction (resorption) by osteoclasts and formation by osteoblasts. In the normal adult skeleton, these two processes are "in sync", maintaining a constant amount of bone. Bone replenishment helps to maintain homeostasis of this "coupled" process, as a function of time (aging).

Bone replenishment responds to shifts in homeostasis, influenced by age, sex, lifestyle and environment. Multiple factors control the bone homeostasis. For example, growth factors (i.e. *IGF* or *TGF*) release during bone resorption to initiate local bone formation. Factors deposited on the bone surface by osteoclasts initiate bone formation. Humoral factors, such as PTH and prostaglandin E, stimulate bone resorption as well as bone formation in tandem. Lactoferrin *(LF)* and Ribonuclease *(RNase)* appear during the early embryonic (ossification and vascularization) stage and play a regulatory role in bone metabolic homeostasis through each phase of human development. These vital factors are continuously depleted by bone metabolism; and their synthesis (physiological levels) gradually decline with aging.

Aging is a progressive decline in homeostasis and reduced adaptability to stress - decrease in BMD is inevitable with age.

Given the dramatic increase in skeletal size during growth, and the need to preserve skeletal mass during adulthood, and the management of bone "bank" with mineral highly deposits and withdrawals – homeostasis takes the center stage. Therefore, it is not surprising that highly complex pathways have evolved for "cross-talk" between bone and other organs to recalibrate metabolic activities in response to continuously changing physiological requirements of the body.

Bone homeostasis is under the influence of both endogenous hormonal changes and external mechanical loads resulting from physical activity. The ability of bone to change its structure and adapt to mechanical loads implies that physical forces can regulate bone turnover. Accordingly, higher loads should increase formation and decrease resorption, whereas unloading should have the opposite effect. Indeed, immobilization stimulates resorption, suppresses formation and provides a clear example of "uncoupling" between the two processes. Muscle contractions serve as one of the two major sources of mechanical loading on bones and directly effect bone homeostasis. For example, acute muscle paralysis induced by "Botox" (neurotoxin) injection rapidly precipitates substantial muscle and causes bone degradation. Furthermore, space flights induce loss of bone mass, especially in weight-bearing bones, a condition similar to *disuse* osteoporosis.

Oxygen homeostasis: The human physiology has evolved under the influence of oxygen, the vital element of the body. Oxygen runs the signaling pathways that control cellular development, differentiation and demise. Oxygen drives the processes of bone homeostasis; specifically by controlling the basal metabolic rate *(BMR)*, the energy reserve for many functions. During the body's resting state, muscular activity is needed to maintain circulation, respiration and skeletal movement; and these functions consume about 20% of the body's energy expenditure. Much of the remainder of the basal metabolism is used to maintain and replace cells throughout the body, including those in bone turnover. Several studies have shown that the amount of oxygen necessary to maintain resting state of the body declines with age. On average, the human body reduces its energy expenditure by about 12 calories per year after the age of 30, which represents a decline of 120 calories every decade. This is probably due to changes in body's composition that occurs with aging. The risk analysis between smoking and bone fractures suggests the underlying mechanism of oxygen deficit in the higher incidence and delayed healing of fractures in smokers compared to nonsmokers. It has been postulated that any disturbance in oxygen homeostasis of bone tissue may lead to bone loss, resulting in the clinical onset of *osteopenia* and *osteoporosis*.

BMR is the average amount of oxygen (energy) used by a body while at rest on a daily basis

Calcium homeostasis: The role of calcium and vitamin-D in bone metabolism are intertwined. Several conditions could affect intestinal calcium absorption. Low exposure to sunlight could reduce vitamin-D levels (synthesis in skin) and affect *trans-cellular* calcium uptake. Decrease in gastric acid production (with aging and/or frequent use of antacids) could affect *para-cellular* calcium absorption. Calcium homeostasis is a net outcome of three factors: i) net calcium input from the gut; ii) net calcium loss in the urine; and iii) the net amount of calcium deposited in bone. In the human body, mainly three hormones regulate the calcium metabolism and the bone turnover: 1)*1, 25-dihydroxycholecalciferol* increases calcium absorption from the intestine and, indirectly, from bone; 2) PTH up regulates calcium levels; and 3) *calcitonin* down regulates calcium levels.

Phosphorus homeostasis: Phosphorus is a critical element in the body for two major reasons: first, for high-energy phosphate bonds *(ATP)* that serve as the primary source of readily available energy; and secondly, for maintaining skeletal integrity. Bone is the largest repository of extracellular phosphate. The deposition and withdrawal of phosphate from bone is under the influence of parathyroid gland and vitamin-D3. Kidney plays a crucial role in the phosphate homeostasis. It maintains serum phosphate levels within a narrow range by modulating phosphate clearance. Phosphate is readily filtered in the glomeruli and subsequently reabsorbed in the proximal tubule.

Aging of bone: Bone mass increases dramatically during childhood and continues to grow even after attaining full height during adolescence. At around 35 years of age, peak bone mass is achieved in both men and women. Ninety percent of bone mass accumulates by age twsenty, and 10% between age twenty and the early thirties. Peak bone mass is about 30% higher in men than in women. Starting at about age 40 in both men and women, a slow bone loss begins when bone resorption surpasses formation. This occurs due to decrease in intestinal absorption of calcium, slow down in the synthesis of vitamin-D needed for calcium absorption, and reduced osteoblast activity. Adult bone loss occurs at a rate of 6-8% per decade. Women experience a rapid bone loss of approximately 2% per year for the first 5 post-menopausal years because of the dwindling estrogen levels. Thereafter, bone mass gradually decreases at a slower pace at 1% per year. This incremental decline results in a 30-40% cumulative loss from peak bone mass by the age of 70. While men lose 25% of both trabecular and cortical bone, women lose approximately 50% of their trabecular bone and 35% of their cortical bone.

Consequences of menopause on bone health are most clearly apparent after ovariectomy

Age-related bone loss is universal, especially among older women and men. A number of other age-related factors are also implicated in both sexes. These include secondary hyperparathyroidism, impaired vitamin-D metabolism, and abnormal osteoblast function.

Milk is a rich biological fluid that contains many growth factors, and provides nutrition at a time of rapid skeletal growth and development in the neonate. Therefore, milk is a natural source of anabolic factors for bone metabolism. The role of such milk factors in bone metabolic homeostasis, under age-related stress conditions and expedited rate of living, are described in the following sections.

Calcium Regulation in the Body

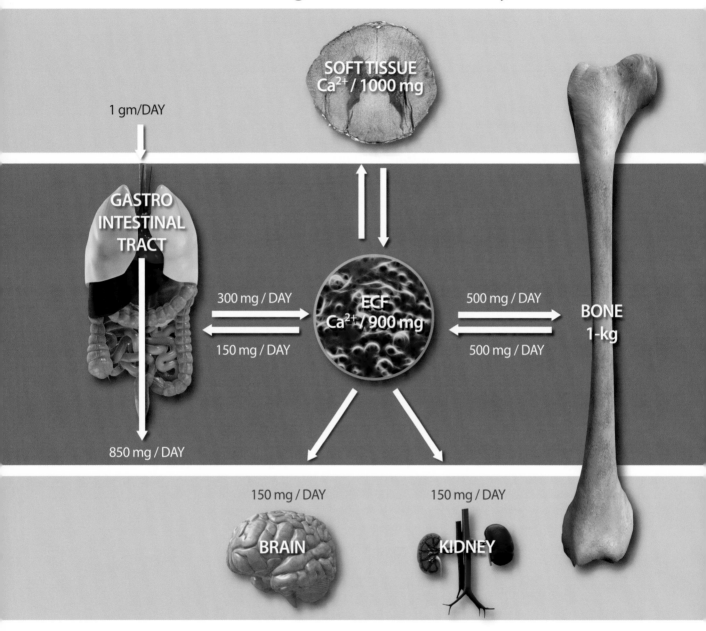

SOFT TISSUE
Ca^{2+} / 1000 mg

1 gm/DAY

GASTRO INTESTINAL TRACT

300 mg / DAY

ECF
Ca^{2+} / 900 mg

500 mg / DAY

BONE
1-kg

150 mg / DAY

500 mg / DAY

850 mg / DAY

150 mg / DAY

150 mg / DAY

BRAIN

KIDNEY

Extracellular fluid *(ECF)* Ca^{2+} levels are regulated by bone, gastrointestinal tract, and kidney (certain extent by the liver and brain). In addition to the intestinal absorption, Ca^{2+} is also released into the intestinal lumen by gastric secretions. Accordingly, the net Ca^{2+} absorption in an average normal individual is about 150 mg/day. The movement of Ca^{2+} in and out of bone in a normal young adult stays in balance, meaning that bone resorption and bone formation remain at equilibrium. Finally, Ca^{2+} is filtered by the kidney but also recycled back into circulation.

Adapted from Mundy and Guise, 1999

6.2 | Bone Replenishment: **Regulation**

Homeostatic mechanisms operate at every inch of the skeletal system. It involves constant monitoring and regulation of numerous factors, including the gases oxygen and carbon dioxide, nutrients, enzymes, hormones, and organic and inorganic substances. The concentrations of these substances in the skeleton remain unchanged, within limits, despite changes in the external environment.

At molecular level – a homeostatic mechanism called *feedback inhibition* operates to limit the amount of chemical produced by an enzyme. An enzyme system consists of several proteins that act sequentially to convert a metabolite into an end product to fulfill the needs of an organism. The functional concentration of an end product is maintained at a fairly constant level.

At cellular level – a homeostatic phenomenon called *contact inhibition* operates, in which cells stop to multiply when the population (contact) becomes intense. An inter-cellular signal from a 'chemical messenger' inhibits further cell division. In contrast, cultured or cancer cells continue to divide even after intense cell density. Thus, cancer cells appear to have lost the homeostatic mechanism of contact inhibition.

Both intrinsic and extrinsic mechanisms control metabolic homeostasis of the bone. In intrinsic regulation, the metabolic pathway self-regulates in response to changes in the levels of substrates or products; for example, a decrease in the amount of calcium or phosphate can increase the flux through a pathway to compensate the loss. This type of regulation often involves interaction of a specific enzyme with an effector ("allosteric regulation") in the pathway. For example, hydronium ion act as an effector for bone-specific alkaline phosphatase *(BAP)* in the enzymatic release of phosphates from the bone matrix; on the other hand, homo-arginine is a negative effector (inhibitor) for BAP enzyme. Extrinsic regulation involves a cell in an organ change its metabolism in response to signals from other cells. These signals are usually in the form of soluble messengers such as hormones and growth factors, which latch to specific receptors on the cell surface. For example, parathyroid hormone *(PTH)* binds to specific receptors on the cell surface of osteoblasts and triggers a response to lay down a brand new bone matrix.

Homeostasis in the skeletal system is regulated by bone-specific enzymes and a myriad of hormones

Mechanostatic regulation from physical stress (i.e. weight bearing) can adjust bone mineral density *(BMD)*. Frost (1992) suggested that an internal skeletal *mechanostat,* initiates changes in bone remodeling to adjust and distribute bone mass to a level appropriate for the biomechanical forces. The higher strain levels associated with growth or extreme physical activity will induce modeling that increases bone mass by accretion on bone surfaces. However, repeated low strain induces a disuse mode of bone remodeling. In this mode, there is an increased bone turnover on all bone surfaces. The bone loss will continue until a new steady state is reached where once again strain is sensed as high enough to return to the conservation mode of bone remodeling. Over time, repeated small stresses on the skeleton can produce areas of defective bone, termed "micro-damage". Replacement of damaged sites by remodeling restores bone strength.

Bone remodeling serves both the structural and metabolic functions of the skeleton. It also repairs any local damage.

Bone remodeling can be stimulated by *hormones* that regulate mineral metabolism, *chemical factors* (e.g. growth factors and cytokines) that control bone growth and *stress factors* (e.g. mechanical and weight bearing). Hormones are chemical substances that serve as messengers, controlling and coordinating activities throughout the body. Upon reaching a target site, a hormone binds to a receptor, much like a key fits into a lock. Once the hormone locks into its receptor, it transmits a message that causes the target site to take a specific action. Ultimately, hormones control the function of an entire organ, affecting such diverse processes as growth, development, reproduction, and sexual characteristics. Extremely low levels of hormone can trigger very large responses in the skeletal system.

Sex hormones – *estrogen (E)* made in the ovary of females, and *testosterone (T)* made by the testes in males, are important for bone strength. Bone development and growth are similar in boys and girls up to the start of puberty. Thereafter, skeletal sexual dimorphism evolves with a greater bone mass in adult males than in adult females. The volumetric or true density of bone is, however, similar in both sexes. After a period of peak bone mass, age-related bone loss occurs in both genders, but men experience less age-related net bone loss, again in contrast to the accelerated bone resorption in women.

Parathyroid hormone (PTH) maintains the level of calcium and stimulates both resorption and formation of bone. *Calcitonin (CT)* inhibits bone breakdown and may protect against excessively high levels of calcium in the blood. Population studies showed a gradual increase in serum PTH levels from about twenty years of age, such that the maximum value at age eighty years may be as much as 50% higher than at the age of thirty. This condition leads to secondary hyperparathyroidism, which can seriously impair calcium homeostasis. Gastro-intestinal health is of pivotal importance to facilitate efficient mineral transport and to maintain calcium homeostasis.

Sex hormones E and T are responsible for differences in skeletal development of males and females

Endocrine glands release more than 20 major hormones directly into the bloodstream where they can be transported to cells in other parts of the body. Although the endocrine glands are the body's main hormone producers, some other organs not in the endocrine system - such as the brain, heart, lungs, kidneys, liver, and skin - also produce and release hormones. The pancreas produces two important hormones, insulin and glucagon. They work together to maintain a steady level of glucose, or sugar, in the blood and to keep the body supplied with fuel to produce and maintain stores of energy.

TABLE: *Hormones – Site of secretion and endocrine function in the human body*

Body Site	Hormone	Endocrine Function
Pituitary	*Vasopressin*	Helps kidneys to retain water
	Corticotropin (ACTH)	Controls hormone secretion by adrena
	Growth hormone (GH)	Controls growth and development
	Luteinizing hormone (LH) & Follicle-stimulating hormone (FSH)	Controls male & female sexual characteristics, reproductive functions & menstrual cycles
	Oxytocin	Causes uterus & breast muscles to contract
	Prolactin	Starts breast milk production
	Thyroid-stimulating hormone	Stimulates hormone secretion by thyroid
Parathyroid	*Parathyroid hormone (PTH)*	Controls bone formation, regulate the release of bone calcium & phosphorus
Thyroid	*Thyroid hormone*	Regulates body function (metabolic rate)
	Calcitonin (CT)	Regulates calcium balance
Adrenal	*Aldosterone*	Helps regulate salt & water balance
	Cortisol	Maintains blood sugar level & blood pressure
	Dehydroepiandrosterone (DHEA)	Has effects on skeletal & immune system
	Epinephrine & Norepinephrine	Stimulates heart, lungs & nervous system
Pancreas	*Glucagon*	Raises the blood sugar level
	Insulin	Lowers the blood sugar level
Kidneys	*Erythropoietin*	Stimulates red blood cell production
	Renin	Controls blood pressure
Ovaries	*Estrogen*	Controls female sex characteristics
	Progesterone	Prepares uterus for implantation of fertilized egg
Testes	*Testosterone*	Controls male sex characteristics
GI tract	*Cholecystokinin*	Controls release of digestive enzymes
	Glucagon-like peptide	Increases insulin release from pancreas
	Ghrelin	Causes sensation of hunger
Fat tissue	*Resistin*	Blocks the effects of insulin on muscle
	Leptin	Controls appetite
Placenta	*Chorionic Gonadotropin*	Controls progesterone release during pregnancy
	Estrogen & Progesterone	Keeps uterus receptive to fetus during pregnancy

Estrogen *(E)*

Estrogens or *oestrogens* are a group of steroid sex hormones. The following three estrogens are the prominent ones: *estrone (E1)*, *estradiol (E2)* and *estriol (E3)*. E is present in both sexes; usually at higher levels in women during reproductive age. E is necessary for normal female sexual development, plays a pivotal role in the early maturation of the vagina, uterus, fallopian tubes and other female organs, as well as secondary sex characteristics such as the enlargement of breasts and hips. E also regulates menstrual cycle and prepares the uterus for pregnancy. In males, estrogen regulates certain functions of the reproductive system important to the maturation of sperm and may be necessary for a healthy libido.

Role in bone metabolism: E has specific functions at the organ, tissue, and cellular levels of the skeleton. At the organ level, E acts to conserve bone mass. At the tissue level, E suppresses bone turnover and maintains balanced rates of bone formation and bone resorption. At the cellular level, E affects the generation, lifespan and functional activity of both osteoclasts and osteoblasts. E decreases osteoclast formation and activity and, by increasing apoptosis, it decreases osteoclast lifespan. Some evidence suggests that E increases osteoblast formation, differentiation, proliferation, and function.

Deficiency: In 1941, Albright and co-workers were the first to relate the causation of postmenopausal osteoporosis to E deficiency and suggested that hormone replacement could improve calcium balance. E deficiency affects remodeling in several ways. First, it increases the activation frequency of bone cells, which leads to higher bone turnover. Second, it induces a remodeling imbalance by prolonging the resorption phase and shortening the formation phase. E is linked to calcium absorption and hence, there is a decreased calcium absorption resulting in increased bone resorption.

Estrogen replacement helps prevent postmenopausal osteoporosis by slowing bone loss and promoting some increase in bone density; reduces the frequency and severity of hot flashes; improves depression and sleep problems related to hormone changes; maintains the lining of the vagina, reducing irritation; increases skin collagen levels, which decline as E levels decline; and reduces the risk of dental problems, such as tooth loss and gum disease. However, long-term hormone therapy for prevention of postmenopausal conditions is no longer routinely recommended.

In 2002, a large clinical trial called the Women's Health Initiative *(WHI)* reported that hormone therapy actually posed more health risks than benefits for women. In 2008, US-FDA imposed restrictions on bio-identical hormone replacement therapy *(BHRT)*, especially medicines compounded with the drug estriol.

Androgen / Testosterone (T)

Androgens, traditionally viewed as 'male' hormones, are sex steroids produced by the testes in men; both by the ovaries and the adrenal glands in women. The major gonadal androgens in male are *testosterone (T)*, and *androstenedione*, other types include *dihydrotestosterone (DHT)*, *dehydroepiandrosterone (DHEA)* and DHEA sulfate *(DHEA-S)*. Androgens induce male sexual differentiation before birth and sexual maturation during puberty. In men, T maintains the male genital function, including spermatogenesis. In women, androgens are important for maintaining strong muscles and bones, positive protein balance, sexual desire and overall well being.

Role in bone metabolism: Androgens affect skeletal growth and adult bone metabolism by interacting with different types of cells located within the bone compartment. As with estrogen, the major action of T at the tissue level is to reduce bone resorption. T also increases the lifespan of both osteoblasts and osteoclasts. T has a modest effect on osteoblast proliferation. Both effects of T contribute to its action on enhancing bone formation.

Deficiency: Androgen deficiency could lead to fatigue, depression, low libido, muscle weakness and bone loss. T deficiency in men induces bone loss similar to estrogen deficiency in postmenopausal women. The histological and biochemical changes induced by T deficiency in men are similar to changes observed in postmenopausal women; the rate of bone remodeling is increased after loss of sex steroids, resulting in enhanced bone resorption and a decline in the number of osteoblasts, with the former exceeding the latter. This imbalance between resorption and formation leads to a decrease in bone volume, thickness and connectivity of the *trabecular* bone. During the onset of menopause, the T levels decline by about 10% to 50%. However, the E levels drop by a steep 70% to 80% at menopause. Thus, the T to E ratio increases substantially at menopause. As a result, some women acquire more facial hair, a deeper voice, and other androgen-accentuated characteristics at menopause.

Androgen replacement: The T replacement therapy been extensively used in *hypogonadal* men. The potential applications of androgen administration extend to young men with delayed puberty, elderly men with partial androgen deficiency, *eugonadal* men and *glucocorticoid*-treated men suffering from osteoporosis, and even postmenopausal women.

The T replacement therapy looks similar to ERT in postmenopausal women, primarily acting as an anti-resorptive. Limited data suggests that combined E and T replacement may result in an additional increase in BMD compared to E alone. However, the potential side effects of long-term T replacement is a growing concern.

Vitamin-D

Vitamin-D, also known as the 'Sunshine Vitamin', is produced by the skin when exposed to sunlight. Ultra-violet *(UV)* rays in sunlight activate cholesterol to form vitamin-D3 or cholecalciferol. Vitamin-D2 or ergocalciferol is found in plants and yeasts. Both vitamin forms are converted to a hormonally active calcitriol by the liver. Calcitriol increases the absorption of calcium and phosphate from the gastrointestinal tract and kidneys and inhibits release of calcitonin.

Vitamin-D levels in the body are influenced by ecological factors (ranging from season, weather conditions to latitude); lifestyle (ranging from clothing patterns to dietary habits); and individual features (ranging from race, pigmentation to age). Factors that contribute to low vitamin D levels include low sunlight exposure, decreased skin activity, low intestinal absorption and inadequate diet.

Role in the body: The role of vitamin-D is closely associated with the maintenance of calcium and phosphate levels in the body. Vitamin-D facilitates calcium and phosphate absorption in the gastrointestinal tract, and mineral re-absorption in the kidney. Vitamin-D plays an important role in several biological systems including skin, immune system, insulin secretion, and drug metabolism.

Due to the skin pigmentation, vitamin-D deficiency is prevalent among black population.

When dietary calcium is low or bio-unavailable, vitamin-D activates resting osteoclasts into a bone resorption mode. Calcium loss from the skeleton during such resorption mode eventually leads to osteoporosis. Vitamin-D depletion could trigger adverse effects on calcium metabolism, new bone formation, matrix ossification, BMD and bone remodeling. Vitamin-D supplementation could reduce the number of fractures and directly improve the neuro-muscular function, thus helps to prevent falls and subsequent fractures.

Deficiency: There is a concern about the inadequate synthesis of vitamin-D due to geographical and seasonal variation in sunlight in different parts of the world. Vitamin production also depends on skin pigmentation. Individuals with darker skin have the more difficulty in vitamin-D synthesis. Clouds, smog, clothing, and even window glass also filter out UV rays. Therefore, indoor-bound individuals, with dark skin, those that

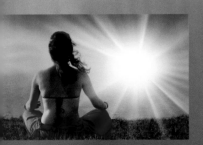

A fair-skinned person makes a sufficient quantity of vitamin-D with only 20 to 30 mins of sun exposure a day. It would take much more time, about 3 hrs, for a dark-skinned person to make an equal amount of the vitamin because skin pigment filters out UV rays.

Vitamin-D from sun exposure can not be overdosed due to its self limiting process. Sunscreens not only filter out the UV rays that burn skin but also block the synthesis of this 'Sunshine Vitamin'.

cover most of their body when outdoors and those who live in cloudy climates are most likely to develop vitamin-D deficiency. Such individuals must get vitamin-D from foods and supplements.

Obese individuals might need higher doses of vitamin-D supplementation than the general population.

Vitamin-D deficiency is common in the elderly and frequently associated with a raised serum parathyroid hormone *(PTH)*, increased bone resorption and low BMD. Generally the negative effect of vitamin-D deficiency on bone has been attributed to a decrease in calcium absorption. Vitamin-D deficiency triggers osteopenia, aggravates osteoporosis, sets off osteomalacia – a painful disease, and increases muscle weakness that worsens the risk of falls and fractures.

There is also a reduction in the ability to synthesize vitamin-D precursor in the skin with aging, and reduced exposure by lifestyle changes and immobility. The elderly population could be at risk of chronic vitamin-D deficiency that leads to osteoporosis or gradual loss of bone. Impaired structural integrity of bones leads to thinner and more porous bones, susceptible to fracture. Vitamin-D supplementation, therefore, is one of the most common treatments for the elderly.

Recent studies suggested a strong link between decreased serum levels of vitamin-D precursor and obesity. Low vitamin-D levels (and elevated PTH) could be the result of decreased sunshine exposure in individuals with high body mass index (obesity). The association of obesity and low vitamin-D levels has been found not only in the morbidly obese, but in all overweight categories.

Breastfed infants are particularly sensitive to vitamin-D deficiency. In general, human breast milk has low vitamin-D content. Rickets is a nutritional disorder that occurs most commonly in the early months of life as a result of decreased availability of vitamin-D, calcium or phosphorus. It is most prevalent among infants whose mothers have vitamin-D deficiency due to inadequate diet, dark skin pigmentation, or religious dress codes that limit/prevent skin exposure.

Vitamin-D is the critical hormone for total bone health.

Parathyroid Hormone *(PTH)*

PTH or parathormone, a polypeptide of 84 amino acids, is the most important endocrine regulator of calcium and phosphorus concentration in extracellular fluid. This hormone is secreted from cells of the parathyroid glands and finds its major target cells in bone and kidney. The parathyroid cell monitors extracellular free calcium concentration via a membrane protein that acts as a calcium-sensing receptor.

PTH is released in response to low extracellular concentrations of free calcium and tightly regulates blood calcium levels within 8.8 and 10.2 mg/dL. As the blood circulates through, the parathyroid glands measure calcium and reacts accordingly by releasing more or less PTH. If the blood calcium level is too low, more PTH is released. This causes the bones to release more calcium into the blood and reduces the amount of calcium released by the kidneys into the urine. If the calcium level is too high, the parathyroid glands release less PTH and the whole process is reversed. The PTH feed-back regulation in a normal healthy individual will turn on and off several times a day, to maintain the calcium homeostasis. PTH also converts vitamin-D to a more active form and facilitates intestinal absorption of calcium and phosphorus.

PTH stimulates the bone cells to release their calcium into the bloodstream

Role in bone metabolism: PTH performs its homeodynamic function by three distinct mechanisms: *i) Calcium mobilization from bone:* PTH stimulates osteoclasts to reabsorb bone minerals and release calcium into blood. *ii) Calcium absorption from the small intestine:* PTH stimulates production of the active form of vitamin-D in the kidney; that in turn, induces synthesis of a calcium-binding protein in intestinal epithelial cells to facilitate efficient absorption of calcium into blood. *iii) Suppression of calcium loss in urine:* PTH prevents the urinary excretion of calcium, which is mediated by stimulating the tubular recovery of calcium in the kidney. The hormone also enhances both the excretion of phosphate by the kidneys and its uptake by the cells. PTH is closely linked to vitamin-D, and both of these substances likely play a role in the long-term regulation of blood pressure.

Abnormal levels: *Hyperparathyroidism*, the result of over secretion of PTH, often leads to the resorption of bone and can only be treated by surgical removal of parathyroid glands. Chronic secretion or continuous infusion of PTH may lead to decalcification of bone and loss of bone mass. However, in certain conditions, PTH treatment can stimulate an increase in bone mass and bone strength. This seemingly paradoxical effect occurs when the hormone is administered in pulses (e.g. by once daily injection), and such treatment appears to be an effective therapy for diseases such as osteoporosis.

The four 'pea-sized' parathyroid glands have a rich blood supply to help monitor calcium levels in the blood – 24 hours a day

Inadequate production of PTH, *hypoparathyroidism*, results in decreased concentrations of calcium and increased concentrations of phosphorus in blood.

Common causes of this disorder include surgical removal of the parathyroid glands and disease processes that lead to destruction of parathyroid glands. The resulting *hypocalcemia* often leads to tetany and convulsions, which are life-threatening. Treatment focuses on restoring normal blood calcium concentrations by calcium infusions, oral calcium supplements and vitamin-D therapy.

PTH replacement: PTH can induce *osteoblasts*, the bone-forming cells, to lay down new collagen and subsequently mineralize that tissue. Early in treatment, PTH therapy raises markers of bone formation, in advance of any change in bone resorption. By 9 months of therapy, PTH increases bone formation both in both men and women. Bone resorption is also activated, but this effect is not seen biochemically until several months into therapy. In this way, bone remodeling is uncoupled: formation increases more than resorption.

PTH is an anabolic agent, thus, bone replenishment with PTH is a valuable weapon in the battle against osteoporosis

A series of bone-specific genes are turned on by intermittent PTH, but not by continuous treatment. This leads to enhanced matrix generation and subsequent mineralization. Bone strength, as measured directly in animals and indirectly in humans, is remarkably enhanced. Thus, PTH has the advantage of not only building bone mass, but also strengthening bone's structural components, resulting in reduced skeletal fragility.

PTH has been given in combination with anti-resorptive therapies in several trials. Preliminary studies have shown that PTH provides an additional increase in BMD of the spine and hip in postmenopausal women on *hormone replacement therapy (HRT)*. Considering the risks associated with the use of HRT, however, patients should be cautioned about HRT for the purpose of preserving bone mass. Combination therapy with PTH and alendronate does not appear to be more effective than PTH monotherapy. However, studies show that PTH followed by alendronate results in greater bone mass than PTH followed by placebo.

Recombinant PTH1-34 *('teriparatide')* has received approval by the US-FDA for treatment of osteoporosis. In clinical trials to date, teriparatide is well tolerated. A few people develop mild *hypercalcemia* and leg cramps, nausea, dizziness, *arthralgias*, general weakness (all about 2% more than in placebo groups), increased uric acid, and increased blood and urine calcium (but no increase in kidney stones or gout).

3-D ribbon structure of PTH

Calcitonin *(CT)*

Calcitonin *(CT)* is a naturally occurring peptide hormone that maintains calcium and phosphorus homeostasis in the body. It acts to reduce blood calcium *(Ca^{2+})*, opposing the effects of PTH. In humans, the major sites for CT production are the *parafollicular* or *C cells* in the thyroid gland, but this hypocalcemic hormone is also synthesized in a wide variety of other tissues, including the lung and the intestinal tract. Elevated levels of extra-cellular and blood calcium strongly stimulates CT secretion, and suppressed when the concentration of ionized calcium falls below normal.

Role in bone metabolism: CT maintains calcium homeostasis in the body through specific activity on three target organs: i) *gut,* where it inhibits trans-cellular calcium absorption; ii) *bone,* where it suppresses resorption by inhibiting the osteoclast activity; iii) *kidney*, where it prevents the urinary loss of calcium and phosphorus by reclamation through kidney tubules.

Furthermore, CT regulates bone mineral metabolism and protects against Ca^{2+} loss from skeleton during periods of Ca^{2+} stress such as pregnancy and lactation CT prevents *postprandial hypercalcemia* resulting from absorption of Ca^{2+} from foods during a meal. As a "satiety" hormone, a role for CT has been suggested on the nerve impulses involving the regulation of feeding and appetite.

CT replacement: CT extracted from the *ultimobranchial* glands (thyroid-like glands) of fish, particularly salmon, resembles human CT and is more active. CT is rapidly absorbed and eliminated in the human system. The benefits of CT may take many weeks to notice, and they often go away soon after the therapy is stopped. Since CT is a polypeptide, oral route is not preferred (due to digestion). Historically, CT was administered as a parenteral injection, but the intranasal formulation is now the most widely used because of its improved tolerance. Intranasal CT has been shown to increase bone mass in postmenopausal women with established osteoporosis. The recommended dose of CT is one spray (200 IU) in one nostril daily, alternating nostrils each day.

CT is used to treat symptoms of *Paget's disease, hypercalcemia* and postmenopausal osteoporosis. CT acts directly on chondrocytes, attenuating cartilage degradation and stimulating cartilage formation; therefore, it may have a protective role in osteoarthritis *(OA)*. CT is often administered to cancer patients experiencing bone pain due to metastasis. CT may be considered as second line of treatment for those at high risk of osteoporosis, but unsuitable for bisphosphonates. The evidence suggests that CT reduces vertebral fractures when compared with placebo in postmenopausal women when given with calcium and vitamin-D supplements. CT is approved only for the treatment, not the prevention, of osteoporosis.

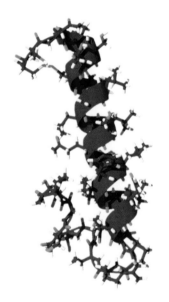

3-D ribbon structure of CT – *contains a disulfide bond, which causes the N-terminus region of the protein to assume the shape of a ring.*

Chemical Factors of Bone Metabolism

Chemical factors are necessary for bone cells to communicate with each other and rest of the body. These groups of chemicals are incorporated into the mineralized bone matrix and release during resorption. There is also increasing evidence that abnormal production of these factors, especially cytokines, in diseases such as RA, OA and osteoporosis.

Growth Factors: *Insulin-like growth factor (IGF)* regulates bone remodeling with potent effects on various phases of skeletal tissue developments; importantly for multiplication of osteoblasts. *Transforming growth factor (TGF)* regulates collagen synthesis and controls the bone mineralization process; also couples the bone formation and resorption activities. *Bone morphogenetic proteins (BMPs)* are the only molecules so far discovered capable of independently inducing ossification (bone growth). BMPs can stimulate bone growth in implants placed under the skin *(subcutaneous)* or between the muscles *(intramuscular)*. BMPs play a pivotal role in procedures such as bone grafts and hip replacement surgery. *Fibroblast growth factor (FGF)* are synthesized by osteoblasts, stored in bone matrix, and released during bone resorption. FGF exists in acidic and basic forms; and the basic FGF *(bFGF)* is important at later stages of bone growth, FGFs stimulate growth of several bone cells, including *mesenchymal* cells responsible for the development of limbs. *Platelet-derived growth factor (PDGF)* is sequestered from the blood circulation and located in bone matrix. PDGF is a growth stimulant for several bone cells, especially, osteoblasts, PDGF increases DNA synthesis in certain bone cells.

Chemical Factors are small soluble molecules produced by cells, which affect growth of other 'local' cells; as well as cells at 'distant' sites when released into blood circulation

Cytokines are necessary for the regulation of bone and cartilage cells. In post-menopausal osteoporosis, when cytokine production is altered, it leads to uncoupling of bone formation from resorption; which is a characteristic of this disease. *Tumor necrosis factor (TNF)* induces formation of new blood vessels; it may also work with other local factors to spread blood capillaries into the bone tissue. *Interleukin (IL)* exists in several types. *IL type-1* stimulates bone resorption, decreases proteoglycan and collagen synthesis. It also regulates enzymes that digest bone proteins. *IL type-6* mediates some of the effects of estrogen on the bone. *IL type-8* mediates inflammation and may have an important role in RA and OA. Interferon *(IFN)* is a family of molecules that are potent inhibitors of cancer cells in the bone. *Colony stimulating factors (CSFs)* are critical for blood cells formation in the bone marrow. CSF injections can reverse *osteopetrosis* (a condition of impaired bone resorption). *Parathyroid hormone related peptide (PTHrP)* is a protein fragment closely related to PTH. It can regulate calcium levels (e.g. hypercalcaemia) associated with some bone cancers. This peptide may also have an important role in skeletal development during the embryonic stage. *Calcitonin gene related peptide (CGRP)* is located in the nerve cells with a potential role in the modulation of nerve impulses to the bone cells. CGRP is important in the local regulation of skeletal tissues and inhibition of bone resorption.

Angiogenin *(ANG)* or Ribonuclease *(RNase)*

Physical growth requires new, functional and durable blood vessels to support an amassing tissue with more oxygen (energy), nutrients and defense. The components that fill the blood vessels – erythrocytes *(RBC)*, leucocytes *(WBC)*, platelets, however, are introduced from the bone marrow. Therefore, the inter-reliance between the cardiovascular and the skeletal system manifests as: i) the bones provide cellular machinery for the circulatory network, whereas, ii) the circulatory portal supports the bone metabolism with mobilization of chemicals to and from the skeletal tissue. Bio-replenishment plays a significant role in maintaining the fine balance between both systems. Malfunction or breakdown of bio-replenishment could impair several vital pathways and lead to homeostatic imbalance.

Angiogenesis: Circulatory system is the first organ that emerges in an embryo and eventually expands into the largest transport network in the body. *Vasculogenesis* refers to the formation of new blood vessels and *angiogenesis* is the process of sprouting blood vessels from pre existing ones. Angiogenesis is a vital process for growth, development and wound healing. Abnormal or insufficient angiogenesis is the cause of many disorders including *arthritis, synovitis, osteomyelitis* and *osteophyte* formation. Osteoporosis and impaired healing of bone fractures are linked to insufficient angiogenesis. Age dependent decline of angiogenesis leads to impaired bone formation, one of the risk factors for osteoporosis. Diminished angiogenesis due to chemical inhibitors prevent fractures from healing. Delayed bone healing and non-fusion of fractures are shown to be associated with low angiogenic activity. During

ANG is a potent replenishment with specific angiogenic activity to promote bone health

fracture healing, a "cartilage callus" is formed to provide initial stability to the fractured zone. Growth of new blood vessels into the callus is critical for the conversion of cartilage scaffold into bone tissue, which is accomplished by angiogenesis.

Angiogenic factors include *vascular endothelial growth factor (VEGF), basic fibroblast growth factor (bFGF), angiogenin (ANG), angiopoietin 2 (Ang-2), platelet-derived growth factor AB (PDGF-AB)* and *pleiotrophin (PTN)*. Among these factors, ANG derived from milk has recently shown very promising results in promoting bone formation with age-related and post-menopausal bone loss.

Angiogenin *(ANG)* is a member of the ***ribonuclease*** super family and a normal constituent of the circulating blood. ANG is a potent inducer of new blood vessel formation, and is involved in the early stages of bone healing. ANG has an important role in the plasminogen-mediated break down of extracellular matrix and basement membranes, which enables formation of new blood vessels. In the fracture healing process, serum concentrations of ANG rise within the 1st week, indicating its anabolic activity during the regeneration process.

ANG is a multi-tasking protein with functions such as RNase activity, basement membrane degradation, signal transduction and nuclear translocation. ANG interacts with endothelial and smooth muscles to induce a wide range of cellular responses including cell migration, invasion, proliferation and formation of tubular structures. In brief, the ANG-induced angiogenic mechanism is as follows: i) ANG binds to cell surface *actin* and the ANG-actin complex dissociates from the cell surface; ii) the complex accelerates the production of plasmin from plasminogen; iii) the basement membrane and the extracellular matrix are degraded; iv) the endothelial cells penetrate into the surrounding tissue to form new tubular structures; and v) the capillary wall protrudes into the lumen and splits a single blood vessel in two. The process of "splitting angiogenesis" by ANG is the basic mechanism to lay new plumbing into a regenerated tissue, such as a newly formed bone. Recent studies have demonstrated that long bones are formed by *osteogenic-angiogenic* coupling.

ANG-replenishment can be designed with highly purified milk proteins; RNases type 2 and 4, with pre-calibrated doses of individual RNase types, for established biological outcomes. Capillaries are designed to provide maximum nutrient delivery efficiency so an increase in the number of capillaries allows the network to deliver more nutrients in the same amount of time. A greater number of capillaries also allows for greater oxygen exchange in the network. ANG-replenishment could help optimize this process.

ANG-replenishment provides an excellent therapeutic target to reverse osteoporosis. Bio-replenishment is a potent, physiological process that underlies the natural manner in which bones respond to any decline in nutrient supply through the circulatory transport. The production of new collateral vessels with ANG-replenishment could overcome the bone metabolic imbalance. Several conditions, such as *cardiovascular diseases, ischemic chronic wounds,* are the result of failure or insufficient blood vessel formation and could be reversed by a local expansion of blood vessels, thus bringing new nutrients to the site, facilitating repair using the ANG-replenishment. Other diseases, such as age-related macular degeneration, could also be reversed with ANG-replenishment that can trigger local expansion of blood vessels, thus promoting normal physiological processes.

ANG-replenishment in the human body declines with age. Osteoporosis is not merely a manifestation of an age-related delayed angiogenesis, but a result of multiple impairments. Mechanical stimulus such as physical exercise (shear stress) could act on capillaries to cause angiogenesis. Muscle contractions are known to increase nitric oxide production and elevate ANG levels. Chemical stimulation of angiogenesis could be accomplished by various angiogenic proteins and growth factors, including ANG. Administration of ANG-replenishment from exogenous route(s) is an effective approach.

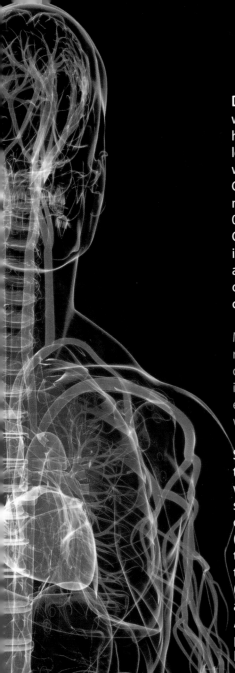

Diffusion is a powerful transport mechanism to facilitate chemical exchange when operating over short distances and through large areas such as the human body. Capillary beds allow huge amount of chemicals to enter and leave blood because they maximize the area across which exchange can occur while minimizing the distance over which the diffusing substances must travel. Capillaries are extremely fine vessels with lumen (inside) diameter of about 5 microns, a wall thickness of about 1 micron and an average length of perhaps 0.5 mm (for comparison a human hair is roughly 100 micron in diameter). Capillaries are distributed in massive numbers in organs and communicate intimately with all regions of the intestitial space. It is estimated that there are about 10 billion capillaries in the systemic organs with a collective surface area of about 100 m². That is roughly the area of one player's side of a singles tennis court.

Most substances cross the capillary walls simply by passive diffusion from regions of high concentration to regions of low concentration. Factors that determine the diffusion rate of a substance between the blood and the interstitial fluid include: i) the concentration difference, ii) the surface area for exchange, iii) the diffusion distance, and iv) the permeability of the capillary wall to the diffusing substance.

Substances are carried between organs within the cardiovascular system by the process of convective transport, the simple process of being swept along with the flow of the blood in which they are contained. The rate at which a substance (X) is transported by this process depends solely on the concentration of the substance in the blood and the blood flow rate (Transport rate = flow rate x concentration). One can extend the convective transport principle to determine a tissue's rate of chemical utilization (eg. bone turnover) by simultaneously considering the transport rate of the substance (eg. calcium) to and from the tissue. The relationship that results is referred to as the "Fick Principle" (after Adolf Fick, a German Physician, 1829-1901 AD). Accordingly, the amount of calcium that goes into a bone matrix in a given period of time, minus the amount of calcium that comes out, must equal the bone utilization rate of calcium.

Transcapillary
Solute Diffusion

Angiogenesis, the regular formation of new blood vessels and an uninterrupted supply of vital chemicals to meet the metabolic demands of bone remodeling are the key for a healthy aging process

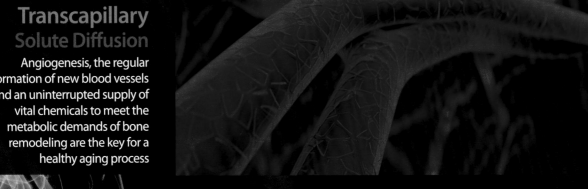

6.2 | Bone Replenishment: **Transport**

Transport and uninterrupted delivery of nutrients, vitamins, minerals, building blocks (amino acids, bio-polymers, etc) and regulatory molecules (enzymes, hormones, etc) to bone matrix is critical for homeostasis of the skeleto-muscular system. Bone transport processes are influenced by diet and lifestyle (i.e. stress, physical activity), environmental exposure (i.e. sunlight, pollutants), age, sex and genetic predisposition of an individual. The health status of other physiological systems in the body, in particular, the gastrointestinal, the circulatory, the neurologic and the endocrine systems are inter-related with the target delivery of bone health chemicals.

Gastrointestinal route: Skeletal system requires food (energy source) to operate its metabolism. Food undergoes three types of processes – digestion, absorption, and elimination; digested to nutrients, ready to be absorbed to fuel the bone metabolism. The GI tract is a remarkable food processing system. Stomach stores all the food from a meal for both mechanical and chemical processing. It is able to digest materials that are more complex in composition tougher than its own structure. *Hydrochloric acid (HCl)* in the stomach provides an acidic milieu needed for enzymes (pepsin) to break down proteins. The stomach's high acidity also serves as a barrier against infection. Acid secretion is stimulated by nerve impulses to the stomach, *gastrin* (a hormone released by the stomach), and *histamine* (a substance released by the stomach). Pepsin is the only enzyme that digests collagen, which is a major polypeptide constituent of bone matrix. The nutrient absorption is facilitated by millions of fingerlike projections called *villi*, which line the inner walls of the small intestine. Beneath the layer of villi, are capillaries (tiny vessels) of blood and lymph that transport nutrients produced by digestion to various cells of the body. Simple sugars and amino acids pass through the capillaries to enter the bloodstream. Fatty acids and glycerol move through the lymphatic system. Finally, the large intestine absorbs water, about 6 liters (1.6 gallons) daily and dissolved salts (electrolytes) from the residue dispatched by the small intestine.

We have to boil food in strong acids at 212°F with cookery what stomach does at body's normal temperature of 98.6°F!

Since, the GI tract provides a continuous source of chemical energy, any interruption to this nutritional gateway could severely affect bone metabolism. Natural levels of HCl and digestive enzymes decrease with age and/or abuse of the GI tract with excesses diet, chemical use, and stress. The most common age-related health problem with the GI tract is *hypochlorhydria*, the underproduction stomach acid. Almost 30% people over the age of sixty develop stomach acid deficiency.

Constipation affects more than 33 million adults in the U.S., accounting for 2.5 million physician visits and 92,000 hospitalizations/year

Hypochlorhydria is a well established risk factor for several metabolic bone diseases, notably, the osteoporosis, resulting in part from decreased calcium absorption; as well as the *iron-deficiency anemia*, due to poor iron absorption. *Helicobacter pylori* infection (peptic ulcers), which occurs more commonly during midlife is associated with a decrease in gastric acid secretion.

Maximal oxygen consumption of the heart declines about 10% per decade after age 25

As the GI tract changes with time, constipation becomes more prevalent. Indigestion promotes an overgrowth of unfriendly bacteria in the small intestine and colon, a condition known as *dysbiosis*. This situation may lead to chronic disease conditions as arthritis, autoimmune disease, vitamin B12 deficiency, chronic fatigue syndrome, eczema, food allergies and food sensitivities, inflammatory bowel disease *(IBD)*, and irritable bowel syndrome *(IBS)*. It is estimated that 80 percent of patients with food allergies suffer from some degree of impaired hydrochloric acid secretion in the stomach. Therefore, digestive tract and its function may be the single most important transport system that determines bone health and disease.

Cardiovascular *(CV)* route maintains homeostasis using its continuous and controlled flow of blood through thousands of miles of capillaries that permeate every tissue and reach every cell in the body. The circulatory functions include assimilation of nutrients from the digestive tract, transport of minerals to and from bone tissue, carry hormones to regulate organ functions, mobilize defense mediators to wade off infections, and regulate temperature, water and ionic balance in the tissues.

After the digestive process, a network of capillaries and fine lymphatic vessels underlying the GI tract, act as efficient exchange sites for of bone nutrients and minerals. Ultimately, the absorbed chemicals are transported to specific skeletal sites of for 'assimilation'. The skeleto-muscular system is highly dependent on the CV route for several critical functions; therefore, any breakdown in the CV system could lead to serious consequences and may eventually compromise the bone health.

Chemical messengers from endocrine route regulate various aspects of skeletal homeostasis, including bone turnover

Cardiovascular health declines as a result of physical inactivity, increased body weight (fat) and progressively deteriorates with age. Cardiovascular aging is characterized by a gradual debility of endothelial function and myocardial performance, which begins to accelerate after mid-life. One of the unavoidable consequences of aging is a decline in the maximal capacity of the CV system to pump blood for delivery of vital chemicals and for removing metabolic waste products.

Endocrine route releases hormones into the bloodstream, which reach different organs in the body, including the skeletal system, with a specific target-delivery mechanism. However, changes naturally occur with aging and affect the endocrine route. Certain target tissues in the bone matrix may become less sensitive to their controlling hormone. Also, blood levels of some hormones increase, some decrease, and some remain unchanged. As individuals age, there is a decline in the peripheral levels of estrogen *(E)* and testosterone *(T)*, with an increase in luteinizing hormone *(LH)*, follicle-stimulating hormone *(FSH)* and sex hormone-binding globulin *(SHBG)*.

Additionally there is a decline in serum concentrations of growth hormone *(GH)*, insulin-like growth factor-I, DHEA and its sulfate-bound form. Even though there are complex changes within the *hypothalmo-pituitary-adrenal/thyroid axis*, there is minimal change in adrenal and thyroid function with aging. The clinical significance of these deficiencies with age are variable and include reduced protein synthesis, decrease in lean body mass and BMD, increased fat mass, insulin resistance, higher cardiovascular disease risk, increase in vasomotor symptoms, fatigue, depression, anemia, poor libido, erectile deficiency and a decline in immune function.

Lymphatic route acts as a secondary circulatory system to maintain bone metabolic homeostasis. It consists of three main components: i) a complex capillary network that carries the lymph; ii) a system of collecting vessels that drain the lymph back into the bloodstream, and iii) lymph glands, or nodes, that filter the lymph as it passes through. In humans, approximately 3 quarts, or 2.83 liters, of lymph is returned to the heart everyday. Unlike the CV sytem, the lymphatic system is not closed and has no central pump. Lymph movement occurs despite low pressure due to peristalsis (propulsion of the lymph due to alternate contraction and relaxation of smooth muscle), valves and compression during contraction of adjacent skeletal muscle and arterial pulsation. Therefore, skeleto-muscular and lymphatic functions are inter-connected.

Neuro-chemical route: Bio-transport operates through nerve conduction with the involvement of neurotransmitters, chemicals that communicate nerve signals. Aging and conditions such as diabetes, cause deterioration of nerve fibers and affect neurotransmission. Also with aging, there is loss of motor neurons and a decrease in the numbers of motor axons available to innervate the muscles. There is also a decrease in the speed of nerve impulses, neurotransmission, and receptor numbers. Consequently, peripheral nerves conduct impulses more slowly, which results in decreased sensation, slower reflexes, and often some clumsiness. Nerve conduction slows, because myelin sheaths (that speed conduction of nerve impulses) degenerate. Such age-related nerve relapse is due to decreased blood flow, overgrowth of nearby bones that put pressure on the nerves, or both. The balance centre in the brain relies on signals from the muscles, particularly of the neck and lower legs, the eyes and ears. If any of the neuro-transmission is defective or delayed, the balance may be affected and increase the risk of falls and fractures.

Lymphatic system is critical for homeostasis, therefore, called "river of life"

Transport is quintessential for homeostasis and bone health. Networks of several physiological routes operate in sync to meet the regular supply-demand of vital chemicals for bone metabolism. Aging is not just "a matter of time," it is a process of gradual deterioration of transportation networks in the body, which varies among individuals based on their genetic backgrounds and/or lifestyle factors. Repair and maintenance of these basic portal systems is the ultimate purpose of bone-replenishment, to achieve bone metabolic homeostasis.

Lactoferrin *(LF)*

Lactoferrin *(LF)* is a metal-binding glycoprotein present in milk and secretions of the exocrine glands located mainly in the gateways of the digestive, respiratory and reproductive systems, to provide mucosal protection against invading microorganisms and toxic insults. It occurs in three different physiological pools: i) the secretory (exocrine) pool, ii) the circulatory pool and iii) the stationary (tissue-borne) pool. In the secretory pool, the normal levels of LF are reported at 1-2 mg/mL in breast milk, tears and gastric mucins; 0.1-1 mg/mL in vaginal, cervical and bronchial mucus; 0.01-0.1 mg/mL in seminal plasma, pancreatic juice, saliva and crevicular fluids; <0.01 mg/mL in plasma, cerebrospinal and synovial fluids. Neutrophils contain LF at about 0.01 mg/10^6 cells, which contributes to the plasma levels of LF in the circulatory pool. In the stationary pool, LF is localized in several tissues. LF regulates a variety of physiological pathways and credited with an impressive list of multifunctional health benefits.

TABLE: *Lactoferrin – Multifunctional Protein for Bone-Replenishment*

Specific Function	Possible Role in Bone Health
Metal binding and transport	Provides essential bone minerals (eg. zinc, chromium)
Anti-microbial activity	Evades bone infections (eg. osteomyelitis)
Anti-oxidant activity	Prevents bone and joints from free radical damage
Anti-tumor activity	Controls metastatic bone conditions (eg. osteosarcoma)
Anti-inflammatory activity	Protects from inflammatory bone diseases (eg. *OA, RA*)
Prebiotic activity	Maintains healthy gut for optimal bone nutrient absorption
Opsonic activity	Scavenges foreign bodies that may harm bone tissue
DNA binding activity	Bone development and growth
Bone growth factor	Stimulates osteoblasts to form new bone matrix
Sperm-coating antigen	Facilitate sexual transfer of genetic (hereditary) information
Intestinal absorption	Maintains healthy gut for bone mineral transport
Immuno-modulation	Protects the bone from antigen-mediated immune responses
Complement activation	Helps combat rheumatoid arthritis
Platelet activation	Participates in bone repair processes (eg. healing of fractures)
Feed-back regulation	Controls various bone homeostatic pathways
Down-regulation of myelopoiesis	Controls blood cell production in the bone marrow
Regulation of collagenase	Maintains healthy cartilage in bone joints

LF – Gastrointestinal system: Healthy function of the digestive tract is critical for nutrient absorption and has an obvious impact on bone metabolism. LF stands out as the primary caretaker for the GI system with following protective functions: *1) Elimination of harmful microbes from the gut:* LF could suppress microbial growth and facilitate fecal excretion of several harmful bacteria and viruses. LF could block colonization of *Helicobacter pylori* (causative agent of peptic ulcers) and detach this pathogen from the gastric epithelium. *2) Enrich the populations of beneficial microbial populations in the gut:* This prebiotic effect by LF in the intestinal milieu is a phenomenon of natural selection to enrich beneficial probiotic flora and affect competitive exclusion of harmful pathogens by bacteriostasis. Certain peptide domains on LF have been identified to stimulate growth of bifidobacteria *in vivo*. *3) Elimination of endotoxins from the GI tract:* LF could effectively neutralize and eliminate endotoxin influx (bacterial lipopolysaccharides) into the bloodstream while toxins are still inside the intestinal lumen. *4) Anti-inflammatory activity* of LF in the gut is primarily associated with its ability to scavenge free iron. It is known that accumulation of iron in inflamed tissues could lead to catalytic production of highly toxic free radicals. During an inflammatory response, neutrophils migrate to the challenged site to release acidic granules that contain LF. This results in the creation of a strong acidic milieu at the inflamed tissue site to amplify iron-sequestering ability of LF. Also, LF plays an important role in the modulation of gastric inflammation, since this protein is also expressed in the gastric mucosa and interacts with receptors localized on gastric intestinal epithelial cells. Furthermore, the expression of LF is elevated in the feces of patients with inflammatory conditions including ulcerative colitis and Crohn's disease. *5) Modulation of mucosal immunity:* Oral administration of LF (60 mg capsule/day) could enhance immune response in healthy human volunteers. Human clinical trials showed a positive correlation of LF consumption with primary activation of host defense. *6) Gut maturation and mucosal repair:* The GI tract matures more rapidly in the newborn during suckling. Oral administration of LF, either at low (0.05 mg/g body wt/d) or high (1 mg/g body wt/d) dosages could function as an immune stimulating factor in the intestinal mucosa. This activation is dependent on LF binding to the intestinal epithelia. *7) Intestinal absorption (transport):* LF plays an important role in the intestinal absorption of iron, zinc, copper, manganese and other essential trace elements. LF also protects the gut mucosa from excess uptake of heavy metal ions. Specific LF binding receptors in the human duodenal brush border are involved in the absorption. An intestinal LF receptor with a cellular density of 430 trillion sites per milligram of solubilized human intestinal brush-border membranes (IBBM) has been identified.

LF – Skeletal system: LF has a multi-functional role in skeletal development and homeostasis. LF is expressed biphasically during embryogenesis, appearing firstly in the 2-4 cell embryo, it expression declines during the post-blastocyst stage, its expression declines, but increases again dramatically in the latter half of gestation. Thus, LF could play a significant role in

3-D ribbon structure of LF

the development and function of chondrocytes and osteoblasts in the fetal skeleton. *LF – Bone formation:* LF stimulates multiplication and differentiation of pre-osteoblastic (precursor) cells. It also reduces the apoptosis (programmed cell death) of precursor cells by up to 50-70%, and acts as their potent survival factor. LF promotes the differentiation of these precursors to produce mature osteoblasts that are capable of promoting bone matrix deposition and mineralization. As a result of its effects on osteoblast growth, LF could produce substantial increases in local bone formation *in vivo*, even with the very short-term exposure. This anabolic potency suggests that LF or its analogs should be explored as bio-replenishment to reverse osteoporosis and restore skeletal strength. This bone-replenishment approach could be of enormous significance, since most current "anti-resorptive" interventions merely block further structural decline. *LF – Bone resorption:* LF inhibits osteoclast formation in a dose-dependent manner with complete arrest of osteoclasto-genesis at a concentration of 0.1 mg/mL. LF inhibits bone resorption by reducing the number of osteoclasts formed from precursor cells; however, it does not affect the activity of fully differentiated osteoclasts to resorb bone. These actions of LF on osteoclasts are strikingly different from those observed with osteoblasts. LF seems to reduce RANKL expression in bone marrow cultures which could in part explain the inhibition of osteoclastogenesis.

LF – Bone joints (articulations): LF stimulates the growth multiplication of *chondrocytes*, cells exclusively limited to bone cartilage. Chondrocytes produce and maintain the cartilage, which consists mainly of *collagen* and *proteoglycans*. Decline in chondrocyte population leads to loss of cartilage "lubrication" of the joints and lead to joint disorders such as osteoarthritis *(OA)*. In experimental animal model, joints with established inflammation, when injected with LF (0.5 mg or 1 mg dosage) could significantly suppress local inflammation for up to 3 days. LF is released from activated neutrophils at sites of inflammation to provide antimicrobial and anti-inflammatory protection. LF is effective in reducing articular inflammation, particularly septic arthritis, in which anti-inflammatory effects may be achieved without promoting bacterial survival. Orally administered LF has both preventive and therapeutic effects on the development of adjuvant-induced inflammation and pain. Immuno-modulatory properties of LF, such as down-regulation of TNF-alpha and up-regulation of interleukin (IL)-10, could be beneficial in the treatment of rheumatoid arthritis *(RA)*. Hydroxy *(OH)* free radical is a major damaging agent in the inflamed rheumatoid joint. Free radical formation is triggered by the release of iron into synovium, the bone joint. Addition of exogenous LF may prevent iron-mediated tissue damage in RA by scavenging "free" synovial iron when inflammatory stimuli have deregulated iron homeostasis.

LF – Cardiovascular system: The main source of LF in the circulation is the secondary granules of neutrophils. Systemic levels of LF can reach concentrations as high as 0.2 mg/mL during inflammation. During these inflammatory states, LF may play a role in counter-balancing the catabolic effects on the skeleton from some of the mediators of the inflammatory response. LF also plays immuno-modulatory function decreasing the secretion of a number of osteolytic cytokines. Therefore, its direct effects on the activity and development of bone cells appear to be complemented by these cytokine-mediated effects.

6.4 | Bone Replenishment: **Bio-ments**

Bio-ments are non-proteinaceous polymers, which are essential for the structure of the cellular matrix. Most of the bio-ments can withstand gastric digestion. Their high-charge molecular property, facilitates diffusion cross the intestinal barrier in their structural entirety. Bio-ments are vital for inter-cellular communication and their physiological concentrations decline with aging.

Glycosaminoglycans *(GAGs)*, phospholipids, DNA and RNA are four major negatively charged biopolymers made by the animal cells. Of these only GAGs plaster the animal cell surface and directly interact with hundreds of extracellular signaling processes. The extended long unbranched polysaccharide conformation imparts high viscosity and low compressibility properties to GAGs. These characteristics make GAG molecules ideal for making the "lubricating fluid" for the bone joint. At the same time, their rigidity provides structural integrity to open up passageways between bone matrices, allowing for cell migration. Hydraulic resistance of the joint lining depends on the concentrations of GAGs and collagen in the synovial (joint) spaces. Both these biopolymers create a hydraulic drag for the skeletal articulations.

GAGs are the most information dense, negatively charged biopolymers found in nature

A majority of GAGs are also linked to proteins and form *proteoglycans* (also called *mucopolysaccharides*). By virtue of their high net negative charge, GAGs and proteoglycans play a pivotal role in several vital functions of the skeleto-muscular system, such as cell-cell and cell-matrix interactions, sequestration of growth factors, activation of chemokines and cytokines. GAGs are especially critical for normal bone joint development and skeletal homeostasis. Since GAGs are abundant in the articular cartilage, these molecules are widely used as indicators of cartilage integrity and chondrocyte activity. GAGs are the building blocks of cartilage and joint (synovial) fluid. GAGs maintain and support collagen, elastin, turgidity (bounce) in the cellular spaces and keep ligaments in balance. They also support collagen and elastin fibers to retain moisture and remain soluble. GAGs are linked to the lymphatic system. Chondroitin sulfate, keratan sulfate, and hyaluronic acid are three classes of GAGs found in the articular cartilage. Approximately 80% of GAGs in the adult articular cartilage and tendons is chondroitin sulfate. Chondroitin protects the bone joints by inhibiting enzymes that destroy cartilage. Keratan sulfate represents 5% to 20% of the GAG chains in articular cartilage. Hyaluronate, as a component of the synovial fluid acts as a lubricant for bone joints. High concentrations of HA are generally found during development and the early stages of wound healing and repair. The molecular mass (density) of hyaluronate declines with aging. As a function of development, age, and disease, GAGs exhibit changes in chain length, chain termination, substitution of sulfate ester and protein core.

Bio-ment can be considered as a biological 'cement' essential for construction, repair and maintenance of bone and joints.

Chondroitin

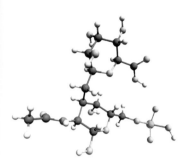

Chondroitin *(shown above)* **is a major bio-polymer of the bone cartilage.**

Chondroitin sulfate occurs naturally in the body and belongs to a class of very large molecules called glucosaminoglycans *(GAGs)*. It is a major component of cartilage, the tough, connective tissue that cushions the bone joints. Chondroitin sulfate may protect the joints by blocking enzymes that break down cartilage, and provide building blocks for the body to make new cartilage. It also helps to keep the cartilage healthy by absorbing fluid (particularly water) into the connective tissue.

Osteoarthritis *(OA)* is characterized by the breakdown and eventual loss of cartilage, either due to injury or to normal wear and tear that occurs with aging. OA is also associated with a local deficiency of chondroitin sulfate, hence its use as a supplement. Chondroitin supplements have been shown to decrease the pain of OA and may slow progression of the disease.

Chondroitin sulfate acts on a number of pathways in patients with OA. In addition to anti-inflammatory (pain reducing) activity, it stimulates the synthesis of proteoglycans and hyaluronic acid, and inhibits the synthesis of proteolytic enzymes, nitric oxide and other substances that could damage cartilage matrix. In some recent studies, chondroitin sulfate has reduced the activity of pro-inflammatory cytokines and shown positive effect on bone micro-structural changes in OA.

Chondroitin sulfate is used as an alternative medicine to treat OA and also approved and regulated as a symptomatic slow-acting drug for this disease *(SYSADOA)* in Europe. It is also a prescription or over-the-counter drug in 22 countries. However, chondroitin sulfate is regulated as a dietary supplement (ingredient) by the US-FDA.

Orally, chondroitin sulfate is used with a typical dose of 200-400 mg 2-3 times daily. It is frequently used in combination with various glucosamine salts and manganese ascorbate. The dosage of oral chondroitin used in human clinical trials is 800-1,200 mg per day. Clinical studies have not identified any significant side effects or overdoses of chondroitin sulfate, which supports its long-term safety.

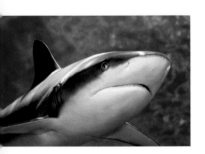

Since chondroitin is not a uniform chemical, it occurs naturally in a wide variety of forms. Most of the dietary chondroitin is obtained from extracts of cartilage tissue of cows (trachea), chicken (sternum), pigs (ear) and fish (shark bone).

Chondroitin protects the bone joints by blocking enzymes that break down the cartilage. It provides building blocks for the body to make new cartilage.

Glucosamine

Glucosamine is a normal constituent of cartilage matrix and synovial fluid. Made of sugar (glucose) and amino acid (glutamine), glucosamine is needed in the synthesis of glycosaminoglycan *(GAG)*. GAG is an essential biochemical in the formation and repair of cartilage. Glucosamine levels slowly decrease with age and also due to excess bone activity, therefore, supplementation with this amino-sugar may support cartilage repair in the joints and promote bone health.

Oral glucosamine is commonly used for the management of osteoarthritis *(OA)*, particularly of the knee. It is believed that the sulfate moiety provides functional benefit in the synovial fluid by strengthening cartilage and aiding GAG synthesis. Some of the benefits include pain relief, possibly due to an anti-inflammatory effect of glucosamine, and improved joint function. In people with osteoarthritis, glucosamine supplementation may reduce pain, may improve their physical function, without any serious side effects. Glucosamine is also extensively used in the veterinary applications as an unregulated but widely accepted supplement.

In the U.S., glucosamine is classified as a dietary supplement; therefore, its safety and efficacy are solely the responsibility of the manufacturer. However, glucosamine is approved as a medical drug in Europe and is sold in the form of glucosamine sulfate. Most studies have used glucosamine sulfate supplied by one European manufacturer (Rotta Research Laboratorium), and it is not known if glucosamine preparations made by other manufacturers are equally effective. More well-designed clinical trials are needed to confirm safety and effectiveness, and to test different formulations of glucosamine.

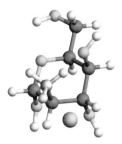

Glucosamine *(shown above)* is a basic building block of the skeletal system.

Glucosamine is commonly used in the form of sulfate and hydrochloride salts. A typical dosage of glucosamine salt is 1,500 mg per day. Glucosamine is often taken in combination with other supplements such as chondroitin sulfate and hyaluronic acid. OsteoArthritis Research Society International *(OARSI)* guidelines for hip and knee osteoarthritis also confirm its excellent safety profile.

Glucosamine reserves in the body decline with regular bone activity, therefore, its supplementation may support cartilage repair in the joints and promote bone health.

Glucosamine is usually derived from crustaceans (crab, lobster or shrimp shells), therefore, individuals allergic to shellfish may wish to avoid it. Glucosamine is also available from fermented grains (corn or wheat).

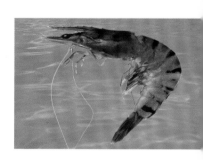

Hyaluronic Acid

Hyaluronic Acid (HLA) is the primary component of synovial fluid that lubricates bone joints. A well-lubricated joint has 100 times less friction than ice skates gliding on the ice. Chemically, HLA is a type of glycosaminoglycan (GAG) that attaches to collagen and elastin to form cartilage. The molecular weight (size) of HLA in cartilage decreases with age, but the amount increases.

HLA is present in every tissue of the body with a role in several important functions. It helps deliver nutrients to and carry toxins from cells that do not have a blood supply, such as those found in cartilage; without adequate amounts of HLA, the joints will become brittle and deteriorate. Not only does it keeps the joints lubricated, but HLA also facilitates water retention in the bone tissue.

HLA plays a positive role in the bone health; it slows down the progressive deterioration of joint function and mobility. Clinical studies have shown HLA to be an effective treatment for both rheumatoid and osteoarthritis, particularly in its injectible form (the only form that has been approved for medical use by the FDA). Injection of HLA into arthritic joints is called visco-supplementation. In a clinical study, over 80 percent of participants had significant relief of their painful arthritic symptoms immediately after treatment with HLA injections. For treating osteoarthritis, HLA dosage of 20 mg once per week for 3-5 weeks has been used.

Oral supplements of HLA are used for various joint disorders, including osteoarthritis (especially of the knee) and preventing the effects of aging. HLA has been touted as a 'fountain of youth', however, there is no evidence to support the claim that oral or topical use can prevent changes associated with aging.

> Hydrogels made from HLA are considered to be the state-of-the-art in bone tissue design. HLA polymers swell in water to form a gel-like material. They interact with growth factors much like the demineralized bone matrix and provide scaffolding for bone cells to proliferate and form new tissue. HLA is also used in bone allografts to repair and reconstruct bone defects.

Hyaluronate (shown above) is a primary polymer of the synovial fluid that lubricates bone joints.

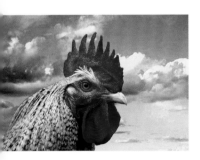

HLA is extracted from rooster comb (a naturally occurring source), purified and enzymatically split into smaller (low molecular weight) pieces for enhanced absorption. Non-animal source of HLA is also available through bacterial fermentation.

An average human body contains about 15-gms of HLA, one-third of which is turned over (degraded and synthesized) daily, to sustain the resilience of cartilage (its resistance to compression).

Anabolic agents directly stimulate bone formation (distinguished from anti-resorptive agents that act by blocking bone resorption) thus, allows the endogenous rate of bone formation to build bone since it is now unopposed by resorption. The difference between the lowered bone resorption rate and the continuing intrinsic bone formation results in an eventual gain in bone mass

Clinical testing of parathyroid hormone *(PTH)*: PTH is naturally an 84-amino-acid polypeptide. The complete PTH1-84 is approved in Europe, for osteoporosis treatment in postmenopausal women at high risk of fracture. In 2002, the US-FDA has approved *recombinant* PTH1-34 – the chemical name *teriparatide*. Teriparatide is an anabolic agent for use in postmenopausal women and men who are at high risk for osteoporotic fractures. Clinical trials indicate that teriparatide increases predominantly trabecular bone in the lumbar spine and femoral neck; it has less significant effects at cortical sites. However, after a maximum of two years of therapy, teriparatide should be discontinued and an anti-resorptive therapy should be initiated to maintain BMD. Teriparatide offers a therapeutic option for patients who are intolerant of or unresponsive to anti-resorptive therapy.

Teriparatide should not used with concurrent bisphosphonates and such combination therapy could attenuate the efficacy of teriparatide. Side effects with teriparatide include nausea, headache, dizziness, leg cramps, hypercalcemia (usually mild), and increased uric acid. *In vivo* experiments showed a development of *osteosarcoma* in about 50% of animals treated with high doses of intermittent PTH. Nevertheless, this drug should not be used in patients with a risk of bone cancer.

New Developments: The first human study of nitroglycerine for bone loss prevention, demonstrated an equivalent efficacy to estrogen. A randomized National Institute of Health *(NIH)*-funded clinical study is currently assessing the effectiveness of topically administered nitroglycerine in the prevention of postmenopausal bone loss. *Strontium ranelate* is a new agent for the treatment of osteoporosis, and an extension of the phase-III trials up to 5 years has shown sustained anti-fracture efficacy. The human monoclonal antibody to the *receptor activator of nuclear factor-kappaB ligand (RANKL)* is known to cause a rapid, high-magnitude, dose-dependent inhibition of bone resorption. A 12-month clinical trial with salmon *calcitonin* nasal spray (200 IU/day) showed a reduction in bone turnover serum markers, loss of further bone density and pain. Additionally, calcitonin promoted the repair of hip fractures and, as a coincidence finding, was associated with a significant reduction in the rate of refractures in postmenopausal elderly women, after total hip arthoplasty.

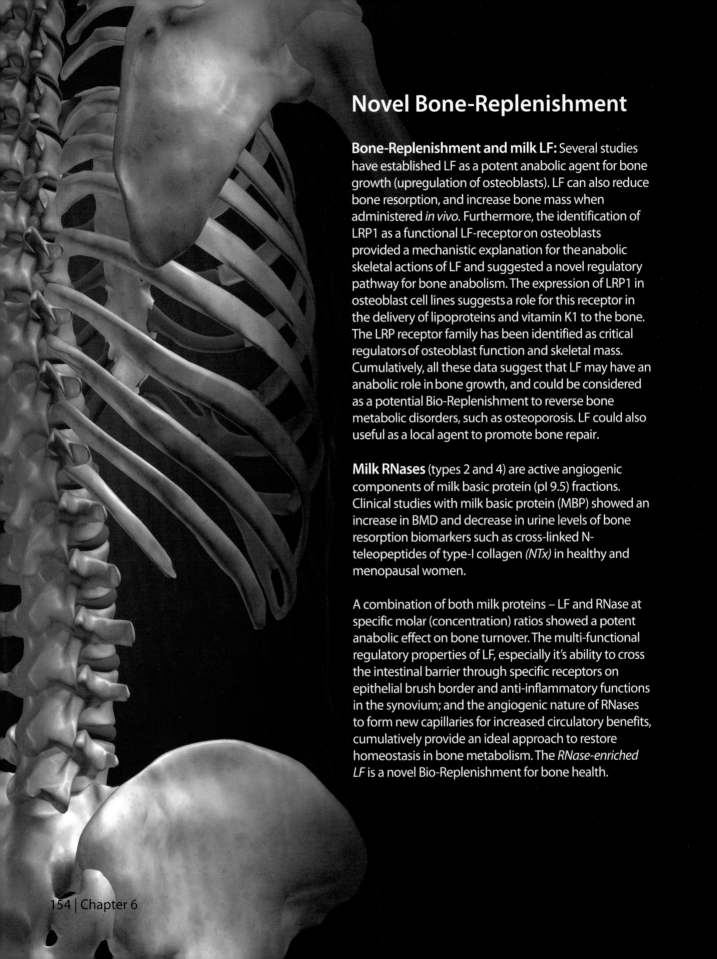

Novel Bone-Replenishment

Bone-Replenishment and milk LF: Several studies have established LF as a potent anabolic agent for bone growth (upregulation of osteoblasts). LF can also reduce bone resorption, and increase bone mass when administered *in vivo*. Furthermore, the identification of LRP1 as a functional LF-receptor on osteoblasts provided a mechanistic explanation for the anabolic skeletal actions of LF and suggested a novel regulatory pathway for bone anabolism. The expression of LRP1 in osteoblast cell lines suggests a role for this receptor in the delivery of lipoproteins and vitamin K1 to the bone. The LRP receptor family has been identified as critical regulators of osteoblast function and skeletal mass. Cumulatively, all these data suggest that LF may have an anabolic role in bone growth, and could be considered as a potential Bio-Replenishment to reverse bone metabolic disorders, such as osteoporosis. LF could also useful as a local agent to promote bone repair.

Milk RNases (types 2 and 4) are active angiogenic components of milk basic protein (pI 9.5) fractions. Clinical studies with milk basic protein (MBP) showed an increase in BMD and decrease in urine levels of bone resorption biomarkers such as cross-linked N-teleopeptides of type-I collagen *(NTx)* in healthy and menopausal women.

A combination of both milk proteins – LF and RNase at specific molar (concentration) ratios showed a potent anabolic effect on bone turnover. The multi-functional regulatory properties of LF, especially it's ability to cross the intestinal barrier through specific receptors on epithelial brush border and anti-inflammatory functions in the synovium; and the angiogenic nature of RNases to form new capillaries for increased circulatory benefits, cumulatively provide an ideal approach to restore homeostasis in bone metabolism. The *RNase-enriched LF* is a novel Bio-Replenishment for bone health.

Milk Ribonuclease-Enriched Lactoferrin *(R-ELF)*

Bio-replenishment with R-ELF demonstrated highly favorable effects on bone turnover. R-ELF replenishment significantly reduced bone resorption (osteoclast activity) while in tandem markedly increased bone formation (osteoblast activity), within six months of oral administration.

A clinical study was conducted with 38 healthy, ambulatory postmenopausal women (age range: 45-60, with no menses for at least 12 months). Of these, 15 women in the control group were given 100% RDA of calcium only and the other 20 women in the test group received R-ELF replenishment along with the calcium supplement, for six months. Bone resorption markers, N-telopeptides *(NTx)* in the serum and free deoxy-pyridinoline crosslinks *(DPD)* in urine; simultaneously, two bone formation markers in serum, bone-specific alkaline phosphatase *(BAP)* and osteocalcin *(OC)* were measured before (baseline) and at the end of 15, 30, 60, 90 and 180 days.

Median bone resorption markers for the placebo group showed an increase (NTx 40%, Dpd 18%) relative to baseline levels, reflecting significant bone resorption while the R-ELF replenishment group showed a relatively smaller rise (NTx 24%, Dpd -15%) during the same period. There was a significant elevation of bone formation markers (BAP 43%, OC 19%) with R-ELF replenishment compared to modest increase (BAP 26%, OC 3%) observed for the placebo group. The duration to achieve 80% of the peak change in bone turnover ranged 25-45 days for R-ELF compared to 45-115 days taken by the placebo group.

Osteoblasts are primarily responsible for turning osteoclast production and activity on and off. They do this via a system of signaling proteins and cytokines. R-ELF replenishment significantly reduced the pro-inflammatory cytokines associated with bone resorption and increased the cytokines that are necessary for osteoblast activity. This clinical study clearly demonstrated that R-ELF replenishment could restore the balance of bone turnover in post-menopausal women.

In view of limitations due to adverse side effects with current anti-resorptive treatments for postmenopausal bone loss, the results of R-ELF supplementation are very promising, since it is based on natural milk proteins which are generally regarded as safe. Stimulation of growth of collateral arteries and capillaries to facilitate supply of nutrients towards restoration of homeostasis in ischemic (inadequate blood supply) conditions, such as metabolic bone diseases is a new concept.

R-ELF could serve as an effective bio-replenishment to restore the balance of bone turnover and maintain homeostasis in bone metabolism.

Hormone Replacement Therapy *(HRT)* is a collective term to describe a variety of sex steroids, estrogens and progestogens, given to postmenopausal women at various doses and administered through different routes. The therapeutic significance of certain large, randomized controlled clinical trials on HRT has changed the risk/benefit perception. HRT appears to decrease coronary disease in younger women, near menopause; yet, in older women, HRT increases risk of a coronary event. Although HRT is a recognized method in the prevention and treatment of osteoporosis, it is not licensed for the prevention of osteoporosis as a first-line treatment. The effectiveness of low estrogen doses has been demonstrated for the treatment of vasomotor symptoms, genital atrophy and the prevention of bone loss, with fewer side-effects than the standard dose therapy.

A major unmet need is the availability of suitable treatments for the ever-increasing incidence of bone metabolic diseases.

The use of bio-identical hormones, including progesterone, estradiol, and estriol, in HRT has sparked intense debate. In 2002, when results of the Women's Health Initiative *(WHI)* randomized controlled trial of HRT showed an increased occurrence of breast cancer and *thromboembolism*; up to two-thirds of women taking HRT stopped the therapy, often without medical consultation. In June 2005, the World Health Organization *(WHO)* classified combined hormone contraception and menopausal therapy as carcinogenic in humans. However, experimental and clinical studies indicate that adverse effects of HRT may largely depend on the estrogen and progesterone -progestin formulation, dosage, mode of administration, patient's age, associated diseases, and duration of treatment.

Selective Estrogen Receptor Modulators *(SERMs)* are "designer" drugs that have many of the same beneficial effects as estrogen especially in stabilizing bone mass, improving lipid profile, reducing hot flashes, etc., however, without some of the risks associated with the HRT (cause breast cancer, stimulate the endometrium). *Tamoxifen*, the first SERM developed, has been used to prevent breast cancer for many years. *Raloxifene hydrochloride* is the first SERM approved by the US-FDA for the prevention and treatment of post-menopausal osteoporosis. Raloxifene has been shown to maintain bone density in the spine, hip and other bones, as well as reduce the incidence of fractures in the spine

The reported side effects with raloxifene include hot flashes or night sweats, leg cramps, muscle and joint aches, weight gain, vaginal dryness and rash. Rare but serious side effects include blood clots in the deep veins, called deep vein thrombosis *(DVT)*, a risk also associated with estrogen therapy. Raloxifene should therefore be used with caution by women who are at risk for blood clots.

> Teriparatide *(PTH1-34)* is the only approved bone anabolic agent available today, unfortunately has a limited use; it is relatively expensive and difficult to administer. Recent studies in bone metabolic regulation have led to the discovery of critical bio-replenishments that may usher in a new wave of innovative treatments for osteoporosis as well as orthopedic and dental indications.

6.1 | PERSPECTIVE

1. Ali M (2000) *Oxygen and Aging*, New York, Canary 21 Press, Aging Healthfully Books
2. Beck W (1971), *Human Design* (New York, NY: Harcourt, Brace, & Jovanovich).
3. Campos Pastor MM, Lopez-Ibarra PJ, Escobar-Jimenez F, et al (2000) Intensive insulin therapy and bone mineral density in type 1 diabetes mellitus: a prospective study. *Osteoporosis International* 11:455-459.
4. Frost HM (1992) The role of changes in mechanical usage set points in the pathogenesis of osteoporosis. *Journal of Bone Mineral Research* 7:253-261.
5. Goldsmith TC (2004) Aging as an evolved characteristic – Weismann's theory reconsidered. *Medical Hypotheses* 62:304-308.
6. Haden, ST, Brown, EM, Hurwitz, S, et al (2000) The effects of age and gender on parathyroid hormone dynamics. *Clinical Endocrinology (Oxford)* 52:329.
7. Ivers RQ, Cumming RG, Mitchell P, Peduto AJ (2001) Diabetes and the risk of fracture. *Diabetes Care* 24:1198-1203.
8. Krakauer JC, McKenna MJ, Buderer NF, et al (1995) Bone loss and bone turnover in diabetes. *Diabetes* 44:775-782.
9. Lu H, Kraut D, Gerstenfeld LC, Graves DT (2003) Diabetes interferes with the bone formation by affecting the expression of transcription factors that regulate osteoblast differentiation. *Endocrinology* 144:346-352.
10. Melton III LJ, Chrischilles EA, Cooper C, et al (1992) Perspective. How many women have osteoporosis? *Journal of Bone Mineral Research* 7:1005-1010.
11. Quarles LD (2008) Endocrine functions of bone in mineral metabolism regulation. *The Journal of Clinical Investigation* 118: 3820-3828.
12. Rapuri PB, Gallagher JC, Balhorn KE, Ryschon KL (2000) Smoking and bone metabolism in elderly women. *Bone* 27:429-436.
13. Speakman JR, Selman C, McLaren JS, Harper EJ (2002) Living fast, dying when? The link between aging and energetics. *The Journal of Nutrition* 132 (6): 1583S–1597S.

6.2 | REGULATION

1. Findlay DM, Sexton PM (2005). Calcitonin. *Growth Factors* 22:217-224.
2. Frost HM (1992) The role of changes in mechanical usage set points in the pathogenesis of osteoporosis. *Journal of Bone Mineral Research* 7:253-261.
3. Lindsay R, Aitken JM, Anderson JB, et al (1976) Long-term prevention of postmenopausal osteoporosis by oestrogen: evidence for an increased bone mass after delayed onset of oestrogen treatment. *Lancet* 1:1038–1041
4. Lindsay R, Nieves J, Formica C, et al (1997) Randomized controlled study of effect of parathyroid hormone on vertebral-bone mass and fracture incidence among postmenopausal women on estrogen with osteoporosis. *Lancet* 350:550-555.
5. Mundy GR, Guise TA (1999) Hormonal control of calcium homeostasis. *Clinical Chemistry* 45:1347-1352.
6. Neer RM, Arnaud CD, Zanchetta JR, et al (2001) Effect of parathyroid hormone (1-34) on fractures and bone mineral density in postmenopausal women with osteoporosis. *New England Journal of Medicine* 344:1434-1441.
7. Poole K, Reeve J (2005). Parathyroid hormone - a bone anabolic and catabolic agent. *Current Opinion in Pharmacology* 5:612-617.

8.   Riggs BL, Khosla S, Melton LJ (2002) Sex steroids and the construction and conservation of the adult skeleton. *Endocrine Reviews* 23:279-302.

9.   Stumpf WE, Sar M, Reid FA, et al (1979) Target cells for 1,25 dihydroxy vitamin D3 in intestinal tract, stomach, kidney, skin, pituitary and parathyroid. *Science* 206:1188-1190.

10. Thomas K (1996) Vascular endothelial growth factor, a potent and selective angiogenic agent. *Journal of Biological Chemistry* 271:603-606.

11. Vanderschueren D, Vandenput L, Boonen S, et al (2004) Androgens and bone. *Endocrine Reviews* 25:389-425.

6.3 | TRANSPORT

1.   Baveye S, Elass E, Mazurier J, et al (1999) Lactoferrin: a multifunctional glycoprotein involved in the modulation of the inflammatory process. *Clinical Chemistry Laboratory Medicine* 37:281-286.

2.   Cornish J (2004) Lactoferrin promotes bone growth. *Biometals*17:331–335.

3.   Cornish J, Callon KE, Naot D, et al (2004) Lactoferrin is a potent regulator of bone cell activity and increases bone formation in vivo *Endocrinology* 145:4366–4374.

4.   Di Mario F, Aragona G, Dal BN, et al (2003) Use of bovine lactoferrin for *Helicobacter pylori* eradication. *Digestive and Liver Disease* 35:706-710.

5.   Erdei J, Forsgren A, Naidu AS (1994) Lactoferrin binds to porins OmpF and OmpC in *Escherichia coli. Infection and Immunity* 62:1236-40.

6.   Grey A, Banovic T, Zhu Q, et al (2004) The low-density lipoprotein receptor-related protein 1 is a mitogenic receptor for lactoferrin in osteoblastic cells. *Molecular Endocrinology* 18:2268–2278.

7.   Hangoc G, Falkenburg JH, Broxmeyer HE (1991) Influence of T-lymphocytes and lactoferrin on the survival- promoting effects of IL-1 and IL-6 on human bone marrow granulocyte-macrophage and erythroid progenitor cells. *Experimental Hematology* 19:697-703.

8.   Kawakami H, Lonnerdal B (1991) Isolation and function of a receptor for human lactoferrin in human fetal intestinal brush-border membranes. *American Journal of Physiology* 261:841-846.

9.   Lonnerdal B, Iyer S (1995), Lactoferrin: molecular structure and biological function. *Annual Review of Nutrition*15:93-110.

10. Lorget F, Clough J, Oliveira M, et al (2002) Lactoferrin reduces in vitro osteoclast differentiation and resorbing activity. *Biochemical Biophysical Research Communications* 296:261–266.

11. Naidu AS (2000) *Lactoferrin: Natural Multifunctional Antimicrobial.* Boca Raton: CRC Press. ISBN 0-8493-0909-3

12. Naidu AS (2000) *Natural Food Antimicrobial Systems.* Boca Raton: CRC Press. ISBN 0-8493-2047-X

13. Naidu AS (2005) Ultra-cleansing of lactoferrin: Nutraceutical implications. *Agro Food Industry hi-tech* 16(2):7-13.

14. Naidu AS, Arnold RR (1994) Lactoferrin interaction with salmonellae potentiates antibiotic susceptibility in vitro. *Diagnostic Microbiology and Infectious Diseases* 20:69-75.

15. Naidu AS, Bidlack WR (1998) Milk lactoferrin - Natural microbial blocking agent for food safety. *Environment and Nutritional Interactions* 2:35-50.

16. Naidu AS, Bidlack WR, Clemens RA (1999) Probiotic spectra of lactic acid bacteria (LAB). *Critical Reviews in Food Science and Nutrition* 39:13-126.

17. Naidu AS, Chen J, Martinez C, et al (2004) Activated lactoferrin inhibits proliferation of *Candida albicans* and *Candida glabrata* clinical isolates *in vitro* and prevents attachment of yeast cells to vaginal epithelial monolayer. *Journal of Reproductive Medicine* 49:859-866.

18. Naidu SS, Erdei J, Czirok E *et al* (1991) Specific binding of lactoferrin to *Escherichia coli* isolated from human intestinal infections. *APMIS* 99:1142-50.

19. Petschow BW, Talbott RD, Batema RP (1999) Ability of lactoferrin to promote the growth of *Bifidobacterium* spp. in vitro is independent of receptor binding capacity and iron saturation level. *Journal of Medical Microbiology* 48:541-549.
20. Rosen, C.J. and Bilezikian, J.P. (2001), Clinical review 123: Anabolic therapy for osteoporosis. *Journal of Clinical Endocrinology and Metabolism* 86:957-964.
21. Sawatzki G, Rich IN (1989) Lactoferrin stimulates colony stimulating factor production in vitro and in vivo. *Blood Cells*15:371–385.
22. Yamauchi K, Wakabayashi H, Hashimoto S, et al (1998) Effects of orally administered bovine lactoferrin on the immune system of healthy volunteers. *Advances in Experimental Medicine and Biology* 443:261-265.

6.4 | BIO-MENTS

1. Altman RD, Moskowitz R (1998) Intra-articular sodium hyaluronate (Hyalgan) in the treatment of patients with osteoarthritis of the knee. A randomized clinical trial. Hyalgan Study Group. *Journal of Rheumatology* 25:2203-2212.
2. Clegg DO, Reda DJ, Harris CL, *et al* (2006) Glucosamine, chondroitin sulfate, and the two in combination for painful knee osteoarthritis. *New England Journal of Medicine* 354:795-808.
3. Herrero-Beaumont G, Ivorra JA, Del Carmen TM, *et al* (2007) Glucosamine sulfate in the treatment of knee osteoarthritis symptoms: a randomized, double-blind, placebo-controlled study using acetaminophen as a side comparator. *Arthritis Rheum* 56(2):555-567.
4. Leeb BF, Schweitzer H, Montag K, *et al* (2000) A meta-analysis of chondroitin sulfate in treatment of osteoarthritis. *Journal of Rheumatology* 27:205-211.
5. Mazieres B, Combe B, Phan Van A, et al (2001) Chondroitin sulfate in osteoarthritis of the knee: a prospective, double blind, placebo controlled multicenter clinical study. *Journal of Rheumatology* 28(1):173-181.
6. McCarty MF (2005) Supplemental arginine and high-dose folate may promote bone health by supporting the activity of endothelial-type nitric oxide synthase in bone. *Medical Hypotheses* 64:1030-1033.
7. Nakamura H, Masuko K, Yudoh K, *et al* (2007) Effects of glucosamine administration on patients with rheumatoid arthritis. *Rheumatology International* 27(3):213-218.
8. Petrella RJ, DiSilvestro MD, Hildebrand C (2002) Effects of hyaluronate sodium on pain and physical functioning in osteoarthritis of the knee. A randomized, double-blind, placebo-controlled clinical trial. *Archives of Internal Medicine* 162:292-298.
9. Pickart L (2008) The human tri-peptide GHK and tissue remodeling. *Journal of Biomaterials Science Polymer Edition* 19:969-988.

6.5 | CLINICAL STUDIES

1. Bharadwaj S, Naidu AG, Betageri GV, Prasadarao NV, Naidu AS (2009) Milk ribonuclease-enriched lactoferrin induces positive effects on bone turnover markers in postmenopausal women. *Osteoporosis International* Jan 27. [Epub ahead of print].
2. Cosman F, Nieves J, Zion M, et al (2005) Daily/cyclic parathyroid hormone in women receiving alendronate. *New England Journal of Medicine* 353:566-575.
3. Eastell R, Nickelsen T, Marin F, et al (2009) Sequential treatment of severe postmenopausal osteoporosis after teriparatide: final results of the randomized controlled European Study of Forsteo (EUROFORS). *Journal of Bone Mineral Research* 24:726-736.
4. Finkelstein JS, Wyland JJ, Leder BZ, et al (2009) Effects of teriparatide retreatment in osteoporotic men and women. *Journal of Clinical Endocrinology and Metabolism* 94:2495-2501.
5. Olevsky OM, Martino S (2008) Randomized clinical trials of raloxifene: reducing the risk of osteoporosis and breast cancer in postmenopausal women. *Menopause* 15:790-796.

6. Rosen CJ, Bilezikian JP (2001) Anabolic therapy for osteoporosis. *Journal of Clinical Endocrinology and Metabolism* 86:957-964.

7. Rubin MR, Dosman F, Lindsay R, Bilezikian JP (2002) The anabolic effects of parathyroid hormone. *Osteoporosis International* 13:267-277.

8. Stepan JJ, Lachman M, Zverina J, Pacovsky V (1989) Castrated men exhibit bone loss: effect of calcitonin treatment on biochemical indices of bone remodeling. *Journal of Clinical Endocrinology and Metabolism* 69:523–527.

9. Stroup J, Kane MP, Abu-Baker AM (2008) Teriparatide in the treatment of osteoporosis. *American Journal of Health System Pharmacy* 65:532-539.

10. Wimalawansa SJ (2007) Rationale for using nitric oxide donor therapy for prevention of bone loss and treatment of osteoporosis in humans. *Annals of New York Academy of Sciences* 1117:283-297.

11. Yamamura J, Aoe S, Toba Y, et al. (2002) Milk basic protein (MBP) increases radial bone mineral density in healthy adult women. *Bioscience Biotechnology Biochemistry* 66:702-7049.

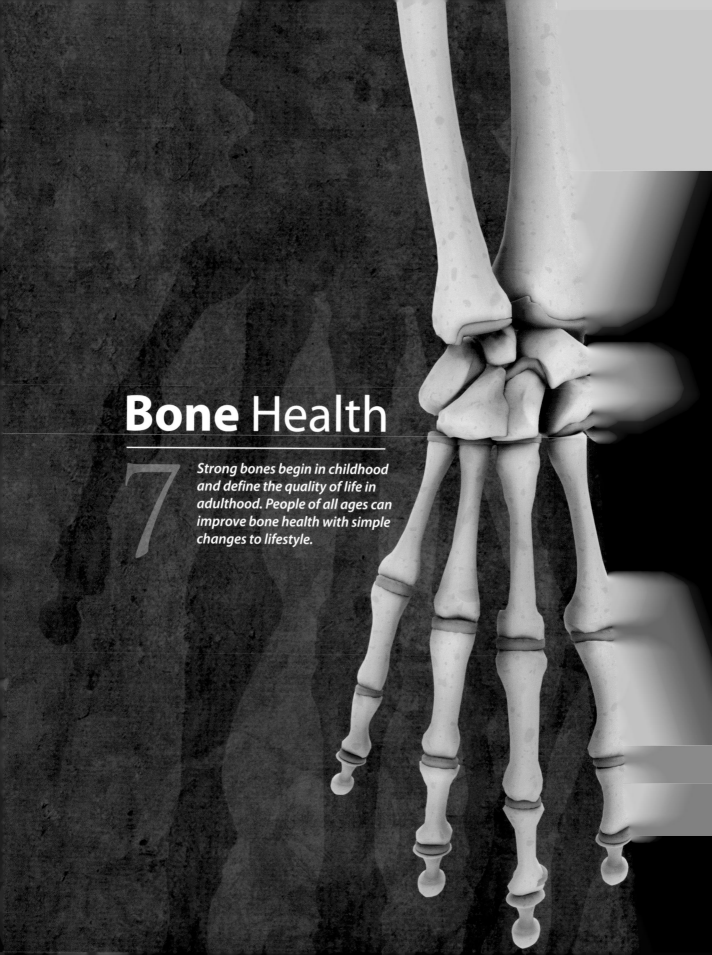

Bone Health

7

Strong bones begin in childhood and define the quality of life in adulthood. People of all ages can improve bone health with simple changes to lifestyle.

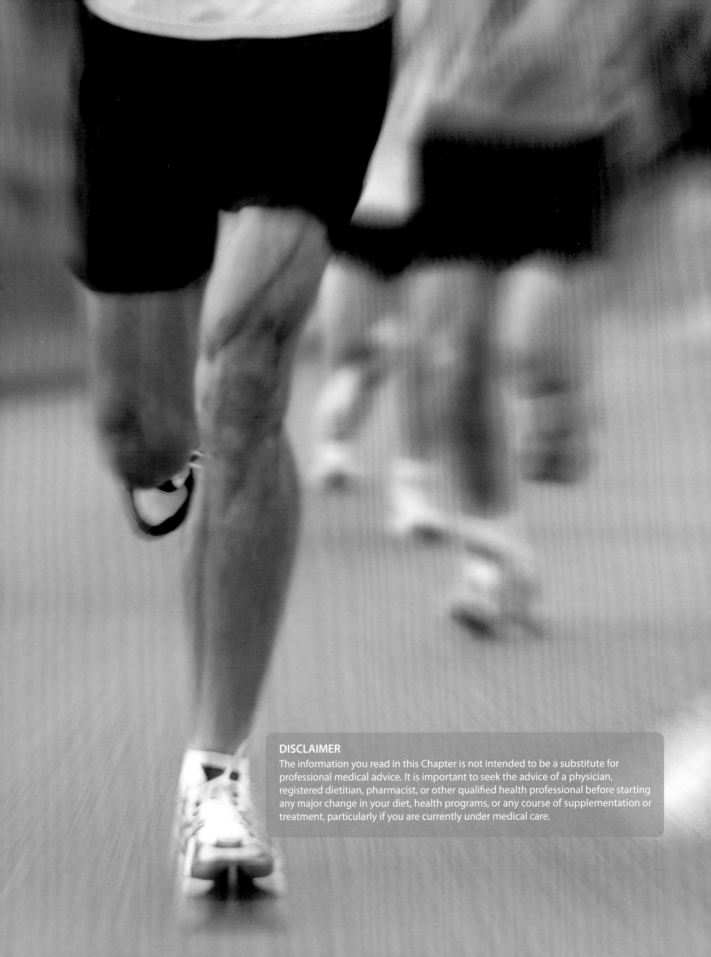

7

7.1 | Bone Health **Management**

Bone Health is achieved during childhood and adolescence, the skeletal forming years; and is established during young adulthood. **Management** and functional up keeping of bone health is dependent on several factors including, nutrition (e.g. minerals, vitamins, and supplements), lifestyle (e.g. physical activity and addiction), environment and the aging process.

Bioavailability and function of bone health nutrients are closely inter-related; the presence or absence of one may influence the uptake of another. For example, a proper ratio of calcium to phosphorus promotes bone mineralization; however, when the ratio is disturbed, it leads to a detrimental bone loss. Dietary habits have a direct role in the overall outcome of bone health. Malnutrition (low calcium, vitamin-D and trace mineral intake) and diabetes, can influence bone health.

Lifestyle, especially addictive habits, such as tobacco consumption, smoking, alcohol, drug abuse, extreme dieting and certain medications can adversely affect bone health. Bones work on the *'use it or lose it'* principle. Therefore, physical activity, especially, the weight-bearing exercises influence the strength and agility of the skeletal system. Indoor living (with little or no exposure to sunlight) and sedentary lifestyle can trigger a rapid bone loss and predispose several disease conditions.

Aging is a regular biological phenomenon. Environmental factors (i.e. polluted air, water and land) and stress can take a cumulative toll on the body and cause rapid aging. Skeletal system is the primary target of an aging process. Sports, occupational and accidental injuries only worsen the aging bone. This *Chapter* will elaborate the most common factors that influence bone function and possible ways to manage bone health.

7.2 | Bone Health **Nutrition**

Nutrition is a critical factor in the management of bone health. Among bone nutrients most attention has focused on the beneficial role of calcium and calcium-rich foods (e.g., dairy products); however, several macro-nutrients (eg. proteins, carbohydrates, fats) and vegetables are necessary for bone health.

Protein: High protein intakes have been associated with reduced bone loss, high BMD, and reduced fracture risk in elderly population. However, excess dietary protein; particularly purified proteins can increase urinary calcium excretion *(calciuric effect)*. This mineral loss could potentially cause negative calcium balance, leading to bone loss and osteoporosis. These effects have been attributed to an increased endogenous acid load created by protein metabolism, which requires neutralization by alkaline calcium salts from the bone. *However, this theory is controversial*. In a 3-year prospective study of more than 30,000 post-menopausal women; it was found that higher protein intake, particularly animal protein, showed a 70% reduction in hip fractures. Protein and calcium act synergistically on bone if both are present in adequate quantities in the diet, but protein can become antagonistic towards the bone *(calciuric effect)* when calcium intake is low.

Protein is part of bone collagen, critical for the skeletal matrix and function; recent studies have shown the role of dietary protein and bone health.

Thus, reasonable amounts of calcium and protein help maintain the skeleton. Dietary calcium to protein ratio equal to or greater than 20:1 (mg/g) can provide adequate protection for the skeleton. Milk is a unique source of protein because its calcium content is high in relation to its protein content. The calcium to protein ratio of cow's milk is approximately 36:1. Thus, the nutrient package of milk has beneficial effects on bone health.

Fats are important for optimum function of hormones; and transport of fat-soluble vitamins A, E, K and D, that are crucial for calcium absorption. Saturated fats also promote calcium homeostasis. Studies have shown that diets rich in the omega-3 fatty acids from fish such as *docosahexaenoic acid (DHA)* and *eicosapentaenoic acid (EPA)* can reduce bone loss.

Vegetables: Fresh vegetables, fruit, nuts, seeds and whole grains need to be included in the bone health diet. Dark-green leafy vegetables such as spinach, broccoli, kale, chard, turnip greens and romaine lettuce are excellent sources for bone health nutrients. Fruit and vegetables help to maintain a healthy alkaline pH balance in body fluids; otherwise, calcium is released from the bones to counter the acidity, which results in gradual bone loss. For optimal bone health, the diet should contain about 70-80% of fruit and vegetables.

The **Food Pyramid** is a guide to help individuals make healthy food choices each day. Start with plenty of whole grains (bread, cereals and rice), vegetables and fruit. Add 3 or more servings from the dairy foods and non-dairy alternatives group. Then choose 2 - 3 moderate portions from the protein group. Fats and oils should be used sparingly. It is important to know that there are many calcium-rich foods available in each food group. The actual calcium content of a food may vary depending upon the brand. It is always important to read the nutrition facts on each food label when selecting a product.

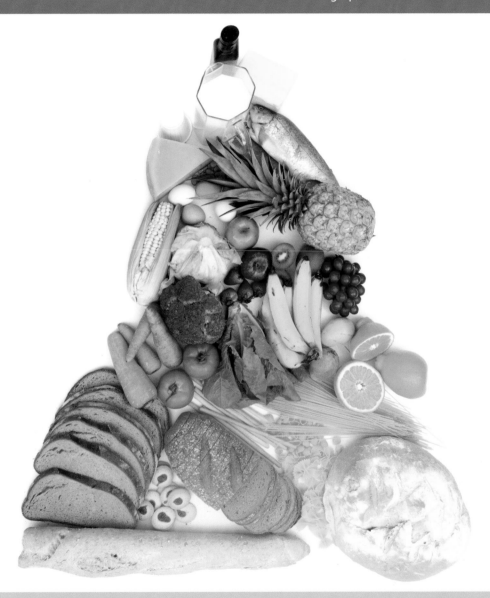

Calcium is a key ingredient for bone health. The best source of calcium is dairy foods. Milk, cheese and yogurt are rich in calcium. And not only are dairy foods naturally rich in calcium, the calcium is more easily absorbed into the body. Three serves of dairy foods a day are recommended for good bone health.

Milk

Milk is the fundamental diet a newborn mammalian receives from the mother. This is the only *Complete Nutrition* designed by *Mother Nature*; enriched with essential macro- and micro-nutrients to support mammalian growth and development. Other milk nutrients include sugars, enzymes, globulins, growth factors, lipids and bioactive peptides. Recent studies have shown that the milk protein, lactoferrin; and milk enzyme, ribonuclease; can affect bone turnover.

Dairy foods have been part of the adult diet (after the age of weaning); only since the domestication of dairy animals. With an average Western diet, individuals consume about half a pint of milk per day. Milk and dairy products provide approximately 19% of the daily intake of protein and approximately 8.5% of the total amount of fat.

Milk Calcium: Milk and milk products provide a unique mix of minerals - calcium, phosphorus and potassium - that all contribute to maximize bone density and slow down the age-related bone loss. Dairy foods represent a distinct group, due to the relatively high calcium content; they provide over 50% of the total calcium in the diet. Calcium in nondairy sources is less concentrated, which makes it difficult to meet the recommended dietary allowance *(RDA)* without concomitant consumption of dairy foods or supplements. The calcium in dairy products, including the processed low-fat and fat-free milk, is easy for the body to absorb and in a form that gives the body easy access to the calcium. Calcium bioavailability can be enhanced even more with fortification of the dairy products with vitamin-D. Certain individuals may get an upset stomach with dairy products due to *milk allergy or lactose intolerance*. However, such conditions are less common in young children.

Clinical Studies: Milk is an important nutrition for optimum bone health in both younger and older population. A number of studies have shown a link between low milk consumption during the childhood and adolescence; resulting in low bone mineral density *(BMD)*. In a recent study of 649 Chinese adolescent girls aged 12-14 years, milk intake was found to be positively associated with *distal radius* and *ulna bone mass*, with milk accounting for 3.2% of the variation in BMD. Milk-supplementation studies have demonstrated a positive relationship with bone health, prevention of osteoporosis, in particular, among pre- and postmenopausal women. In a recent clinical study, a total of 200 Chinese women aged 55-59 years were randomly assigned to receive 50 g of milk powder (containing 800 mg of calcium) per day. The results showed that the milk-supplementation group had a significantly reduced height loss as well as reduced BMD loss compared to control group. Bone health in children who habitually avoid milk tend to be short and overweight, with higher rate of bone fractures at a young age due to poor calcium intake than milk-drinkers.

Soybean (*Glycine max*) contains all three *macro-nutrients*, protein, carbohydrates and fat; and several *micro-nutrients*, including vitamins and minerals. Soy is rich in vitamin-D, folate, vitamin-A, riboflavin, vitamin-B12, calcium, potassium, iron and high-quality protein that have a significant role in bone nutrition. In addition, soybean and other beans contain *genistein*, a plant *estrogen (phytoestrogen)* that acts like the female sex hormone in the body. Accordingly, soy beans, soy milk, meat substitutes made with soy, tofu, and products made with soy flour can also provide good source of nutrients for bone health.

Soy Calcium: Soy provides an excellent source of calcium (300 mg per 8-oz serving), and its bioavailability is equivalent to that of milk. Approximately 30 to 40% of the calcium from various soy products such as soy milk, tofu and soybeans is absorbed. Soy is also rich in high quality protein, which unlike the meat proteins, causes less calcium loss in the urine. Recent studies show soy consumption can improve both bone density the overall quality of the bone.

Soy Isoflavones: Over the past decade, growing evidence suggests that a component of soy foods, called *isoflavones*, may benefit bone health. Soy isoflavones can act like a weak *estrogen* in the body and control the activities of bone-dissolving *(osteoclast)* and bone-building *(osteoblast)* cells. As a result, bone loss slows and BMD improves. The isoflavones found in soy are *genistein, daidzen* and *glycitein,* which exhibit the same effects as the potent anti estrogen *tamoxifen,* in protecting bones against osteoporosis. A single cup (8-oz) of soy milk may contain 20 to 40 milligrams of isoflavone. Therefore, soy milk can be particularly valuable for post-menopausal women when natural estrogen production tapers off. Studies show that post-menopausal women who consume higher amounts of soy have less bone loss and fewer bone fractures.

Clinical Studies: Some, but not all, clinical trials have shown significant protective effects on bone in post-menopausal women, who are supplemented with soy isoflavones and/or soy protein. Soy isoflavones demonstrated protective effect on bone in animals with surgical removal of *ovaries* (female reproductive organs that produce *estrogen* and *progesterone*). In humans, however, the results are conflicting. Recent human studies found that isoflavone-rich soy intake may prevent bone loss from the lumbar spine in post-menopausal women, who may otherwise are expected to lose 2 to 3% yearly.

> *Clinical data suggest that 60–90 mg/d of isoflavones may be effective. This translates into about 2–3 servings of traditional soyfoods. Several soyfood products are also enriched with calcium to provide an additional benefit for bone health.*

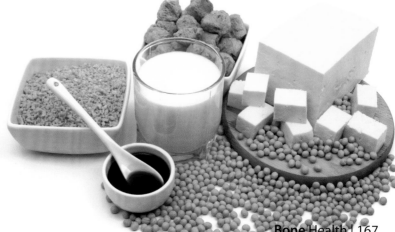

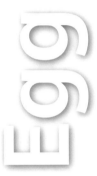

Eggs are an excellent source of nutrition for bone health. With significant protein, vitamin, mineral content and relatively low saturated fat content, egg is a valuable healthy diet. A medium egg has an energy value of 78 kilocalories *(kCal)* and consumption of one egg daily would contribute about 3% of the average energy requirement of an adult man; 4% for an adult woman. On a nutrient evaluation scale, most commonly used for assessing protein, egg has the highest score, 100, and is used as the reference standard against other foods.

Both egg white and yolk provide protein, plus assorted amounts of all needed vitamins, (except vitamin-C), and an array of important minerals. Altogether, these nutrients maintain the bones, repair tissues and ensure that body processes function properly. For 140 calories, a serving of two eggs provides all the following nutrients: protein (20%), vitamin-A (12%), vitamin-B12 (16%), vitamin-B6 (8%), vitamin-D (12%), vitamin-E (6%), folate (12%), thiamine (4%), phosphorus (16%), riboflavin (30%), zinc (8%), and iron (8%).

Egg Minerals: Eggs contain many essential minerals, in particular phosphorus, essential for healthy teeth and bones; iron, which is essential for red blood cell formation; and zinc, important for wound healing, growth and fighting infection.
Trace elements are also present in eggs, especially iodine, required to make thyroid hormones, and selenium, important for antioxidant activity. Antioxidants work by preventing the damage caused by uncontrolled free radicals in the body and are believed to help protect against diseases such as *arthritis*.

Egg Vitamins: Eggs contain most of the essential vitamins with the exception of vitamin-C. Egg is one of the very few foods for good source of natural vitamin-D. Egg yolk contains significant amounts of vitamin-D, necessary for absorption of calcium and phosphorus and critical for bone metabolism. They also contain vitamin-A, essential for normal growth and development; vitamin-E that is important for protecting cells from free radical damage. Eggs are also rich in B vitamins that perform many vital functions in the body; especially, riboflavin *(B2)*, important for release of energy in the body; finally, cobalamin *(B12)* is needed for normal blood formation.

It has been found that ½ a cup of egg substitute provides up to 130 mg of calcium. Some studies have shown that calcium obtained from eggshell is beneficial for bone health. It probably reduces acidity in the stomach and also helps in digestion. Even calcium supplements are made using crushed eggshell to help overcome calcium deficiency. However, calcium carbonate obtained from eggshell is insoluble and requires vitamin-D and other nutrients to facilitate bioavailability.

7.3 | Bone Health **Vitamins**

Vitamin is an organic substance that a human body can not synthesize in sufficient quantities, therefore, must be obtained through diet. The term *vitamin* excludes other essential nutrients such as dietary minerals, fatty acids, or amino acids, also it does not encompass other micro-nutrients that promote health.

Human body needs at least 13 different vitamins (A, D, E, K, C and 8 different B vitamins). The body can produce 4 of these vitamins; biotin, pantothenic acid, and vitamin-K are made in the human intestine. Sunlight exposure on the skin can trigger vitamin-D synthesis. Remaining vitamins need to be obtained through diet. Vitamins are classified as either water-soluble or fat-soluble based on dissolution and absorption properties.

Water-soluble vitamins include the B-complex group and vitamin-C. These vitamins easily dissolve in body fluids, readily enter the blood stream and rapidly used by the body. Water-soluble vitamins that are not used (excess) are eliminated by urinary excretion. Vitamin-B12 is the only water-soluble vitamin that can be stored in the liver for many years. Since, most of these vitamins are not stored, deficiency can easily occur.

The body is able to store some vitamins, such as vitamin A (up to a year's supply is stored in the liver). The body needs other vitamins on a regular basis.

Fat-soluble vitamins include types A, D, E and K that are absorbed through the intestinal tract with the help of lipids (fats). Individuals with digestive disorders and pancreatic insufficiency (e.g. cystic fibrosis) who can not digest or store fats properly, need a continuous supply of fat-soluble vitamins. Since these vitamins are stored (or accumulated) in the body for a few days to up to months, they are more likely to cause *hypervitaminosis*.

Vitamin Deficiency occurs when the body doesn't get a particular vitamin for an extended period of time. Such deficiency may induce diseases including beriberi, pellagra, rickets and scurvy. Before the onset of a vitamin deficiency disease, signs of a subclinical deficiency include fatigue, irritability, nervousness, depression, allergies, insomnia, frequent minor colds or illnesses. During pregnancy, any lack of essential vitamins can cause birth defects.

Vitamin Toxicity: Conversely, too much of some vitamins can create a toxic condition known as *'hyper-vitaminosis'*, with symptoms like nausea and vomiting. In some cases, ingesting too much of certain vitamin supplements can lead to death.

There is also strong evidence that diets low in antioxidants – particularly vitamins A, C and E may predispose some individuals to joint problems. Some studies claim that following a vegetarian diet and losing any extra body weight can relieve several of the symptoms of arthritis.

Function: Vitamins perform a wide range of biochemical functions, including acting as hormones (e.g. vitamin-D), antioxidants (e.g. vitamin-E), and regulators of cell and tissue growth (e.g. vitamin-A). Finally, the B-complex, the largest group of vitamins, acts as catalyst and substrate in metabolism. Certain basic functions of all 13 essential vitamins are listed in the following TABLE:

Vitamin	Function
A	Helps in the formation and maintenance of healthy teeth, bones, soft tissue, mucous membranes, and skin.
B1 (Thiamine)	Helps convert carbohydrates into energy. It is also essential for heart function and healthy nerve cells.
B2 (Riboflavin)	Helps form red blood cells and promotes healthy skin and normal vision.
B3 (Niacin)	Helps lower cholesterol; maintains healthy skin and digestive system.
B6 (Pryidoxin)	Helps protein metabolism, forms red blood cells, antibodies, insulin and maintains brain function.
B12 (Cobalamin)	Important for metabolism, functioning of nervous system and is required for DNA synthesis.
Pantothenic acid	Helps stabilize blood sugar levels, defends against infection, produces hormones and cholesterol.
Folate	Necessary for the production of DNA. Plays a role in bone tissue growth, cell division and forming red blood cells.
Biotin	Essential for protein and carbohydrate metabolism; plays a role in the production of hormones, cholesterol and helps prevent fat deposits.
C (Ascorbate)	As an antioxidant promotes healthy bones, teeth, muscle and gums. Helps wound healing, resists infection and plays a role in hormone production and iron absorption
D (Calciferol)	Promotes calcium absorption for healthy teeth and bones. Helps regulate blood levels of calcium and phosphorus.
E (Tocopherol)	As an antioxidant plays a role in lipid metabolism, formation of blood cells and cardiovascular health.
K (Menadione)	Important for blood coagulation. Helps promote strong bones and prevents fractures in the elderly.

To get the best of vitamins from the diet, refrigerate fresh produce and keep milk and grains away from strong light. Vitamins are easily destroyed and washed out during food preparation and storage. Vitamin supplements should be stored at room temperature in a dry place free of moisture.

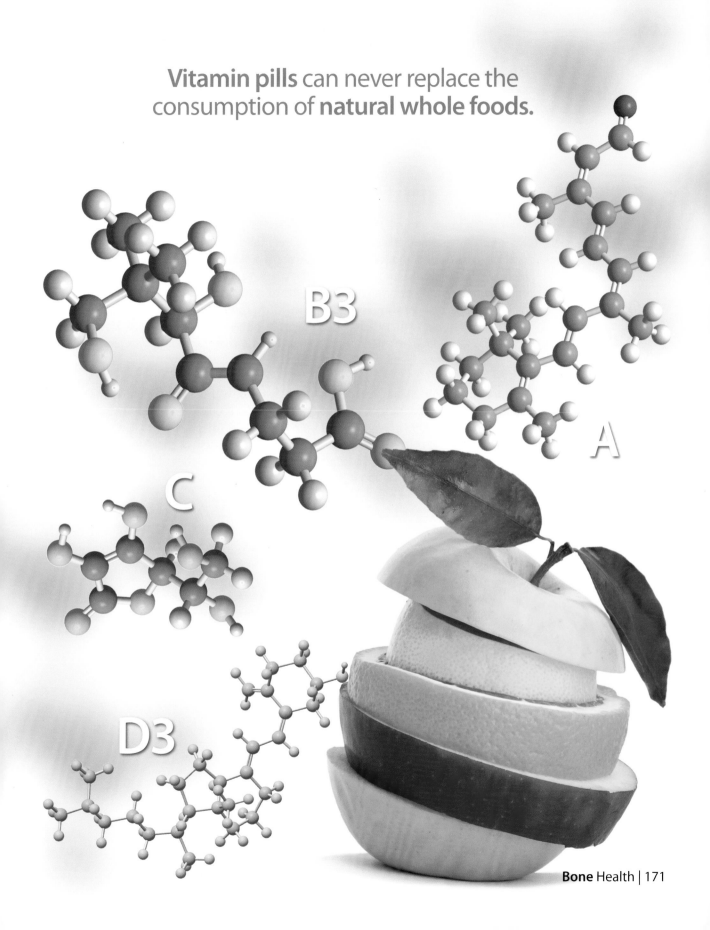

Vitamin pills can never replace the consumption of **natural whole foods.**

B3

A

C

D3

Vitamin-D

Vitamin-D: Early 20th century scientists discovered that *rickets*, a childhood bone disease could be prevented by a compound isolated from cod liver oil referred to as *'fat-soluble factor D'*, now known as vitamin-D. This vitamin is also called *'calciferol,'* since it can boost calcium deposits in the bone. There are two basic types of vitamin-D, one derived from *ergosterol* (plant-based), and the other from *cholesterol* (animal-based). When UV light from the sun hits the leaf of a plant, ergosterol converts to *ergocalciferol* (or vitamin-D2); similarly, exposure of skin to UV light transforms cholesterol to *cholecalciferol*, a form of vitamin-D3.

Vitamin-D is found naturally in very few foods. Foods containing vitamin-D include some fatty fish (salmon, mackerel, sardines), and fish liver oils. Vitamin-D is also found in beef liver, cheese and egg yolk. Some mushrooms provide D2 (ergocalciferol) in variable amounts. Fortified foods provide most of the vitamin-D in the diet. In the US, milk and infant formula are fortified with vitamin-D (400 IU or10 *mcg* per quart). In the 1930s, a milk fortification program implemented in the US to combat rickets, then a major public health problem, has virtually eliminated that bone disease. Ready-to-eat breakfast cereals, breads, yogurt, margarine and orange juices also contain added vitamin-D. Maximum levels of added vitamin-D are specified by the law.

Dietary Source: Most vitamin-D supplements available without prescription contain D3-form, which is more potent than the D2. Vitamin-D2 is produced by the UV irradiation of ergosterol in yeast; and vitamin-D3 is synthesized by the irradiation of 7-dehydrocholesterol from lanolin and the chemical conversion of cholesterol. The two forms have traditionally been regarded as equivalent based on their ability to cure rickets; however, D3-form is about 3 times more effective than D2.

Adverse Effects: Vitamin-D toxicity *(hypervitaminosis D)* can cause nonspecific symptoms such as nausea, vomiting, poor appetite, constipation, weakness, and weight loss. More seriously, it can raise blood levels of calcium *(hypercalcemia)* and calcify organs like heart and kidneys if untreated over a long period of time.

Drug Interactions: Vitamin-D supplements may interact with several types of drugs. *Corticosteroids*, often prescribed to reduce inflammation, can impair vitamin-D metabolism. Both the weight-loss and cholesterol-lowering drugs can reduce vitamin-D absorption. Heparin, an anticoagulant, may also interfere with vitamin-D activation. Individuals taking such medications on a regular basis should discuss vitamin-D intakes with their healthcare providers.

TABLE: *The RDA values for vitamin-D intake in the U.S.*

Infancy - 50 years	200 IU / day
Adults (51-70 years)	400 IU / day
Adults (above 70 years)	600 IU / day

TABLE: *Foods Rich in Vitamin-D Content*

Food	Serving Size (Average)	Vitamin-D (mcg)	Vitamin-D (IU)
Herring	85 g (3 oz)	34.6	1383
Pure Cod liver oil	1 Tbs (15 mL)	34.0	1360
Tuna, blue fin (cooked)	75 g	17.2	690
Catfish	85 g (3 oz)	10.6	425
Salmon (cooked)	3½ oz	9.0	360
Mackerel (cooked)	3½ oz	8.6	345
Oyster	3 oz	6.8	272
Shitake mushrooms (dried)	4 pieces	6.2	249
Tuna fish (canned in oil)	85 g (3 oz)	5.0	200
Sardines (canned in oil)	1¾ oz	5.0	200
Shrimp (steamed/boiled)	4 oz	4.1	162
Fortified Sources			
Butter (fortified)	100g	17.5	700
Tofu (fortified)	1/5 block	3.0	120
Milk (fortified)	1 cup	2.5	100
Orange juice (fortified)	8 oz	2.5	100
Margarine (fortified)	1 tbsp	1.5	60
Egg (boiled)	1 whole	0.6	23
Liver, beef (cooked)	3½ oz	0.4	15

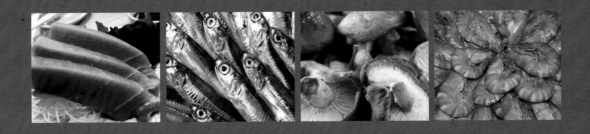

Folate

Folate, the name derived from the Latin word for *'folium'* for leaf, refers to the water-soluble B-vitamin present in green leafy vegetables like spinach. The words 'folate' and 'folic acid' are often used interchangeably but there are important differences. *Folate* is a naturally-occurring form of the vitamin, whereas, *folic acid* is a synthetic form of the vitamin commonly used in supplements and fortified foods.

Folates play an important role in bone metabolism. Elevation of *homocysteine* levels, prevalent in post-menopausal women, is associated with an increased risk in bone fractures. Folic acid supplementation reduces homocysteine levels in post-menopausal women, thereby reduces the risk of osteoporosis. It blocks the cross-linking of bone collagen, which otherwise could lead to a defective bone matrix and an increased risk of bone fractures.

Folate also substitutes for a cofactor of *nitric oxide synthase*, and preserves the enzyme activity that stimulates bone formation by osteoblasts. Folate is needed to make DNA and RNA, the building blocks of cells. This vitamin is critical for cell division, development of nervous system in the fetus, therefore, recommended during pregnancy.

Dietary Source: Leafy green vegetables (like spinach and turnip greens), fruits (like citrus fruits and juices) are natural sources for folate. Other good sources of folic acid include several kinds of beans (e.g. black eye peas, lentils, garbanzo beans and soybeans etc.), asparagus, broccoli, almonds and avocados etc. Citrus fruit juices, legumes, and fortified cereals are also excellent sources of folate.

It is recommended *(RDA)* that adults take a 400 *mcg* supplement of folic acid daily, in addition to folate and folic acid consumed in the diet. In 1996, the US-FDA published regulations requiring the addition of folic acid to enriched breads, cereals, flours, corn meals, pastas, rice, and other grain products. Since cereals and grains are widely consumed in the U.S., these products have become important contributors of folic acid to the diet. Folate supplementation should also include Vitamin-B12 (400-1000 *mcg*/day).

Adverse Effects: Folate intake from food is not associated with any health risk. It is a water-soluble vitamin, so any excess intake is usually excreted in urine. However, intake of supplemental folic acid should not exceed 1,000 *mcg* per day to avoid any symptoms of vitamin-B12 deficiency. Permanent nerve damage can occur if vitamin-B12 deficiency is not treated.

Drug Interactions: There is also some evidence that high levels of folic acid can provoke seizures in patients taking anti-convulsant medications. Individuals taking such medications should consult a physician before taking any folic acid supplement. Other medications that interfere with folate utilization include diuretics, *metformin* (to control blood sugar in type-2 diabetes), *sulfasalazine* (to control Crohn's disease and ulcerative colitis), and barbiturates (used as sedatives).

TABLE: *Recommended Daily Allowance (RDA) for Folic Acid*

Age Group	Folic *(mcg)*
Male (15+ years)	200
Female (15+ years)	180
Female (Pregnant or Postmenopausal)	400

TABLE: *Foods Rich in Folic Acid Content*

Food	Serving (average)	Folate *(mcg)*
Fortified breakfast cereal	1 cup	200-400
Orange juice *(from concentrate)*	6 oz	83
Spinach *(cooked)*	½ cup	132
Asparagus *(~ 6 spears, cooked)*	½ cup	134
Lentils *(cooked)*	½ cup	179
Garbanzo beans *(cooked)*	½ cup	141
Okra *(cooked)*	½ cup	135
Mustard greens *(cooked)*	½ cup	90
Brussels sprouts *(cooked)*	½ cup	80
Lima beans *(cooked)*	½ cup	78
Pasta *(cooked)*	1 cup	60 (Folic acid)
Rice *(cooked)*	1 cup	60 (Folic acid)
Broccoli *(cooked)*	½ cup	50

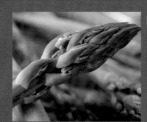
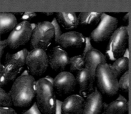
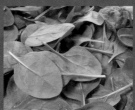
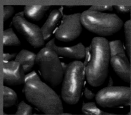

Vitamin-C

Vitamin-C, also known as ascorbic acid, is critical for several body functions, including tissue repair, strengthening blood vessels, and calcium absorption to assist in the formation of bones and teeth. It also helps to resist infections and lower cholesterol.

Vitamin-C is important for bone matrix formation through its role in collagen synthesis. Collagen is the most abundant protein in the body; it forms the connective tissue to support the skeletal system. A complex series of cellular events occur when collagen is produced. Vitamin-C adds hydrogen and oxygen to two amino acids: *proline* and *lysine*. This helps to form a precursor molecule called *procollagen*, which allows the collagen molecule to form its triple helix structure. This makes vitamin-C critical in the repair and maintenance of scar tissue, blood vessels and cartilage. Vitamin-C can also convert vitamin-D to an active form in the body to promote calcium absorption and prevent bone loss. Vitamin-C is useful in preventing osteoporosis and maintaining bone health. Long term supplementation with vitamin-C can increase BMD in women who had never used estrogen replacement therapy.

Dietary Source: Unlike most mammals, humans do not have the ability to make their own vitamin-C. Furthermore, it's water-soluble nature and rapid excretion from the body; warrants a regular dietary intake. Vitamin-C is found in citrus fruits such as oranges, limes, and grapefruit; vegetables including tomatoes, green pepper, potatoes and many others. Vitamin-C is easily damaged during food processing, including chopping, submerging in water, cooking, and boiling. However, vitamin-C levels are high enough in most foods that the residual quantity after food processing is usually enough to meet the DRI.

The DRI for vitamin-C is 60 to 90 mg/day. Men should consume more vitamin-C than women; and individuals who smoke cigarettes need to take 35 mg more of vitamin-C than average adults, since smoking depletes vitamin-C levels in the body.

Adverse Effects: Relatively large doses of vitamin-C may cause indigestion, particularly when taken on an empty stomach. When taken in large doses, vitamin-C causes diarrhea in healthy subjects. The signs and symptoms include nausea, vomiting, diarrhea, flushing of the face, headache, fatigue and disturbed sleep.

Drug Interactions: A number of drugs are known to lower vitamin-C levels, requiring an increase in its intake. Estrogen-containing contraceptives (birth control pills) and aspirin can lower vitamin-C levels if taken frequently. For example, taking 2 aspirin tablets every 6 hours for a week can lower vitamin-C levels by 50%, primarily by increasing urinary excretion. There is some evidence, that vitamin-C interacts with anticoagulant medications (blood thinners) like *warfarin (Coumadin)*.

TABLE: *Dietary Reference Intake (DRI) for Vitamin-C/day*

Life Stage	Age	Males (mg)	Females (mg)
Children	4-8 years	25	25
Children	9-13 years	45	45
Adolescents	14-18 years	75	65
Adults	19 years and older	90	75
Breastfeeding	18 years and younger	-	115
Breastfeeding	19 years and older	-	120

TABLE: *Food Rich in Vitamin-C*

Food	Serving	Vitamin-C (mg)
Rose hip extract	1 cup (8 oz)	1000+
Black Currant juice	1 cup (8 oz)	200
Guava	2 medium	180
Sweet red pepper *(raw chopped)*	½ cup	141
Orange juice	1 cup (8 oz)	100
Strawberries *(whole)*	1 cup	82
Grapefruit juice	1 cup (8 oz)	80
Orange	1 medium	70
Lemon	1 medium	60
Broccoli *(cooked)*	½ cup	58
Grapefruit	½ medium	44
Clementine	2 medium	40
Potato *(baked)*	1 medium	26
Tomato	1 medium	23

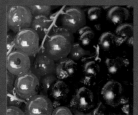
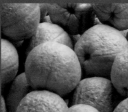
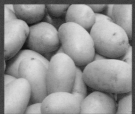
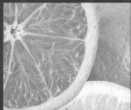

Vitamin-K

Vitamin-K, a fat-soluble vitamin, is essential for blood coagulation or clotting (named after the German term – *koagulation*). It is required for the activation of 7 proteins, involved in the chain of *"coagulation cascade"* in clot formation. There are 2 main forms of vitamin-K: i) phylloquinone *(vitamin-K1)* and ii) menaquinone *(vitamins-K2 or MK)*. Most vitamin-K in the body is in K1 form, found in green leafy vegetables. Vitamin-K2 is a group of compounds synthesized by bacteria, among which, MK-4 is derived from dietary K1. MK-4 is found in animal meat and MK-7 is found in fermented foods like cheese and *natto*.

Recent studies have identified a role for vitamin-K in bone metabolism. Three different bone proteins, *osteocalcin (OC), matrix Gla protein (MGP)*, and *protein-S*, are dependant on vitamin-K. Osteocalcin, synthesized by *osteoblasts*; has a critical role in bone mineralization. Bone protein MGP facilitates normal bone growth and prevents accumulation of calcium in soft tissue and cartilage. Protein-S is important for building bone density.

Vitamin-K also positively affects calcium balance in the bone. Human clinical studies have reported that low dosage of vitamin-K1, in combination with vitamin-D, can improve bone health. This vitamin combination not only increases BMD in osteoporotic individuals, but also reduces the fracture rate. A recent meta-analysis of MK-4 supplementation studies showed an increase in BMD and a consistent reduction of all fracture types.

Vitamin-K deficiency leads to impaired blood clotting. Symptoms include easy bruising and bleeding that manifests as nosebleeds, bleeding gums, blood in the urine, bloody or tarry black stools, or heavy menstrual bleeding. Exclusively breast-fed infants are at higher risk of vitamin-K deficiency, which may result in life-threatening bleeding within the skull (intracranial hemorrhage).

Dietary Source: Green leafy vegetables and some vegetable oils (soybean, cottonseed, canola, and olive) are major contributors of phylloquinone *(vitamin-K1)*, the major dietary form. Hydrogenation of vegetable oils may decrease the absorption and biological effect of dietary vitamin-K. Some of the good sources for vitamin-K are listed in the following TABLE. Individuals at risk for fracture should be encouraged to consume diets rich in green leafy vegetables and vegetable oils.

Multivitamin supplements generally contain 10 to 25 *mcg* of vitamin-K, while bone health supplements may contain 100 to 200 *mcg*. It is sufficient to eat about half a cup of chopped broccoli or a large salad of mixed greens every day, to obtain the same amount of vitamin-K (about 250 *mcg*/day) to decrease risks of hip fracture, according to the Framingham Heart Study. Replacing the dietary saturated fat-like butter and cheese with mono-unsaturated fats found in olive oil and canola oil can increase dietary vitamin-K intake and reduce the risk of cardiovascular diseases.

This recommendation is especially important for the elderly (above 65 years) and patients at higher risk of osteoporosis and hip fractures. Current dietary recommendation for vitamin-K is 90-120 *mcg*/day. The body could store only small amounts of vitamin-K, while most of it is rapidly depleted in the absence of regular dietary intake.

Vitamin-K supplements reduced hip fractures by 77%, vertebral fractures by 60% and all non-vertebral fractures by 81%.

Adverse Effects: Consumption of dietary or supplemental vitamin-K is required in individuals taking anticoagulant medication. These patients are cautioned to avoid consuming excessive or highly variable quantities of vitamin-K in their diets. High doses of *phylloquinone (vitamin-K1)* or *menaquinone (vitamin-K2)* are not known to have toxic effects. However, synthetic *menadione (vitamin-K3)* and its derivatives interfere with the antioxidant function of glutathione, leading to oxidative damage to cell membranes; it could also induce liver toxicity, jaundice and rupture of RBC *(hemolysis)* when given by injection. Therefore, menadione is no longer in use to treat vitamin-K deficiency.

Drug Interactions: Large doses of vitamin-A and vitamin-E interfere with the bioavailability of vitamin-K. Individuals using *warfarin* (anticoagulant) are recommended to take a high and consistent dose of dietary or supplemental vitamin-K. Use of anticoagulants and anticonvulsants by pregnant women can interfere with vitamin-K synthesis and cause deficiency in the newborn. Adequate vitamin-K in conjunction with vitamin-D may prevent arterial calcification and maintain bone health. Prolonged use of broad spectrum antibiotics may also decrease vitamin-K synthesis by intestinal bacterial flora.

Natto intake may help prevent post-menopausal bone loss through the effects of MK-7 or isoflavones, which are more abundant in natto than in other soybean products.

Pregnant and nursing mothers should limit vitamin-K intake to 65 *mcg*/day. Individuals who have experienced stroke, cardiac arrest, and those prone to blood clotting should not take vitamin-K without consulting their physician.

TABLE: *Dietary Reference Intake (DRI) of vitamin-K for healthy individuals*

Age group		Males (*mcg*/day)	Females (*mcg*/day)
Infants	0-6 months	2.0	2.0
	7-12 months	2.5	2.5
Children	1-3 years	30	30
	4-8 years	55	55
	9-13 years	60	60
Adolescents	14-18 years	75	75
Adults	19 years or older	120	90
Pregnancy	18 years and younger	-	75
	19 years and older	-	90
Breast-feeding	18 years and younger	-	75
	19 years and older	-	90

TABLE: *Foods Rich in Vitamin-K Content*

Food	Serving (g)	Vitamin-K *(mcg)*
Kale, frozen *(cooked)*	130	1,147
Collards *(frozen, chopped)*	170	1,059
Spinach *(frozen, chopped)*	190	1,027
Turnip greens *(frozen)*	165	851
Collards *(cooked, boiled)*	190	836
Beet greens *(cooked, boiled)*	145	697
Mustard greens *(cooked)*	140	419
Amaranth leaves	28	319
Brussels sprouts *(frozen)*	155	300
Broccoli *(cooked, boiled)*	155	220
Onions *(spring or scallions)*	100	207
Lettuce *(raw)*	165	167
Parsley *(raw)*	10	164
Spinach *(raw)*	30	145
Asparagus *(frozen)*	180	144
Sauerkraut *(canned)*	240	135
Lettuce, iceberg *(raw)*	540	130
Endive *(raw)*	50	116
Celery *(cooked, boiled)*	150	57
Cucumber, with peel *(raw)*	300	49
Soybeans *(sprouted steamed)*	94	31

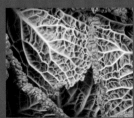
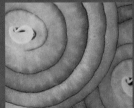
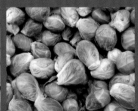
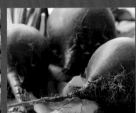

7.4 | Bone Health **Minerals**

Minerals are integral part of bones, teeth, soft tissue, muscle, blood, and nerve cells. They perform several vital functions in the body - from building strong bones to transmitting nerve impulses. Some minerals are involved in the biosynthesis of hormones or maintaining a normal heartbeat

Minerals essential for bone health are of two types, (i) *Macro-minerals*, which include Calcium *(Ca)*, Phosphorus *(P)*, Magnesium *(Mg)*, Sodium *(Na)*, Potassium *(K)*, and Chloride *(Cl)*; (ii) *Trace elements*, which include Iron *(Fe)*, Copper *(Cu)*, Zinc *(Zn)*, Manganese *(Mn)*, Selenium *(Se)*, Iodine *(I)*, Chromium *(Cr)*, Cobalt *(Co)*, Nickel *(Ni)*, Molybdenum *(Mb)*, Fluoride *(F)*, Arsenic *(As)*, Silicon *(Si)* and Boron *(B)*.

All tissue and internal fluids contain varying quantities of minerals. Unlike vitamins, some of which the body can manufacture, not a single mineral can be manufactured by the body. Therefore, dietary intake is the only means for the body to acquire both macro- and micro-minerals.

Bone is made of both living cells and mineral deposits. Hardness and strength for the bone comes from minerals; without these the bone would be soft and fragile.

Vitamins cannot be assimilated without the aid of minerals. Also, certain minerals and vitamins are necessary for the bioavailability or absorption of calcium. Such minerals and vitamins include phosphorus, magnesium, boron and zinc plus vitamins-D3 and A. Dietary uptake of *folic acid* is necessary to maintain *homocysteine* levels in the blood; which not only helps heart health, but also promotes strong bones. Increased intakes of potassium, in addition to vitamin C, fiber and alkaline-producing fruit and vegetables favor adult bone health. Potassium and magnesium help maintain BMD. Potassium plays a role in calcium balance and this regulatory effect may influence bone resorption. Also, silicon-rich foods, such as parsnips, celery, lettuce, unpeeled cucumber, carrots, strawberries, brown rice and other whole grains encourage calcium assimilation.

Diets rich in particular mineral or nutritional factors can also adversely affect the utilization of another nutrient in the body. Such an effect has been observed with the increased excretion of calcium due to sodium-rich and protein-rich diets. Presence of increased calcium with synergistic bone minerals in these diets may compensate for calcium loss from the bones. Finally, for achieving good bone health with an optimum BMD, the body requires a continuous supply of both minerals and vitamins. No mineral or vitamin acts alone in the body; all work in synergy to ensure smooth and normal functioning of the total skeletal system.

Diets high in fruits and vegetables produce more alkaline urine due to a variety of minerals that accept hydrogen ions during metabolism, and increase the BMD.

Deficiencies of certain trace minerals, such as chromium and manganese, have been connected to BMD and weaker bones. Supplementation of calcium with trace minerals can increase BMD. Therefore, calcium alone is not enough!

Calcium

Calcium *(Ca)* is an essential mineral for the whole body, in particular, for providing strength and integrity to the skeletal system. Its absorption, however, is highly dependant on other minerals (e.g. magnesium) and vitamins (e.g. vitamin-D); otherwise calcium is either flushed out or dangerously absorbed into the body, which may trigger calcification of arteries and tissues. Therefore, mineral/vitamin factors are needed in proper ratios for proper calcium assimilation.

A healthy and balanced diet constitutes the basic foundation for daily calcium intake. Milk, butter, ice cream, cheese and other dairy products are among the best sources of calcium in bio-available form. Consumption of calcium-rich (or –fortified) foods is vital for bone health, especially for attaining peak bone mass among children and adolescents. A typical serving size (200-mL) of milk could provide about 22% of the current US recommended daily allowance *(RDA)* of 1000 mg, for 19 to 50 year age group.

Calcium-fortified foods are also a preferred choice because additional nutrients (e.g. vitamin-D in juices) can contribute to bone development and prevention of osteoporosis. For individuals who are unable to attain sufficient calcium through diet; it is recommended to take supplements such as calcium citrate or calcium carbonate. If the diet is low in phosphorus, calcium supplementation alone will not be adequate. Both calcium and phosphorus are needed to increase bone mass.

Strict vegans, who do not consume dairy products, are at high risk of calcium deficiency and osteoporosis. Therefore, it is important for vegans to include adequate amounts of non-dairy sources of calcium in their daily diet. Many plant-based foods such as green leafy vegetables, Chinese cabbage, kale, broccoli, Brussel sprouts, beans, fruits, nuts and seafood are rich sources of calcium. Vegetables, however, contain smaller quantities of calcium per serving with limited bio-availability than dairy foods.

Influencing Factors: Calcium absorption is affected by several factors including, calcium levels in the body, vitamin-D status, age, pregnancy, and plant substances in the diet. The degree of mineral solubility, acidic levels of the ingested food, and diets high in fat (e.g. tofu, sunflower or rapeseed) can impede calcium absorption. Unesterified long-chain saturated fatty acids, i.e. palmitic acid, have a melting point above body temperature and, can interact with calcium in the intestinal lumen and form insoluble calcium soaps.

Certain plant-based foods can interfere with calcium absorption in the intestinal tract due to their fiber and acid content. *Phytic acid* and *oxalic acid* found naturally in some plants, bind to calcium and block its absorption. Phytic acid (or phytate) is present in whole grain bread, beans, seeds, nuts, grains, wheat bran and soybeans. Foods high in oxalic acid include spinach, collard greens, sweet potatoes, rhubarb, and beans. Benefits derived from other nutrients (i.e. vitamin-C, folate, magnesium) in green foods, however, outweigh their negative effect to block calcium absorption.

Dietary intake of phosphorus affects calcium absorption. A 1:1 ratio of calcium to phosphorus is optimum for bioavailability of both minerals. However, if the phosphorus levels are higher than calcium, this condition could seriously interfere with the intestinal calcium absorption; and may increase calcium withdrawal from the bone. Phosphate-rich diet such as soda, soft drinks and foods with preservatives can impede calcium intake.

Dietary Source: It should be noted that calcium in its pure form is a highly reactive metal, therefore, cannot be taken directly into the human body. All calcium supplements, whether in tablet, liquid or powder form are made as salts or chelates of calcium. Thus, an individual can take calcium carbonate, calcium phosphate, calcium gluconate, calcium lactate, but never *'pure'* calcium. Different derivatives of calcium have varying amounts of elemental calcium. Elemental refers to the actual amount of pure calcium in a specific formula. This information is essential for knowledge of how much calcium supplement one must take to get the desired amount of this essential mineral. Calcium carbonate, for example, has about 40% elemental calcium. Thus, if 1 gram (1000 mg) of calcium (elemental) is recommended daily, one must take 2.5 grams (2500 mg.) of this form of calcium to obtain the desired amount. Other sources of calcium usually have less elemental calcium, e.g. (tricalcium salt, 38%; Ca-citrate, 21%; Ca-lactate, 13%; and Ca-gluconate, 9%) and one must take correspondingly more of the calcium salt.

Net calcium absorption can be as high as 60% in infants and young children, when the growing body needs calcium to build strong bones. Absorption slowly decreases to 15-20% in adulthood and even more with aging.

Adverse Effects: Calcium has no known toxic effects. While low intakes of calcium can result in deficiency and undesirable health conditions, excessive intake of calcium may trigger adverse effects such as *hypercalcemia* (elevated levels of calcium in the blood), and impaired kidney function in certain individuals. Furthermore, high calcium intake, at levels above 2500 mg per day has the potential to interfere with the absorption of other minerals, iron, zinc, magnesium, and phosphorus. Excess consumption of calcium may also be associated with the risk of kidney stone formation.

Drug Interactions: Calcium supplements may interfere with the efficacy of certain drugs such as bisphosphonates, calcium channel blockers, fluoroquinolones, tetracyclines and therapeutics for thyroid treatment. Calcium should be taken several hours before or after taking such medications. On the other hand, these medications can interfere with the absorption and utilization of calcium. When medications such as antibiotics, oral contraceptives, anticonvulsants and laxatives are taken, calcium intake needs to be increased.

Estrogen levels in the body are diminished after menopause. Calcium absorption is reduced due to estrogen deficiency after menopause, resulting in increased bone resorption, with the most rapid of bone loss occurring within the first 5 years of menopause. Increased calcium intake alone will not completely offset postmenopausal bone loss.

In 1993, the US-FDA authorized a health claim stating that – *Adequate calcium intake throughout life is linked to reduced risk of osteoporosis through the mechanism of optimizing peak bone mass during adolescence and early adulthood and decreasing bone loss later in life.*

TABLE: *Recomons for Daily Calcium Intake for Various Age Groups*

Calcium

Group	Dairy Foods	Calcium-Rich Foods	RDA
Infants: <6 months 6-12 months	Breast milk/Formula Breast milk/Formula		210 mg 270 mg
Children: 1-3 years 4-6 years	2 2-3	2-3 2-3	500 mg 800 mg
Adolescents: 8-13 years 14-18 years	2-3 2-3	4-5 4-5	1300 mg 1300 mg
Adults: 19-30 years 31-50 years after 51 years	2-3 2-3 2-3	3-4 3-4 4-5	1000 mg 1000 mg 1200 mg
Pregnant/ Nursing: <6 months 6-12 month	2-3 2-3	4-5 3-4	1300 mg 1000 mg

*Source: Standing Committee on the Scientific Evaluation of Dietary Reference Intakes, Food and Nutrition Board, Institute of Medicine. Dietary Reference Intakes for Calcium, Phosphorus, Magnesium, Vitamin D, and Fluoride. NationalAcademy Press, Washington DC, 1999.

> *The recommended daily allowance (RDA) of calcium is 1000-1200 mg depending on age and gender. In general, women need more calcium than men. The peak bone mass is reached before age 30, therefore, it is important that individuals consume optimum amounts of calcium from an early age.*

TABLE: *Foods Rich in Calcium Content*

Calcium-rich Food	Serving Size (average)	Calcium (mg)
Milk and Milk Products:		
Milk *(whole, 2%, 1% skim)*	1 cup, 200 mL	300
Parmesan *(fresh)*	portion, 30 g	308
Cheddar	medium chunk, 40 g	296
Yoghurt *(low-fat, plain)*	¾cup, 150 g	290
Mozzarella *(fresh)*	portion, 56 g	203
Meats, Fish, and Poultry:		
Sardines in oil *(tinned)*	portion, 100 g	500
Anchovies *(canned with bones)*	100 g	300
Sardines *(canned with bones)*	75 g	286
Salmon *(canned with bones)*	75 g	208
Fruit and Vegetables:		
Figs *(ready to eat)*	4 fruit, 220 g	506
Spinach	1 cup	150
Curly Kale	serving, 95 g	143
Apricots *(raw, no stone)*	4 fruit, 160 g	117
Turnip greens	½ cup	104
Grains and Nuts:		
Oats *(instant, regular)*	1 pouch	165
Tahini *(sesame seed butter)*	2 tbsp	130
Almonds *(dry roast)*	1/4 cup	93
Non-Dairy Products:		
Tofu *(medium firm or firm)*	150 g	347
Fortified rice or soy beverage	1 cup	320
Orange juice *(fortified)*	½ cup	165

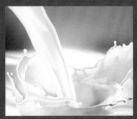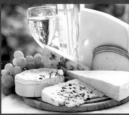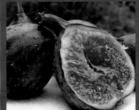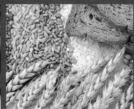

Phosphorus

Phosphorus *(P)* is an essential mineral needed by every cell in the body for normal function. Most phosphorus in the body exist in the form of phosphate (PO_4). About 85% of adult body phosphorus is found in the bones, with the remaining 15% in the soft tissues.

Calcium and phosphorus are co-dependent. If the diet is low in phosphorus, calcium supplementation alone is inadequate, and may aggravate a phosphorus deficiency. Phosphorus is abundant in most foods due to its ubiquitous presence in every living organism. Most inorganic forms of phosphorus, such as those found in health supplements and as preservatives in several foods, are readily assimilated into the human body.

Dietary Source: A diet that provides adequate amounts of calcium and protein also provides sufficient amount of phosphorus. The main sources of phosphorus are the proteins in food, mainly meat and milk. Milk contains significant levels of phosphorus – 200 mL milk can provide about 25% the current US RDA. Scientists have noted that calcium phosphate from milk is absorbed preferentially in children and is utilized for bone accrual. A varied diet could easily provide adequate phosphorus for most people including older adults. Dairy products, meat and fish are particularly rich sources of phosphorus. Phosphorus is also a component of many polyphosphate food additives and is present in most soft drinks as phosphoric acid. The average phosphorus intake in the US is 1,495 mg/day in men and 1,024 mg/day in women, well above the recommended 700 mg/day for adults. The Food and Nutrition Board *(FNB)* estimates phosphorus consumption in the U.S. has increased 10% to 15% over the past 20 years, due to increased use of phosphate salts as food additives and consumption of cola beverages.

Influencing Factors: Aluminum-containing antacids reduce the absorption of dietary phosphorus by forming aluminum phosphate. Such interactions can result in abnormally low blood phosphate levels and increased urinary calcium loss. High doses of *calcitriol*, the active form of vitamin-D, or its analogs may also block phosphate uptake. Calcium carbonate has been reported to interfere with the absorption of phosphorus.

Adverse Effects: Serious adverse effect of elevated blood levels of phosphate *(hyperphosphatemia)* is the calcification of non-skeletal tissues, most commonly the kidneys. Such calcium phosphate deposition can lead to organ damage, especially kidney damage. Also diets high in fructose (20% of total calories) can increase urinary loss of phosphorus.

Drug Interactions: Potassium-sparing diuretics taken together with phosphates may result in high blood levels of potassium *(hyperkalemia)*. Hyperkalemia is a serious health issue; which leads to life threatening heart rhythm abnormalities. Individuals taking such a combination must inform their health care provider and check their serum potassium levels on a regular basis.

TABLE: *Recommended Daily Allowance (RDA) for Phosphorous*

Age Group	Phosphorus (mg/day)
0 to 6 months	100
7 to 12 months	275
1 to 3 years	460
4 to 8 years	500
9 to 18 years	1,250
Adults	700

TABLE: *Foods Rich in Phosphorus Content*

Food	Serving (average)	Phosphorus (mg)
Sesame seeds	100 g	700
All bran cereal	100 g	700
Sunflower seeds	100 g	650
Baking powder	1 tbsp	456
Barley *(pearled raw)*	1 cup	442
Yogurt *(plain nonfat)*	8 oz	385
Fish, salmon *(cooked)*	3 oz	252
Milk *(skim)*	8 oz	247
Fish, halibut *(cooked)*	3 oz	242
Lentils *(cooked)*	½ cup	178
Beef *(cooked)*	3 oz	173
Chicken *(cooked)*	3 oz	155
Almonds *(23 nuts)*	1 oz	134
Carbonated cola drink	12 oz	40

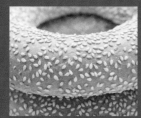
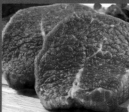
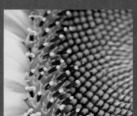
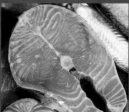

Magnesium

Magnesium *(Mg)* is present in every living cell; approximately 50% of the total body magnesium is found in bones. Magnesium interacts with vitamin-B6 to regulate absorption of calcium into the bone. In other words, without magnesium, calcium will not be deposited into the bone. Accordingly, a 2:1 ratio of calcium to magnesium is considered optimum for gaining an optimum BMD.

Magnesium is abundant in both plant and animal foods. Green vegetables are good sources of magnesium because the center of chlorophyll molecule (which gives green color to the vegetables) contains this mineral. Some legumes (beans and peas), nuts and seeds, and whole, unrefined grains are also good sources of magnesium. Tap water can provide magnesium, but the amount varies according to the water supply. *'Hard'* water contains more magnesium than *'soft'* water.

Dietary Source: Dietary supplements are made of different salts of magnesium, in the form of oxides, sulfates, and carbonates. The amount of elemental magnesium in a compound and its bioavailability influence the effectiveness of a magnesium supplement. The Food and Nutrition Board *(FNB)* has set the tolerable upper intake level *(UL)* for magnesium at 350 mg/day. Milk is a good source of magnesium, a regular serving (200-mL) provides about 6% of the DRI. The current DRI for magnesium is cited in the following TABLE.

Adverse Effects: Dietary magnesium does not pose a health risk; however, signs of excess magnesium can be similar to magnesium deficiency and include changes in mental status, nausea, diarrhea, appetite loss, muscle weakness, difficulty breathing, extremely low blood pressure and irregular heartbeat. Very large doses of magnesium-containing laxatives and antacids also have been associated with risk of kidney failure.

Drug Interactions: A number of common medications drain the body reserves of magnesium. Groups of drugs that deplete or increase elimination of magnesium include diuretics, corticosteroids, hormone replacement therapy *(HRT)*, and oral contraceptives. Drinking alcohol in excess also depletes magnesium from the body. Finally, large doses of calcium intake can impede absorption of magnesium from the gut.

Magnesium deficiency can affect virtually every organ system of the body. Symptoms with the skeleto-muscular system include twitches, cramps, muscle tension and soreness, back aches, neck pain, tension headaches and jaw joint dysfunction. Affected individuals may also experience chest tightness or difficulty in breathing. Symptoms involving impaired contraction of smooth muscles include constipation; urinary spasms; menstrual cramps; difficulty swallowing or a lump in the throat, usually provoked by eating sugar; photophobia, especially difficulty in adjusting to oncoming bright headlights; and sensitivity to loud noise due to muscle tension in the ear. Finally, some evidence suggests that magnesium deficiency may be an additional risk factor for postmenopausal osteoporosis. Magnesium deficiency can alter hormones that regulate calcium homeostasis.

TABLE: *Recommended Daily Allowance (RDA) for Magnesium*

Age Group	Magnesium (mg)
Female (19-50 years)	310-320
Male (19-50 years)	400-420
Children (4-8 years)	130
Pregnant and Lactating women	310-360

TABLE: *Foods Rich in Magnesium Content*

Food	Serving (average)	Magnesium (mg)
Buckwheat flour	1 cup	301
Halibut	½ fillet	170
Spinach *(cooked)*	1 cup	157
Seeds, pumpkin and squash	1 oz	151
Beans, black	1 cup	120
Okra *(frozen)*	1 cup	94
Plantain *(raw)*	1 medium	66
Nuts, peanuts	1 oz	64
Whole grain cereal *(cooked)*	1 cup	56
Scallop	6 large	55
Rockfish	1 fillet	51
Oysters	3 oz	49
Soy milk	1 cup	47
Tofu	¼ block	37
Whole grain cereal *(ready-to-eat)*	¾ cup	24

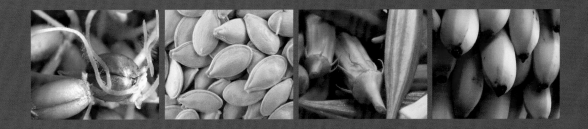

Zinc *(Zn)* is a multi-functional nutrient with a broad range of metabolic activities in the bone. *Alkaline phosphatase*, the enzyme required for deposition of calcium into the bone (bone calcification); *collagenase*, the enzyme necessary for bone resorption and remodeling are zinc *metallo-enzymes*. Accordingly, zinc plays an important role in maintaining the quality of bone matrix.

Zinc is an important (and often underestimated) nutrient for the prevention of osteoporosis. Zinc is often deficient in the diet. Furthermore, zinc levels in the body can run low, in times of physiological need such as during pregnancy or menopause or strenuous exercise. Absorption of zinc is often affected by other minerals (e.g. iron and copper) and supplements, especially when taken together. Calcium in combination with phytic acid may reduce zinc absorption. This effect is particularly relevant among individuals who frequently consume tortillas made with lime (i.e., calcium oxide).

A wide variety of foods contain zinc. Oysters contain more zinc per serving than any other food, but red meat and poultry provide most of the zinc through diet. Other good food sources include beans, nuts, certain types of seafood (such as crab and lobster), whole grains, fortified breakfast cereals, and dairy products. Nuts and legumes are relatively good plant sources of zinc.

Dietary Source: Supplements contain several forms of zinc, including salts of gluconate, sulfate, picolinate and acetate. The amount of elemental zinc varies by form. For example, approximately 23% of zinc sulfate consists of elemental zinc; thus, 220 mg of zinc sulfate contains 50 mg of elemental zinc.

During pregnancy, zinc requirement increases by 50%, particularly, the last 15-10 weeks. Zinc sulfate be avoided or used with caution during pregnancy, since safety is not established when it crosses the placenta.

Adverse Effects: Zinc toxicity can occur in both acute and chronic forms. Acute adverse effects of high zinc intake include nausea, vomiting, loss of appetite, abdominal cramps, diarrhea, and headaches. Intakes of 150–450 mg/day of zinc is associated with chronic effects such as low copper status, altered iron function, reduced immune function, and reduced levels of high-density lipoproteins (HDL or "good cholesterol").

Drug Interactions: Zinc supplements interact with several types of medications. Zinc inhibits antibiotic activity and affects its own absorption in the gut. Taking the antibiotic at least 2 hours before or 4–6 hours after having a zinc supplement minimizes this interaction. Zinc can also reduce the efficacy of *penicillamine*, a drug used in the treatment of rheumatoid arthritis. Diuretics increase urinary zinc excretion by as much as 60%. Prolonged use of diuretics could deplete zinc tissue levels, so clinicians should monitor zinc status in patients taking these medications.

TABLE: *Recommended Daily Allowance (RDA) for Zinc*

Life Stage		Males (mg/day)	Females (mg/day)
Infants	0-6 months	2	2
	7-12 months	3	3
Children	1-3 years	3	3
	4-8 years	5	5
	9-13 years	8	8
Adolescents (14-18 years)		11	9
Adults (above 19 years)		11	8

TABLE: *Foods Rich in Zinc Content*

Food	Serving (average)	Calcium (mg)
Meat, Sea Foods		
Oysters	3.5 oz	25+
Shellfish	3.5 oz	20
Brewers yeast	3.5 oz	17
Beef *(cooked)*	3 oz	6.0
Chicken, broiler	3 oz	6.0
Turkey *(dark meat, cooked)*	3 oz	3.8
Grains, Beans		
Wheat germ	3.5 oz	17
Wheat bran	3.5 oz	14
Beans *(baked)*	3.5 oz	16
All bran cereal	3.5 oz	6.8
Fruits and Nuts		
Pine nuts	3.5 oz	6.5
Pecan nuts	3.5 oz	6.4
Cashew nuts	3.5 oz	5.7

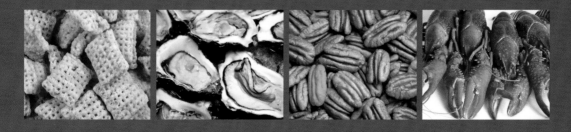

Bone Health
MINERAL

Chromium

Chromium *(Cr)* is an essential micro-nutrient for optimal bone health, and a critical component of the *Glucose-Tolerance Factor*. Chromium acts synergistic with insulin to facilitate cellular uptake of blood glucose. It may also have a role in other insulin-dependent activities such as protein and lipid metabolism.

Chromium promotes insulin efficiency, which may indirectly improve BMD by increasing collagen production by osteoblasts. Insulin also reduces activation of osteoclasts by parathyroid hormone *(PTH)*; thereby, may contribute to reduction in bone resorption.

Chromium levels in the body may be reduced under several conditions. Diets high in simple sugars (comprising more than 35% of calories) can increase chromium excretion in the urine. Infection, acute exercise, pregnancy and lactation, and stressful states (such as physical trauma) increase chromium losses and can lead to deficiency, especially if chromium intakes are already low.

Chromium is widely distributed in the food supply, but most foods provide only small amounts (less than 2 *mcg* per serving). Dietary sources of chromium include whole grains, potatoes, oysters, liver, seafood, cheese, chicken and meat. Brewer's yeast is a rich source of organic chromium complexes. In contrast, foods high in simple sugars (like sucrose and fructose) are low in chromium.

Dietary Source: Chromium supplements are available as chromium chloride, chromium nicotinate, chromium picolinate, high-chromium yeast, and chromium citrate. However, given the limited data on chromium absorption in humans, it is not clear which forms are best to take. Recommended Daily Allowance *(RDA)* for dietary intake of chromium in US and Scandinavia is about 50 *mcg* or lower and, consequently, at or below. The US National Academy of Sciences has established a safe and adequate daily dietary chromium intake range of 50–200 *mcg*/day.

Adverse Effects: Few serious adverse effects have been linked to high intakes of chromium, so the Institute of Medicine *(IOM)* has not established a Tolerable Upper Intake Level (UL) for this mineral. An UL is defined as the *maximum* daily intake of a nutrient that is unlikely to cause adverse health effects. The UL value (together with the RDA and AI) comprises the Dietary Reference Intakes *(DRIs)* for each nutrient.

Drug Interactions: Certain medications may interact with chromium, especially when taken on a regular basis. Antacids, coticosteroids, H2 blockers and proton pump inhibitors alter stomach acidity and may impair chromium absorption or enhance excretion. Also chromium may enhance the effects of beta-blockers, insulin, nicotinic acid, nonsteroidal anti-inflammatory drugs *(NSAIDS)* and prostaglandin inhibitors (e.g. ibuprofen). Therefore, it may be necessary to adjust the dosages of these medications when taken together with chromium.

TABLE: *Dietary Reference Intake (DRI) for chromium*

Age Group	Chromium *mcg*/day
Male (19-50 years)	35
Male (51-70 years)	30
Female (19-50 years)	25

TABLE: *Foods Rich in Chromium Content*

Food	Serving (average)	Calcium *(mcg)*
Onions *(raw)*	1 cup	24.8
Broccoli *(cooked)*	1 cup	22.0
Tomatoes	1 cup	9.0
Romaine lettuce	1 cup	7.9
Potatoes *(mashed)*	1 cup	2.7
Green beans *(cooked)*	1 cup	2.2
Garlic *(dried)*	1 tsp	3
English Muffin, whole wheat	1	4
Cookies, chocolate chip	1 large	3.4
Waffle, egg	1 medium	6.7
Bagel, egg	1	2.5
Milk	200 mL	0.4
Red wine	5 oz	1-13
Orange juice	1 cup	2.2
Grape juice	1 cup	7.5
Turkey leg	3 oz	10.4

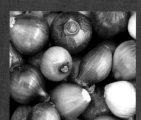 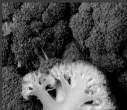 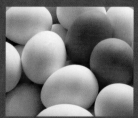 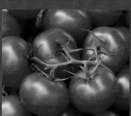

Boron

Boron *(B)* plays an integral part in bone metabolism. It supports the functions of calcium, phosphorus, magnesium, and vitamin-D, all of which are crucial in promoting a healthy dense bone tissue. Highest concentration of boron in the body is in parathyroid glands, which can affect the mineral movement and building of the bones by regulating the hormones, mainly the *parathyroid (PTH)* that controls the bone turnover functions. Boron may also protect already brittle bones from fractures by facilitating calcium absorption.

Boron is involved in hormone regulation; in particular, it raises *testosterone* levels in men and helps to build muscle. Boron also regulates estrogen levels and helps to convert vitamin-D to an active state. Boron is also involved in processes that build and repair joints; prevents arthritis and tooth decay. Boron can alleviate the detrimental effects of vitamin-D deficiency on calcium metabolism. Boron can preserve bone mass and prevent osteoporosis in post-menopausal women.

Because of its involvement in several biochemical pathways, boron deficiency can result in several health problems. Signs of boron deficiency include problems with bone disease (osteoporosis, arthritis), depression, decreased ability to handle stress, carpal tunnel syndrome, joint problems, hormonal imbalance, muscle pain or weakness, memory problems, tooth decay and receding gums. Boron deprivation may produce changes similar to those seen in osteoporosis, and that adequate boron supplementation can reverse demineralization and bone loss.

Dietary Source: Boron occurs most widely in fruits, nuts, legumes and green leafy vegetables, including raisins, prunes, pears, apples, grapes, almonds, soybeans and kale. These sources depend, however, boron content in the cultivation soil. A correlation exists between the soil boron levels and the prevalence of arthritis. In Israel, boron levels in the soil are high, which coincides with the low rate of arthritis (less than 1 percent); in contrast, Jamaica has low boron soil levels with high prevalence of arthritis.

Although there is no established dietary reference intake *(DRI)* for boron, based on scientific evidence suggests the optimal boron intake at 2-3 mg/day (or higher). Due to its low toxicity and possible benefits, elderly people and anyone at risk of osteoporosis should eat boron-rich foods. Adequate boron is necessary to increase bone density and prevent bone loss, especially among post-menopausal women and others at a high risk for osteoporosis. Some athletes are now taking boron to promote better muscle growth, energy metabolism, and hand-eye coordination.

Adverse Effects: Orally, boron appears to have low toxicity. Adverse reactions at doses below 10 mg/day are unlikely. However, it should also be noted that boron is potentially toxic in doses greater than 100 mg. Symptoms of boron toxicity include rash, nausea, vomiting, diarrhea, and circulatory problems. In extreme cases, boron toxicity can result in shock followed by coma. Concomitant administration with estrogenic drugs may increase serum estrogen levels.

TABLE: *Foods Rich in Boron Content*

Food	Boron (mg/100 g)
Raisins	4.5
Almond	2.8
Hazel nuts	2.8
Apricots *(dried)*	2.1
Avocado	2.1
Peanut Butter	1.9
Brazil nuts	1.7
Walnut	1.6
Beans *(red kidney)*	1.4
Cashew nuts *(raw)*	1.2
Prunes	1.2
Dates	1.1
Chick peas	0.7

Normal levels of boron in soft tissues, urine, and blood generally range from less than 0.05 – 10 mg/kg.

In the late 18th century, borate was being used for preserving foods such as fish, shellfish, meat, cream, butter and margarine. Following a report of toxicity in the mid-1950s, use of borates and boric acid as food preservatives was essentially forbidden throughout the world. The maximum acceptable concentration for boron in drinking water in the USA is 0.3 mg/L. Some groundwater bodies in the Mediterranean basin in Cyprus, Greece and the Cornia River basin in Tuscany, Italy contain exceptionally high levels of boron (>1 mg/L) and are unusable. High boron concentrations have also been reported for ground waters in southeastern Spain, Israel, Gaza strip and western Turkey.

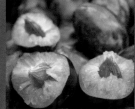 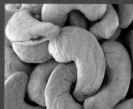 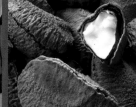 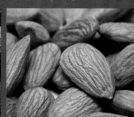

7.5 | Bone Health **Supplements**

Ancient civilizations have acknowledged the medicinal properties of several foods and herbs. Recent advances in food technology, have identified the bioactive compounds in such foods, and made possible the usage of such functional isolates (or enriched fractions) as potent ingredients to alleviate symptoms of various ailments. These supplemental ingredients include phytochemicals, and functional isolates.

Phytochemicals are active chemical compounds from plants, widely used as active ingredients to promote bone health. *Resveratrol* from red wine has a direct stimulating effect on bone formation, and can therefore be a helpful supplement in prevention and treatment of osteoporosis. *Polyphenols* from red grapefruit pulp can slow down bone resorption; increase calcium absorption and bone mineral build up. *Flavonoids* derived from the Chinese herb *Epimedium* may increase BMD of the hip and lower back, and provide benefits against osteoporosis. *Dietary lipids* can alter the fatty acid composition and local production of skeletal growth factors in different compartments of bone. Black pepper *(Piper nigrum)* contains four phytochemicals with anti-osteoporotic activity. Cabbage contains 145 ppm (parts per million) boron on a dry-weight basis, which helps raise estrogen levels.

Functional Isolates: A number of functional isolates such as melatonin, carnitine, polyunsaturated fatty acids *(PUFAs)*, and conjugated linoleic acid *(CLA)* are also widely used to improve bone health. *Betaine* in the stomach, or in the form of betaine hydrochloride supplement, can help proper absorption of calcium and all nutrients. *Phenylalanine* is an amino acid found naturally in the breast milk of mammals. It is structurally related to *dopamine*, and *epinepherine (adrenaline)*, thus, endowed with potent analgesic and antidepressant effects. Phenylalanine is widely used in nutritional supplements, in particular, for the pain management of the bone. *L-lysine* is required for collagen synthesis and helps the body to absorb calcium more efficiently while improving bone health. Lysine is important for bone formation in children; it may be particularly helpful for post-menopausal women at risk of osteoporosis. Lysine is one of the eight essential amino acids, which can not be produced in the body and must be obtained from the diet. Lysine is abundant in brewer's yeast, dairy products, and wheat germ; fish and other meats; and legumes, specifically soybeans, lima, and kidney beans. A supplement of 500 mg may be taken 1 or 2 times a day, 30 minutes before meals.

Supplements have emerged as major segment of the bone healthcare. They work synergistically with critical pathways of bone metabolism and may reduce risk of bone diseases.

The following section elaborates three extensively studied functional ingredients widely used as functional ingredients in bone health supplements.

Inulin-type fructans *(ITFs)* include inulin, oligofructose, fructooligo-saccharides (FOS), derived from sucrose are one of the best studied functional food ingredients. In humans, there is increasing evidence that the colon can absorb nutritionally significant amounts of calcium, and this process may be susceptible to dietary manipulation by fermentable substrates, especially ITFs.

ITFs have been shown to increase the absorption of several minerals (calcium, magnesium, in some cases phosphorus) and trace elements (mainly copper, iron, zinc), thereby enhance bone health. In recent studies both ITF and calcium prevented loss of *trabecular* bone area induced by estrogen deficiency, this, however, occurred at different *trabecular* shapes. The effects of ITF on mineral metabolism can be attributed to its ability to enhance passive and active mineral transport across the intestinal epithelium, mediated by an increase in certain metabolites of the intestinal flora. ITFs can resist hydrolysis in the gastric lumen *(therefore, also called as non-digestible oligosaccharides)*; and are exclusively fermented in the large intestine. This fermentation produces short-chain fatty acids (in particular, butyric acid), which in turn reduce the luminal pH that modifies calcium solubility, and exerts a direct effect on the mucosal transport pathway. Other mechanisms of ITF-mediated effects include acidification of the lumen, enlargement of the intestinal absorption surface, increased expression of *calcium-binding proteins* mainly in the large intestine, modulated expression of *bone-relevant cytokines*, suppression of bone resorption, increased bioavailability of *phytoestrogens*, and, via stimulation of beneficial commensal microorganisms, increase of calcium uptake by *enterocytes*. ITFs stimulate mineral absorption and bone mineral deposition when combined with *probiotic lactic acid bacteria*.

Intestinal absorption is more pronounced when the body's demand for calcium is high, such as, during stages of rapid growth and in conditions of impaired calcium absorption. Even a small stimulation of calcium absorption may result in the increase of mineral accumulation in the skeleton. Direct comparison of different ITFs revealed that a mixture of a long-chain inulin and fructooligosaccharide *(FOS)* is most effective in enhancing mineral absorption.

Fructans

Probiotics (according to the currently adopted definition by the FAO/WHO) are: live microorganisms which when administered in adequate amounts confer a health benefit on the host. Lactic acid bacteria (LAB) are the most common type of probiotics. LAB have been used in the food industry for many years, due to their ability to ferment sugars (lactose, in particular) and other carbohydrates into lactic acid. This not only provides the characteristic sour taste of fermented dairy foods such as yogurt, but also by lowering the pH may create possible health benefits on preventing gastrointestinal infections. Strains of Lactobacillus and Bifidobacterium, are the most widely used probiotic bacteria.

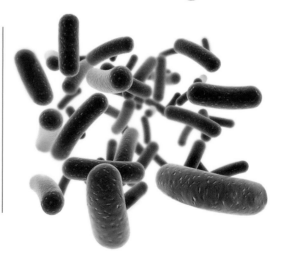

Turmeric

Turmeric comes from the underground stem (rhizome) of the *Curcuma longa* plant, is a powerful medicine that has long been used in the Chinese and Indian systems of medicine. As a natural anti-inflammatory, anti-septic agent, turmeric is widely used in the treatment of several clinical conditions, including flatulence, jaundice, menstrual difficulties, bloody urine, hemorrhage, toothache, bruises, chest pain, and colic.

Curcumin (a volatile yellow oil fraction), 1 of the 3 major phenolic compounds that constitute 3–5% of turmeric, is the primary pharmacological agent. Because of its potent anti-inflammatory properties, curcumin has emerged as a natural treatment for osteoarthritis *(OA)* and rheumatoid arthritis *(RA)*. Several studies have confirmed the anti-inflammatory effects of curcumin, comparable to the potent over-the-counter anti-inflammatory agents. Unlike the drugs, which are associated with significant toxic effects (ulcer formation, decreased white blood cell count, intestinal bleeding), curcumin has no toxicity. As a potent antioxidant, curcumin also has ability to neutralize free radicals that damage various tissues including bone. Free radicals are responsible for the painful joint inflammation and eventual damage to the joints in arthritis. The synergistic combination of antioxidant and anti-inflammatory effects of curcumin can provide relief to most patients with joint disease. Curcumin showed an efficacy comparable to certain *corticosteroids*; accordingly, curcumin treatment has shortened the duration of morning stiffness, improved the walking time, and reduced the joint swelling in rheumatoid arthritis.

A recent study has documented the *in vivo* mechanism of action for the anti-arthritic properties of curcumin-containing extracts. A highly purified curcuminoid containing fraction of turmeric (called *IC-50*) has been reported to be highly potent anti-arthritic compound. This curcuminoid extract can inhibit a *transcription factor* (protein that controls the *switch on and off* of the genes) in the joint. Transcription factor, when turned on (activated), enhances the production of inflammatory chemicals that can destroy the joint. In addition to preventing joint inflammation, this curcuminoid fraction also blocked the metabolic pathway that affects bone resorption. Just as the willow bark provided relief for arthritis patients before the advent of aspirin, it would appear that the underground stem (rhizome) of a tropical plant, turmeric, may also hold promise for the treatment of joint inflammation and destruction.

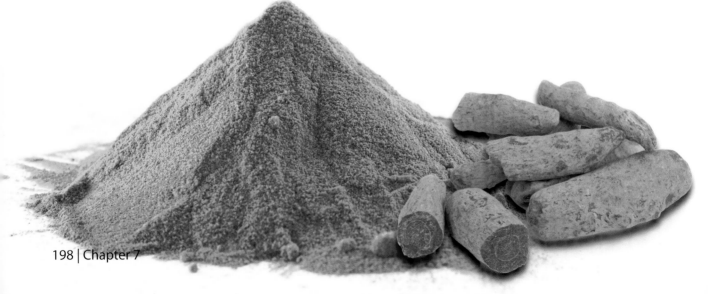

Bromelain is a crude, aqueous extract obtained from both the stem and fruit of the pineapple plant *(Ananas comosus)*, which contains a number of proteolytic enzymes. Bromelain has shown several beneficial effects due to its anti-inflammatory and analgesic properties.

Bromelain seems to work via two different mechanisms: i) it inhibits the release of chemicals that cause inflammation and pain; and ii) it stimulates the breakdown of *fibrin* (a protein-complex that contributes to blood clotting). Fibrin clots reduce blood circulation and prevent the draining of injured tissue. Bromelain's enzyme activity can dissolve fibrin clots, and improve blood flow to clear damaged tissue from the injured body site. Apart from rapid wound healing, the anti-inflammatory action of bromelain is also useful in reducing the pain. Currently, bromelain is used for acute inflammation and sports injuries.

Bromelain has been used as an intervention for a number of medical conditions: to alleviate the symptoms of osteoarthritis *(OA)*, relieve joint stiffness in rheumatoid arthritis *(RA)*, ease the swelling associated with gout, and help sufferers of carpal tunnel syndrome. As an anti-inflammatory agent, bromelain can also be used for sports injury, trauma, and other kinds of swelling. An open study with bromelain intervention *(2 doses x 200 and 400 mg)* for 1-month, in 77 individuals with acute knee pain, showed a significant clinical improvement. Furthermore, mean improvements in total symptom score, stiffness and physical function and psychological well-being were significantly improved.

The many benefits of bromelain come with low risk of side effects, even at high dosages. It has been used in the daily dosage range of 200–2000 mg, with therapeutic action shown at 160 mg/day. Clinical trials assessing bromelain in osteoarthritis have used doses in the range of 540–1890 mg/day. Safety and tolerability at the lower dose appears to be good; data indicates that bromelain at this dose appears to be as effective as standard treatment with at least similar safety and tolerance profiles. Bromelain has been suggested to provide an alternative treatment to non-steroidal anti-inflammatory drugs *(NSAIDs)* for patients with osteoarthritis *(OA)*.

Bromelain can cross the intestinal barrier intact, therefore, its anti-inflammatory effects can be observed outside the digestive tract. Bromelain may be useful in treating minor muscle injuries such as sprains and strains. It's one of the most popular supplements in Germany, where it is approved by the Commission E for the treatment of inflammation and swelling after surgery or injury.

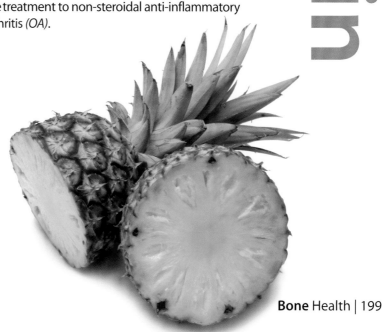

7.6 | Bone Health with **Physical Activity**

Physical activity or routines that cause bones and muscles to work against gravity are called weight-bearing exercises. Resistance exercises such as weight training are also important to improve muscle mass and bone strength. Examples of weight bearing exercises are walking, running, dancing, aerobics and skating. Non-weight bearing exercise include swimming, cycling and water aerobics.

In addition to adequate calcium and vitamin-D intakes, weight bearing exercises are critical to the development, repair and maintenance of healthy bones. Higher bone mass is evident among athletes than non-athletes, and in highly active children compared to those who are sedentary. A similar trend can be observed in retired dancers and gymnasts. Reaching the peak bone mass during early years of life, is likely to offset future development of osteoporosis and bone fragility.

Weight-bearing exercise strongly influences bone health. An astronaut in space can develop osteopenia within 6 weeks due to lack of weight bearing stimulus to the bone.

At the outset, physical activity appears to increase the risk for injury from falls as it involves skeletal muscle movement that displaces the body's center of gravity and balance. Statistically, among the elderly, walking and climbing stairs are the two most common causes of non-fainting falls, which makes up 39% and 20% of falls, respectively. However, physical exercises done with proper training can improve bone density and strength.

Several clinical trials have shown that exercise in elderly women may prevent bone loss and increase BMD significantly. Brisk walking, stepping block training, resistance and strength training provide positive benefits to the BMD of spine. Physical activity in younger elderly population show that not only quantity, but a variety of exercises would help preserve resistance to fractures.

Bone-healthy diet and supplements that help maintain bone mass are not enough. It is also important to engage in weight-bearing exercise to maximize bone strength and bone density to prevent osteoporosis later in life.

Mechanical stresses such as enduring weight or bending are essential aspects of physical activity. These activities mobilize hormones and nutrients to the regions of the body that are undergoing stress. Studies have shown mineral accumulation in such regions of the bone, which eventually increase the bone mass. Therefore, physical activity is crucial in the prevention or even reversal of post-menopausal bone loss.

Weight-bearing activities such as brisk walking and resistance exercises are effective in increasing bone mass and strength. But this effect also declines with age; therefore it is advised to establish an exercise schedule while young and make it a part of the lifestyle. Weight-bearing exercises seem to enhance bone mineral accrual in children, particularly during early puberty.

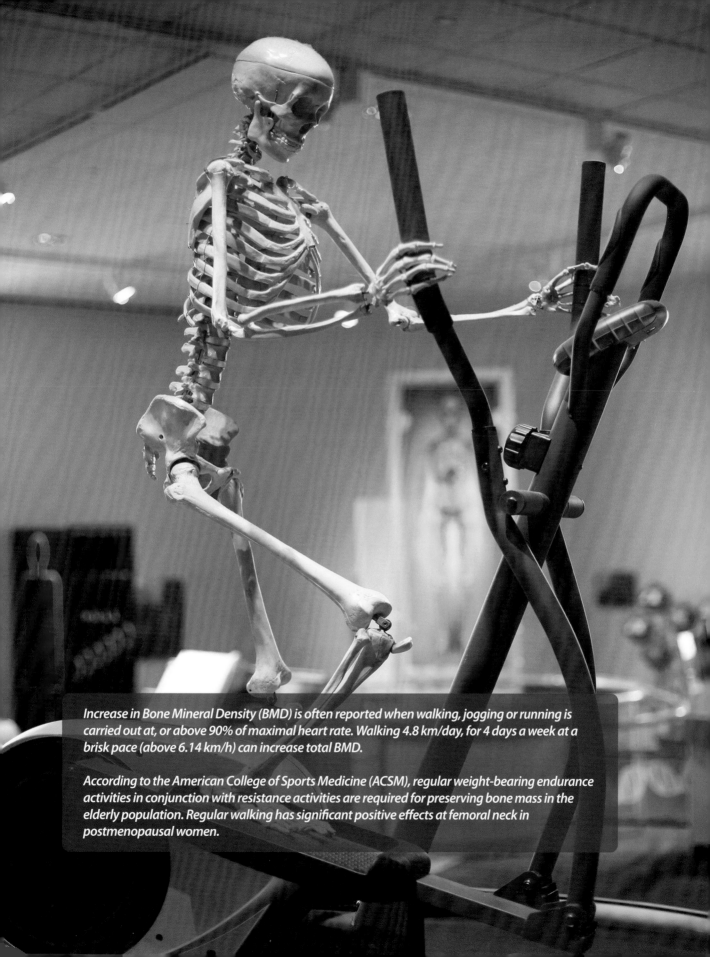

Increase in Bone Mineral Density (BMD) is often reported when walking, jogging or running is carried out at, or above 90% of maximal heart rate. Walking 4.8 km/day, for 4 days a week at a brisk pace (above 6.14 km/h) can increase total BMD.

According to the American College of Sports Medicine (ACSM), regular weight-bearing endurance activities in conjunction with resistance activities are required for preserving bone mass in the elderly population. Regular walking has significant positive effects at femoral neck in postmenopausal women.

Lifestyle factors strongly influence bone health. Sedentary lifestyle will result in bone thinning. The current generation is 'immobilized' in front of a computer screen; a severe compromise with bone function. The human race, in the name of comfort, is gradually leaning towards a sedentary lifestyle with remote controls, mechanical devices that drive, fly and float. The Nature's law of *'use it or lose it'*, with its enforcement (or forced adaption) will cripple the human skeletal system, the one and only bipedal on this Blue Planet.

Dieting habits (e.g. weight loss diets, semi-starvation diets, crash diets) mostly among women, and also some men, attempting to be fashionably thin, can cause serious bone health problems. Patterns of self-imposed undernourishment often begin early in life as adolescents become weight conscious. Body weight is the best predictors of BMD. Low body weight is associated with low peak bone mass development in the young, which eventually poses the risk of increased bone loss and fragility fractures in the adulthood. Body mass index *(BMI)* denotes the relationship between body weight to height and is used to classify individuals as being below or over a healthy range. The risk for hip fractures has almost doubled in people with BMI of 20 kg/m^2, compared to those with BMI of 25 kg/m^2. Overweight adults on a calorie-restricted diet to lose weight, should take proper care to prevent bone loss. Sufficient intake of calcium and vitamin-D, and weight bearing physical activity are highly recommended to individuals on weight loss diets. It is also important to avoid 'fad' diets that eliminate whole foods.

Thin individuals have thin bones. Usually, underweight persons do not consume enough calories to maintain proper body weight; which can result in low BMD.

Anorexia is a form of self-imposed starvation; an extreme end of the current *'slim-fashion mania'.* This eating disorder is also seen as a chronic psychiatric illness. Anorexic youngsters are at high risk of compromised peak bone mass. The extreme body thinness among women can lead to estrogen deficiency and irregular menstruation. In addition, specific nutrient deficiencies and multiple hormonal and metabolic disturbances also enhance the risk for low BMD and fragility fractures.

Anorexic individuals commonly experience a gradual loss of *trabecular* bone at a rate of about 3% per year. The bone loss is even greater during periods of hospitalization and tube-feeding; following such condition a woman might lose about 17% *trabecular* bone. Anorexic patients have an annual fracture rate 7 times higher than healthy individuals of the same age. Young female athletes, gymnasts, and fashion models, who indulge in

Excessive bone loss, similar to menopause; is one of the several health problems that stems from anorexia. Even after recovery, normal bone density is not gained and fracture risk will remain throughout life.

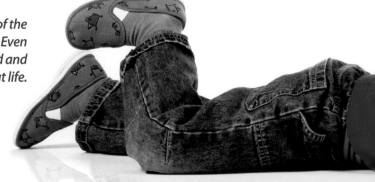

extreme dieting are prone to fractures, tend to become osteoporotic, and jeopardize the skeletal integrity. Adolescence is the time of life when peak bone mass is achieved. Early diagnosis of anorexia and corrective measures are necessary for prevention of bone health issues later in life.

Lactose Intolerance is a disability to digest the milk sugar, *lactose*, in the diet due to the deficiency of an enzyme called *'lactase'*, present in the small intestine. Lactase, produced in the small intestine, is responsible for breaking down lactose into simple sugars for absorption in the body. Lactose intolerance is a potential risk factor for bone loss and osteoporosis, due to non-consumption of dairy products and reduced bioavailability of calcium. About 30 and 50 million Americans are lactose intolerant and this condition is more prevalent among Asian, African, and American Indian populations. Secondary lactase deficiency can also occur due to injury to the small intestine or certain digestive disorders.

Diets for lactose or milk intolerant population should consume non-dairy foods that are rich in calcium, mostly dark green vegetables such as broccoli, or fish with soft, edible bones, such as salmon and sardines. Their dietary regimen should also include an adequate supply of vitamin-D from sources such as eggs and liver; and/or with enough exposure to sun light. Another alternative is to take the lactase enzyme (in caplet or droplet form) to aid the digestion of lactose. These pills are either chewed before eating a dairy product or added to milk before drink

Fast food, typically a meal with burger, fries, drink and dessert; provides almost a daily recommended intake of calories and fats in one serving. Eating too many acid-forming foods (protein, refined flours and sugars) and inadequate alkalizing foods (fruits, vegetables, seaweeds) to counter balance the acidity can trigger bone loss. The high calories and amounts of fat content can contribute to weight gain and obesity, which in turn an affect bone health. High sodium in fast food increases excretion of calcium from bones, and refined sugar also predisposes the risk of bone loss.

Fast foods contain large amounts of fat, sodium and sugar; three ingredients that earned the notoriety as the 'bone robbers'.

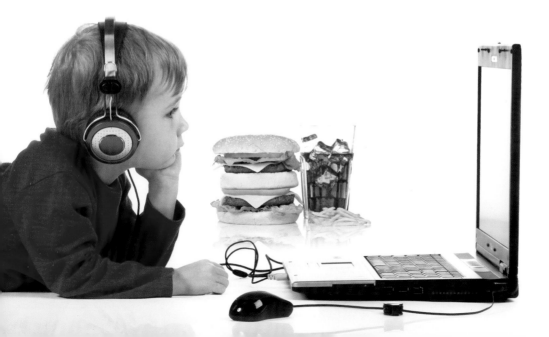

Oral Health defines the true qualitative aspect of a human wellbeing. After all, mouth is the *'bony gateway'* to process a wide range of chemicals, including nutrients to sustain life. Human teeth reflect a myriad of characteristics: body size, disease, stress, nutritional status, climate, age, eating behavior, cause and time of death, and evolution. Dental pattern is strongly associated with social behavior; whereas facial display reflects aggression, happiness, class, and status.

Oral bone, like rest of the skeleton, consists of both *trabecular* and *cortical* bone; it also undergoes bone formation and bone resorption throughout the life span. The portion of jaw bone that anchors teeth is known as the *alveolar* process. However, when the oral bone loss exceeds gain, jaw bone becomes less dense. The loss of alveolar bone is linked to an increase in loose teeth (tooth mobility) and tooth loss. The upper jaw is more susceptible to bone loss than the lower jaw. Low alveolar bone density can create other dental problems. The extent of alveolar bone changes with normal aging are similar to that occur with other bones in the skeletal system. Dental bone loss and subsequent tooth loss is associated with periodontal diseases, estrogen deficiency and osteoporosis.

Prevalence of oral bone loss is significant among adult populations worldwide, and it increases with age for both sexes. As much as 94% of women in the US over 65 years of age, have dental bone loss.

Periodontitis is a chronic infection that affects gums and bones that anchor teeth. Bacteria and body's own immune system break down the bone and connective tissue that hold teeth in the oral cavity. Periodontitis involves progressive loss of the alveolar bone around the teeth, and if untreated, can lead to loosening and subsequent loss of teeth. It is possible that the loss of alveolar bone mineral density *(BMD)* leaves bone more susceptible to periodontal bacteria, increasing the risk for periodontitis and tooth loss. Periodontitis is the leading cause of tooth loss among adults.

Osteoporosis and oral bone loss, both are asymptomatic with diagnosis usually made after the problem has established. Both conditions cause significant bone loss in middle-aged or older persons. These two diseases have many similar pathological mechanisms that initiate bone resorption. Women with osteoporosis are three times more likely to experience tooth loss than without the disease.

It is not known whether osteoporosis treatments have similar beneficial effect on oral health. Of concern are *bisphosphonates*, a group of medications widely used for osteoporosis treatment, have been linked to the clinical onset of *osteonecrosis of the jaw (ONJ)*. The risk of ONJ has been high among patients administered with large doses of intravenous bisphosphonates, commonly used in cancer therapy. The occurrence of ONJ is rare among individuals taking oral forms of medication to treat osteoporosis.

The current grocery practices tend to pick fruits and nuts in a *'green'* (or unripen) state for convenient transport. This 'green' state grocery is highly acidic, which can leach minerals from the body and create deficiencies that affect dentition (including tooth enamel). Full ripening of fruit is required for delignification of secondary cell walls and access to nutrients.

Damage to the enamel occurs through exposure to acidic diets and bacterial infection. When the damaged enamel is not repaired, the dentin is prone to mechanical injury or erosion. Eventually, the dentin will be perforated and expose the pulp cavity to infection. Oral infection can spread to the surrounding jaw bone and cause tooth loss.

A number of essential minerals and trace elements are leached out of the food by cooking. Our paleolithic ancestors consumed twice the calcium and far more potassium than we do today, which may have actively protected them against dental diseases.

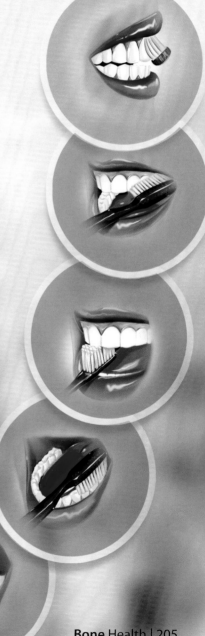

Oral bone health management includes proper care of the teeth, jaw bones and mouth on a regular basis. Maintenance of good oral health requires that the teeth are free from cavities and the gums free from disease. To maintain healthy teeth and a healthy oral cavity, one needs to take the following steps:

- *Floss* the teeth prior to brushing. This can remove particles that a toothbrush cannot reach. About 90% of problems arise from areas between the teeth.
- *Brush* at least twice a day - for at least 5 minutes - first thing in the morning and last thing at night. The best toothbrush is one with a small head and soft bristles.
- *Rinse* the mouth twice a day, after brushing. Choose an alcohol-free mouthwash and be sure to pick an anti-cavity option.
- *Drink* fluorinated water and use fluoride toothpaste. Fluoride's protection against tooth decay is well documented for all ages.
- Chew sugar-free gum in between brushing after meals. This can help remove plaque, and it is beneficial to oral health.
- If medications produce a dry mouth (e.g. diabetes); drink plenty of water, chew sugarless gum, and avoid tobacco and alcohol.
- *Eat wisely*. Adults should avoid snacks full of sugars and starches.
- Visit the dentist regularly. Check-ups can detect early signs of oral health problems and can lead to treatments that can prevent further damage, and in some cases, reverse the problem.
- Dental plaque when hardens on the teeth, is called *tartar* or *calculus*. This needs a professional cleaning (scaling the tartar off) from a Dental Hygienist or Dentist.

7.9 | Bone Health **Disruptors**

Due to human ignorance it seems that for the luxuries of modern life we will have to accept increased outbreaks of new diseases, including the emergence of bone metabolic disorders. Addictive factors, such as alcohol, narcotics, tobacco and caffeine can take major toll on the skeletal system.It has been reported that exhaled tobacco smoke contains more than 3800 chemicals, including numerous carcinogens.

Many bone metabolic disruptors have been implicated in the emerging bone disorders: hormones in food, hormone-mimicking pollutants in the waterways, and pesticides in the environment. When precocious puberty entered the radar screen in the early 1990s, the first suspects were hormones in milk and meats, particularly the recombinant bovine growth hormone *(rBGH)*. Bones can be considered older in individuals with early puberty beyond actual age of individual. Early puberty is marked by growth hormone problems, which may lead to an array of skeletal disorders

By 2020, predictions are that tobacco will cause 10 million deaths per year worldwide.

Prevalence of endocrine disrupting chemicals in our environment, especially, in our potable water supplies is a serious threat. The resulting hormonal disorders can also affect the skeleton in multiple ways. Several other factors can also interfere with the development of a strong and healthy skeleton. Genetic abnormalities can produce weak, thin bones, or bones that are too dense. Nutritional deficiencies can result in the formation of weak, poorly mineralized bone. The diet-repulsive, "thin body-craze" anorexic individuals are at high risk of contracting bone metabolic disorders. Lack of exercise, immobilization, and smoking can also have negative effects on bone mass and strength.

Certain foods and beverages interfere with calcium absorption. The list includes heavily salted foods such as bacon, salami, smoked salmon, prepared soups, salty snacks and other processed food. It is recommended to consume less than 4,000 mg of sodium a day. Cola beverages contain phosphoric acid that impairs calcium absorption, while caffeine can actually deplete calcium from the body. Alcohol in excess has adverse effects on bone health, either, because it damages bones or it could increase the risk trip over and falls

The theory that chemicals in the environment may be disrupting hormones and causing health problems in humans was first published in 1992. Since that time, the general concept of endocrine disruption has gone from a radical theory to an accepted fact. Endocrine disruptors are chemicals in our environment that interfere with hormones. Endocrine disruptors include natural phytoestrogens (estrogen-like chemicals that are made by plants) or synthetic chemicals used in medications, dietary supplements, cosmetics, and household products. Endocrine disruptors can interfere with bone regulatory hormones (i.e. estrogen, testosterone, PTH, calcitonin, thyroxin, etc); which may lead to severe bone disorders.

Alcohol can cause several detrimental effects on the bone. Alcohol inhibits liver enzymes that convert vitamin-D into active form; which can hamper calcium absorption. As a result, chronic alcoholism leads to poor mineral absorption and increased excretion of important bone-building nutrients like calcium, magnesium, vitamin-C, zinc and copper. Alcohol can also block vitamin-B6 function. Alcohol is directly toxic to bone cells, and cause a decline in the spongy inner matrix of the *trabecular* bone.

Currently, there is conflicting evidence on beneficial effects of moderate alcohol consumption on the bone health. Alcohol derived from wine has favorable effects on the level of *high-density lipoprotein (HDL) cholesterol* and inhibition of platelet aggregation. In the elderly population, there seems to be a direct correlation between wine consumption and preservation of BMD. Red wine has high levels of phenolic compounds that positively influence multiple biochemical systems, such as increased HDL cholesterol, antioxidant activity, decreased platelet aggregation and endothelial adhesion, suppression of cancer cell growth, and promotion of nitric oxide production.

In contrast, higher levels of alcohol intake – more than two standard units of alcohol per day, can significantly increase the risk of hip and other osteoporotic fractures. Excess alcohol intake has direct detrimental effects on bone-forming cells and on hormones that regulate calcium metabolism. In addition, chronic, heavy alcohol consumption is associated with reduced food intake (including low calcium, vitamin-D and protein intakes) and overall poor nutritional status, which in turn have adverse effects on skeletal health. Excess alcohol use can influence body balance and predispose the dangers of trip over, thereby increases the risk of fractures. However, available data is insufficient to indicate the precise range of alcohol consumption that would maximize bone density and minimize hip fracture risk.

According to the CDC National Health Interview Survey, overall, 61% of US adults were current drinkers, about 15% were former drinkers and about 5% were heavier drinkers. Current drinking was most prevalent among adults aged 25-44 years for both men (76%) and women (63%).

Alcohol

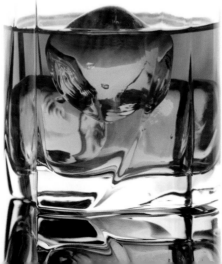
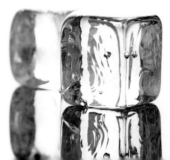

Smoking

Smoking and its relation to the onset of bone disease is complex; also various risk factors often co-exist. Body wise, smokers are thinner than non-smokers, physically less active and consume poor diet. Women smokers tend to reach early menopause than non-smokers. Among smokers, fractures take longer time to repair with several complications during the healing process. Regular tobacco use and smoking cause a significant decrease in blood total alkaline phosphatase *(ALP)*, an indicator of bone metabolism. Although not confirmed yet, exposure to second-hand smoke during youth and early adulthood may increase the risk of acquiring low bone mass.

Smoking elevates nicotine levels in the body that cause blood vessels to constrict by approximately 25% of the normal diameter. Due to this constriction, the blood flow is reduced; consequently the supply of nutrients, minerals, and oxygen to bone tissue is diminished, which may slow down the production of bone-forming cells. In post-menopausal women, it reduces the protective effect of estrogen replacement therapy and may double the risk of rheumatoid arthritis.

Nicotine and other harmful chemicals in cigarettes affect bone health in several ways. Cigarette smoke generates huge amounts of free radicals with devastating effects on the body's natural defenses. Free radicals trigger a chain-reaction that damage tissue, organs, and hormones (e.g. estrogen) that regulate bones health. Other bone-damaging effects of smoking include elevation of the *cortisol* levels (hormone that regulates bone breakdown); and slowing down the *calcitonin* (hormone that helps to build bones). Nicotine and free radicals generated by smoking also kill the *osteoblasts* (bone making cells). Nicotine can also damage nerves in toes and feet, which may increase the risk of falls and fractures.

Smoking increases the body's toxic burden of cadmium, lead, nicotine, and other toxic substances that interfere with calcium absorption and directly damage bone. Bone building is a slow process; it may take several years to lower the risk for bone loss even after an individual quits smoking. Some of the nicotine-induced damage may also be irreversible.

Caffeine is a stimulant present in a wealth of drinks such as tea and coffee. It has been linked to a number of possible health benefits for heart and memory as well as certain detrimental effects.

Caffeine is often implicated in the development of osteoporosis, due to its effect on calcium absorption. It can temporarily increase calcium excretion and may modestly decrease calcium absorption, but these effects are easily offset by increasing calcium consumption in the diet. Controlled clinical studies show that although caffeine ingestion results in a small, temporary increase in calcium excretion, it has no effect on 24-hour urinary calcium loss. One cup of regular brewed coffee causes a loss of only 2-3 mg of calcium which is easily offset by adding a tablespoon of milk. Moderate caffeine consumption, (1 cup of coffee or 2 cups of tea per day), in young women who have adequate calcium intakes would not have any negative effects on their bones. Studies that examined the effects of caffeine on rates of bone loss in post-menopausal women showed that caffeine intake had no detrimental effects, as long as calcium intake is sufficient (above 800 mg/day). However, if calcium intake is low, caffeine intake equivalent to about 3 cups of brewed coffee per day is associated with significant bone loss.

A standard can of Cola drink contains 34-38 mg of caffeine. The potential for acute caffeine toxicity may be greater with the consumption of "energy drinks" (stimulants and boosters) than conventional dietary sources of caffeine, like coffee and tea. Caffeine intoxication has been linked to a number of symptoms like nervousness, anxiety, restlessness, insomnia, gastrointestinal upset etc. which closely resemble symptoms of anxiety and mood disorders.

Caffeine

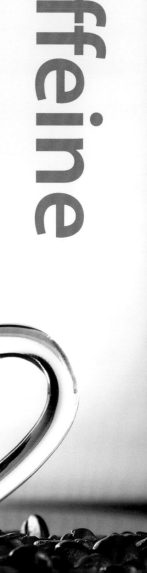

Bone Health
DISRUPTORS

Soda Drinks

Soda drinks, high in phosphate content, are perhaps the most pervasive habit that promotes a calcium drain in the body. Phosphorus, an acid-forming mineral in the cola drinks, can interfere with calcium absorption by the bone and set off calcium loss through urinary excretion. Some studies have reported that high carbonated soft drink consumption either increased the fracture risk or decreased the bone mineral density (BMD). A recent study of soft drink consumption in adolescents suggested that teenage girls who drink lots of soda are predisposed to the risk of developing bone fractures and osteoporosis. These drinks also contain large amounts of refined sugar or equally dangerous sugar substitutes, which can trigger bone loss. During the teenage years, 40 to 60 per cent of peak bone mass is built, and therefore, it is very important to avoid or limit soda intake and change to a natural calcium-rich diet.

On the other hand, studies done with controlled calcium-metabolic methods indicated that the net effect of carbonated soft drinks, including those colas with phosphoric acid on calcium retention is low. An "acidic diet" causes minerals to be drawn from the bones to neutralize the impact of the acid on blood pH. The body normally produces 50 to 100 mEq of acid a day during metabolism. The acid load imposed by a 20-ounce cola is only about 4.5 to 5.0 mEq, substantially less than the amount produced by eating a moderate protein breakfast.

Phosphorus is a key constituent of bone mineral along with calcium, and there is no evidence for detrimental effects of phosphorus intake on bone health or osteoporosis risk in healthy individuals. The possible adverse effect of carbonated beverages may be due to substitution of milk in the diet by these drinks, which reduces calcium intake. Carbonation itself is also not responsible for the calcium depletion, as many commercial mineral waters are carbonated, and some are rich in calcium and other minerals.

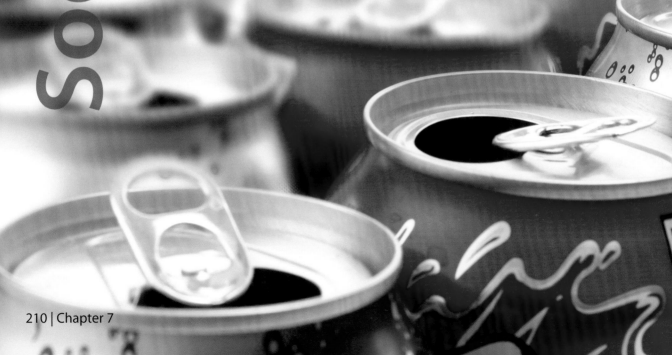

In conclusion, several intrinsic and extrinsic factors play a cumulative role in the management of bone health. Bio-replenishment is undoubtedly the most critical of the intrinsic factors necessary for maintaining the bone metabolic homeostasis.

Diet has a significant impact on the overall health outcomes. Sufficient amounts of calcium and phosphorus, components of hydroxyapatite, the primary salt that makes bones hard, must be included in the diet. Because of the rapid bone development during early childhood, children need adequate calcium intake to reach peak bone mass and decrease their risk of osteoporosis and skeletal fractures in later life. While calcium has found a strong voice in the bone health campaign, the elemental role of magnesium in calcium transport has been ignored. Epidemiologic studies have clearly shown a direct correlation between magnesium intake and increased BMD

Vitamins (especially, A, C, D, E, and K) play a major role in the homeostasis of bone building in different ways. The ever growing indoor activities in our society and the widespread use of sunscreens have already led to a global pandemic of vitamin-D deficiency. There is a dire necessity to revise the current RDA for vitamin-D supplementation and bring global awareness to this health concern.

In the milk-smeared upper lips of its celebrities, the industry campaign to cure osteoporosis is a far fetched reality. It will be of interest to evaluate the effects of newer anabolic agents that enhance formation as well as resorption, such as the R-ELF replenishment and injections of teriparatide (PTH) hormone. Finally, physicians need to remember that interventions in the home to prevent accidents for patients with poor vision, sensory and motor neuropathy, and orthostatic hypotension may well contribute more to reducing the risk for serious fractures than any metabolic intervention.

Decade of the Bone and Joint

Musculoskeletal conditions are the most common causes of severe long-term pain and physical disability, affecting hundreds of million of people across the world. The impact from bone and joint disorders on society, the healthcare system and on the individual led to a proposal for the *Decade of the Bone and Joint from 2000-2010*. The goal of this global program is to improve the health-related quality of life for people with musculoskeletal disorders by raising awareness, empowering patients to participate in their health care, promoting cost-effective prevention and treatment.

7.1 | BONE HEALTH MANAGEMENT

1. Food and Nutrition Board, National Research Council, National Academy of Science (1989) Recommended daily allowances, (10th ed). Washington, DC: National Academy Press.
2. U.S. Department of Agriculture, Human Nutrition Information Service (1992) Food Guide Pyramid (Home and Garden Bulletin Number 252, supersedes HG-249.)
3. U.S. Department of Health and Human Services. Healthy People 2010. Washington (DC): January 2000.
4. Wright JD, Wang CY, Kennedy-Stevenson J, Ervin RB (2003) Dietary intakes of ten key nutrients for public health, United States: 1999-2000. *Advanced Data* 334:1-4.

7.2 | BONE HEALTH NUTRITION

1. Committee on Nutrition, American Academy of Pediatrics (1992) The use of whole cow's milk in infancy. *Pediatrics* 89:1105.
2. Palacios C (2006) The role of nutrients in bone health, from A to Z. *Critical Reviews in Food Science and Nutrition* 46(8):621-628.
3. Chan GM, Hoffman K, McMurry M (1995) Effects of dairy products on bone and body composition in pubertal girls. *Journal of Pediatrics* 126(4):551-556.
4. Merrilees MJ, Smart EJ, Gilchrist NL, et al (2000) Effects of dairy food supplements on bone mineral density in teenage girls. *European Journal of Nutrition* 39(6):256-62.
5. Heaney RP (2000) Calcium, dairy products and osteoporosis. *Journal of American College of Nutrition*19:83S-99S.
6. Cadogan J, Eastell R, Jones N, Barker M (1997) Milk intake and bone mineral acquisition in adolescent girls: randomized controlled intervention trial. *British Medical Journal* 315:1255-1260
7. Lau EMC, Woo J, Lam V, Hong A (2001) Milk supplementation of the diet of postmenopausal Chinese women on a low calcium intake retards bone loss. *Journal of Bone and Mineral Research*16:1704-1709.
8. Alekel DL,Germain AS, et al (2000) Isoflavone-rich soy protein isolate attenuates bone loss in the lumbar spine of perimenopausal women. *American Journal of Clinical Nutrition* 72(3):844-852.
9. Wangen KE, Duncan AM, et al (2000) Effects of soy isoflavones on markers of bone turnover in premenopausal and postmenopausal women. *Journal of Clinical Endocrinology and Metabolism* 85(9): 3043-3048.
10. Arjmandi BH, Smith BJ (2002) Soy isoflavones' osteoprotective role in postmenopausal women: mechanism of action. *Journal of Nutritional Biochemistry* 13(3):130-137.
11. Lydeking-Olsen E, Beck-Jensen J-E, Setchell KDR, Holm-Jensen T (2004) Soymilk or progesterone for prevention of bone loss: A 2 year randomized, placebo-controlled trial. *European Journal of Nutrition* 43:246-257.
12. Sellmeyer DE, Stone, KL, Sebastian A, Cummings SR (2001) A high ratio of dietary animal to vegetable protein increases the rate of bone loss and the risk of fracture in postmenopausal women. Study of the Osteoporotic Fractures Group. *American Journal of Clinical Nutrition* 73(1):118-122.
13. New SA, Robins SP, Campbell MK, et al (2000) Dietary influences on bone mass and bone metabolism: Further evidence of a positive link between fruit and vegetable consumption and bone health? *American Journal of Clinical Nutrition* 71(1):142-151.

14. Rizzoli R, Bonjour JP. Dietary protein and bone health (2004) *Journal of Bone and Mineral Research* 19(4):527-531.
15. Hannan MT, Tucker KL, Dawson-Hughes B, et al (2000) Effect of dietary protein on bone loss in elderly men and women: the Framingham Osteoporosis Study. *Journal of Bone and Mineral Research* 15(12):2504-2512.
16. Dawson-Hughes B, Harris SS, Rasmussen H, et al (2004) Effect of dietary protein supplements on calcium excretion in healthy older men and women. *Journal of Clinical Endocrinology and Metabolism* 89(3):1169-1173.
17. Roughead ZK, Johnson LK, Lykken GI, Hunt JR (2003) Controlled high meat diets do not affect calcium retention or indices of bone status in healthy postmenopausal women. *Journal of Nutrition* 133(4):1020-1026.

7.3 | BONE HEALTH VITAMINS

1. Bischoff-Ferrari HA, Dawson-Hughes B, Willett WC, et al (2004) Effect of Vitamin D on falls: A meta-analysis. *Journal of American Medical Association* 291(16):1999-2006.
2. Dawson-Hughes B, Harris SS, Krall EA, Dallal GE (1997) Effect of calcium and vitamin D supplementation on bone density in men and women 65 years of age or older. *New England Journal of Medicine* 337(10):670-676.
3. Gartner LM, Greer FR, Section on Breastfeeding and Committee on Nutrition (2003) Prevention of rickets and vitamin D deficiency: New guidelines for vitamin D intake. *Pediatrics* 111:908-910.
4. Ooms ME, Roos JC, Bezemer PD, et al (1995) Prevention of bone loss by vitamin D supplementation in elderly women: A randomized double-blind trial. *Journal of Clinical Endocrinology and Metabolism* 80(4):1052-8.
5. Rejnmark L, Vestergaard P, Hermann AP, et al (2008) Dietary intake of folate, but not vitamin B2 or B12, is associated with increased bone mineral density 5 years after the menopause: results from a 10-year follow-up study in early postmenopausal women. *Calcified Tissue International* 82(1):1-11.
6. Sugiyama T, Tanaka H, Taguchi T (2005) Folate and vitamin B12 for hip fracture prevention after stroke. *Journal of American Medical Association* 294(7):792.
7. Sato Y, Honda Y, Iwamoto J, et al (2005) Effect of folate and mecobalamin on hip fractures in patients with stroke: a randomized controlled trial. *Journal of American Medical Association* 293(9):1082-1088.
8. Bügel S (2008) Vitamin K and bone health in adult humans. *Vitamins and Hormones* 78:393-416.
9. Francucci CM, Rilli S, Fiscaletti P, Boscaro M (2007) Role of vitamin K on biochemical markers, bone mineral density, and fracture risk. *Journal of Endocrinological Investigation* 30(6 Suppl):24-28.
10. Cockayne S, Adamson J, Lanham-New S, et al (2006) Vitamin K and the prevention of fractures: systematic review and meta-analysis of randomized controlled trials. *Archives of Internal Medicine* 166(12):1256-1261.
11. Cashman KD (2005) Vitamin K status may be an important determinant of childhood bone health. *Nutrition Reviews* 63(8):284-289.
12. Sahni S, Hannan MT, Gagnon D, et al (2008) High vitamin C intake is associated with lower 4-year bone loss in elderly men. *Journal of Nutrition* 138(10):1931-1938.
13. Turan B, Can B, Delilbasi E (2003) Selenium combined with vitamin E and vitamin C restores structural alterations of bones in heparin-induced osteoporosis. *Clinical Rheumatology* 22(6):432-436.

7.4 | BONE HEALTH MINERALS

1. Heany RP, Recker RR, Inders SM (1988) Variability of calcium absorption. *American Journal of Clinical Nutrition* 47:262-264.
2. Johnston CC, Miller JZ, Slemenda CW, et al (1992) Calcium supplementation and increases in bone mineral density in children. *The New England Journal of Medicine* 327:82-87.
3. Lloyd T, Andon MB, Rollings N, et al (1993) Calcium supplementation and bone mineral density in adolescent girls. *Journal of the American Medical Association* 270:841-844.
4. Recker RR, Bammi A, Barger-Lux MJ, Heany RP (1988) Calcium absorbability from milk products, an imitation milk, and calcium carbonate. *American Journal of Clinical Nutrition* 47:93-95.
5. Heaney RP (2001) Constructive interactions among nutrients and bone-active pharmacologic agents with principal emphasis on calcium, phosphorus, vitamin D and protein. *Journal of American College of Nutrition* 20(5 Suppl):403S-4039S.
6. Heaney RP (2004) Phosphorus nutrition and the treatment of osteoporosis. *Mayo Clinical Proceedings* 79(1):91-97.
7. Institute of Medicine (1997) Dietary reference intakes for calcium, phosphorus, magnesium, vitamin D, and fluoride. Washington, DC: *National Academy of Sciences*; pp. 432.
8. Lee WT, Leung SS, Leung DM, et al (1995) A randomized double blind controlled calcium supplementation trial and bone and height acquisition in children. *British Journal of Nutrition* 74(1):125-39.
9. Beverley S, Wells G, Cranney A, et al (2002) Meta-analysis of calcium supplementation for the prevention of postmenopausal osteoporosis. *Endocrinology Reviews* 23:552-559.
10. Tucker KL, Hannan MT, Chen H, et al (1999) Potassium, magnesium, and fruit and vegetable intakes are associated with greater bone mineral density in elderly men and women. *American Journal of Clinical Nutrition* 69(4):727-36.
11. Nielsen FH, Milne DB (2004) A moderately high intake compared to a low intake of zinc depresses magnesium balance and alters indices of bone turnover in postmenopausal women. *European Journal of Clinical Nutrition* 58(5):703-710.
12. Merialdi M, Caulfield LE, Zavaleta N, et al (2004) Randomized controlled trial of prenatal zinc supplementation and fetal bone growth. *American Journal of Clinical Nutrition* 79(5):826-830.
13. O'Flaherty EJ, Kerger BD, Hays SM, Paustenbach DJ (2001) A physiologically based model for the ingestion of chromium(III) and chromium(VI) by humans. *Toxicological Sciences* 60(2):196-213.
14. Travers RL, Rennie GC, Newnham RE (1990) Boron and arthritis: the result of a double-blind pilot study. *Journal of Nutritional Medicine* 1:127–132.
15. Newnham RE (1994) Essentiality of boron for healthy bones and joints. *Environmental Health Perspectives* 102 (Suppl 7):83-85.

7.5 | BONE HEALTH SUPPLEMENTS

1. Abrams SA, Griffin IJ, Hawthorne KM (2007) Young adolescents who respond to an inulin-type fructan substantially increase total absorbed calcium and daily calcium accretion to the skeleton. *Journal of Nutrition* 137(11 Suppl):2524S-2526S.
2. Abrams SA, Griffin IJ, Hawthorne KM, et al (2005) A combination of prebiotic short- and long-chain inulin-type fructans enhances calcium absorption and bone mineralization in young adolescents. *American Journal of Clinical Nutrition* 82(2):471-476.

3. Coxam V (2005) Inulin-type fructans and bone health: state of the art and perspectives in the management of osteoporosis. *British Journal of Nutrition* 93 (Suppl 1):S111-23.

4. Coxam V (2007) Current data with inulin-type fructans and calcium, targeting bone health in adults. *Journal of Nutrition*137(11 Suppl):2527S-2533S.

5. Griffin IJ, Hicks PMD, Heaney RP, Abrams SA (2003) Enriched chicory inulin increases calcium absorption mainly in girls with lower calcium absorption. *Nutrition Research* 23:901–909.

6. Weaver CM (2005) Inulin, oligofructose and bone health: experimental approaches and mechanisms. *British Journal of Nutrition* 93 (Suppl 1):S99-103.

7. Naidu AS, Xie X, Leumer DA, et al(2002) Reduction of sulfide, ammonia compounds, and adhesion properties of Lactobacillus casei strain KE99 in vitro. *Current Microbiology* 44(3):196-205.

8. Naidu AS, Bidlack WR, Clemens RA (1999) Probiotic spectra of lactic acid bacteria (LAB). *Critical Reviews in Food Science and Nutrition* 39(1):13-126.

9. Walker AF, Bundy R, Hicks SM, Middleton RW (2002) Bromelain reduces mild acute knee pain and improves well-being in a dose-dependent fashion in an open study of otherwise healthy adults. *Phytomedicine* 9:681-686.

10. Brien S, Lewith G, Walker AF, et al (2006) Bromelain as an adjunctive treatment for moderate-to-severe osteoarthritis of the knee: a randomized placebo-controlled pilot study. *Quarterly Journal of Medicine* 99(12):841-850.

11. Brien S, Lewith G, Walker A, et al (2004). Bromelain as a Treatment for Osteoarthritis: a Review of Clinical Studies. *Evidence-based Complementary and Alternative Medicine: eCAM* 1(3):251–257.

12. Taussig SJ, Batkin S (1988) Bromelain, the enzyme complex of Pineapple (Ananas comusus) and its clinical application. An update. *Journal of Ethnopharmacology* 22:191-230.

13. Cohen A, Goldman J (1964) Bromelain therapy in rheumatoid arthritis *Pennsylvania Medical Journal* 67:27-30.

14. Funk JL, Frye JB, Oyarzo JN, et al (2006) Efficacy and mechanism of action of turmeric supplements in the treatment of experimental arthritis. *Arthritis and Rheumatology* 54(11):3452-3464.

15. Funk JL, Oyarzo JN, Frye JB, et al (2006) Turmeric extracts containing curcuminoids prevent experimental rheumatoid arthritis. *Journal of Natural Products* 69(3):351-355.

16. Anand P, Thomas SG, Kunnumakkara AB, et al (2008) Biological activities of curcumin and its analogues (Congeners) made by man and Mother Nature. *Biochemical Pharmacology* 76(11):1590-1611.

7.6 | PHYSICAL ACTIVITY AND BONE HEALTH

1. Bass SL, Saxon L, Daly RM, et al (2002) The effect of mechanical loading on the size and shape of bone in pre, peri, and post-pubertal girls: A study in tennis players. *Journal of Bone and Mineral Research* 17(12):2274-2280.

2. Bassey E, Ramsdale S (1994) Increase in femoral bone density in young women following high-impact exercise. *Osteoporosis International* 4(2):72-75.

3. Kelley GA, Kelley KS, Tran ZV (2001) Resistance training and bone mineral density in women: A meta-analysis of controlled trials. *American Journal of Physical Medicine and Rehabilitation* 80(1):65-77.

4. Specker BL (1996) Evidence for an interaction between calcium intake and physical activity on changes in bone mineral density. *Journal Bone and Mineral Research* 11(10):1539-1544.

5. Wolff I, van Croonenborg JJ, Kemper HC, et al (1999) The effect of exercise training programs on bone mass: A meta-analysis of published controlled trials in pre- and

postmenopausal women. *Osteoporosis International* 9(1):1-12.

6. Wallace BA, Cumming RG (2000) Systematic review of randomized trials of the effect of exercise on bone mass in pre- and postmenopausal women. *Calcified Tissue International* 67(1):10-18.

7.7 | LIFESTYLE AND BONE HEALTH

1. Kiebzak GM (1991) Age-related bone changes. *Journal of Clinical Experimental Gerontology* 26:171-187.
2. Wardlaw G (1988) The effects of diet and lifestyle on bone mass in women. *Journal of the American Dietetic Association* 44:283-286.
3. Wild RA, Buchanan JR, Myers C, Demers LM (1987) Declining adrenal androgens: An association with bone loss in aging women. *Proceedings of Society of Experimental Biology and Medicine* 186(3):355–360.
4. Salamone LM, Cauley JA, Black DM, et al (1999) Effect of a lifestyle intervention on bone mineral density in premenopausal women: A randomized trial. *American Journal of Clinical Nutrition* 70(1):97-103.

7.8 | ORAL BONE HEALTH

1. Loza J, Carpio L, Dziak R (1996) Osteoporosis and its relationship to oral bone loss. *Periodontology* 3:27-33.
2. Kresci C (1996) Osteoporosis and periodontal disease: Is there a relationship? *Periodontal Abstracts,* 44(2):3742.
3. Southard K (2000) Bone density changes in the jaw. *Journal of Dental Research* 79(4): 964-969.
4. Wynn R (2000) Osteoporosis, alvelar bone loss and drug development. *Journal of General Dentistry,* 48(3): 218-222.
5. Geurs NC, Lewis CE, Jeffcoat MK (2003) Osteoporosis and periodontal disease progression. *Periodontology 2000* 32:105-110.

7.9 | DISRUPTORS

1. Felson DT, Zhang Y, Hannan MT, et al (1995)Alcohol intake and bone mineral density in elderly men and women: The Framingham Study. *American Journal of Epidemiology* 142(5):485-492.
2. Sampson HW (2002) Alcohol and other factors affecting osteoporosis risk in women. *Alcohol Research and Health* 26(4):292-298.
3. Schapira D (1990) Alcohol abuse and osteoporosis. *Seminars in Arthritis Rheumatism* 19(6):371–376.
4. Brot C, Jorgensen NR, Sorensen OH (1999) The influence of smoking on vitamin D status and calcium metabolism. *European Journal of Clinical Nutrition* 53(12):920-926.
5. Kanis JA, Johnell O, Oden A, et al (2005) Smoking and fracture risk: A meta-analysis. *Osteoporosis International* 16(2):155-162.
6. Krall EA, Dawson-Hughes B (1999) Smoking increases bone loss and decreases intestinal calcium absorption. *Journal of Bone and Mineral Research* 14(2):215-220.
7. Law MR, Hackshaw AK (1997) A meta-analysis of cigarette smoking, bone mineral density and risk of hip fracture: Recognition of a major effect. *British Medical Journal* 315(7114):973-980.
8. Heaney RP (2002) Effects of caffeine on bone and the calcium economy. *Food Chemistry and Toxicology* 40(9):1263-1270.

9.   Massey LK (2001) Is caffeine a risk factor for bone loss in the elderly? *American Journal of Clinical Nutrition* 74(5):569-570.
10. Sakamoto W, Nishihira J, Fujie K, et al (2001) Effect of coffee consumption on bone metabolism. *Bone* 28:332-336.
11. Heaney RP, Rafferty K (2001) Carbonated beverages and urinary calcium excretion. *American Journal of Clinical Nutrition* 74(3):343-347.
12. Fitzpatrick L, Heaney RP (2003) Got soda? *Journal of Bone and Mineral Research* 18(9):1570-1572.

Bone Health Facts

- The amount of daily calcium intake varies at different stages of life. The body can not absorb more than 500 mg of calcium at a time, therefore, it is recommended to wait 4 to 6 hours between doses or dairy servings.

- Some sun is good for you and your bones, so don't always sit in the shade. About 15 minutes of daily sunlight without sunscreen will produce all the Vitamin-D that the body need. Because the sun doesn't shine everyday, make sure that the calcium supplement contains enough Vitamin-D.

- About 42% of the total body bone mass is achieved between the ages of 12 and 18. Yet, a majority of teenagers (7 out of 10) are not eating their recommended calcium intakes. One in four of all teenage girls (11-14 years) are not achieving the bare minimum of calcium needs for bone health. Therefore, beginning at age nine, children (both boys and girls) should include 1,300 mg. of calcium in their diet.

- Some medications reduce bone mass, such as glucocorticoids used to control arthritis and asthma, some antiseizure drugs; certain sleeping pills, some hormones used to treat endometriosis, and some cancer drugs. Certain medical conditions also increase the risk of brittle bones, including an overactive thyroid gland, kidney disease, and lupus.

- Finally, the following three steps that may prevent osteoporosis:
  i) a balanced diet rich in calcium, vitamin D and phosphorous,
  ii) weight-bearing exercises,
  iii) a healthy lifestyle with no smoking and limited alcohol intake.

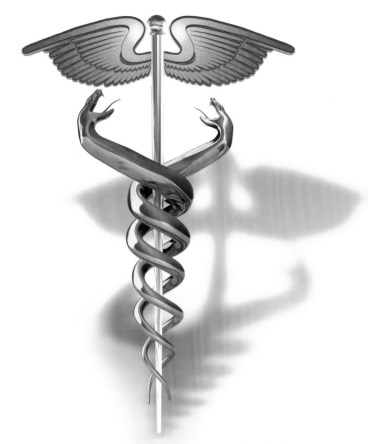

Factors Influencing Bone Health

Genetics	Some ethnic groups may have stronger bones than others
Gender	Men tend to have a greater bone mass than women
Physical Activity	Regular exercise is important for strong bones and weight-bearing exercise, such as brisk walking, running and climbing stairs, can help to increase peak bone mass
Body Weight	Heavier people typically have stronger bones as weight stimulates deposition of bone
Hormones	Irregular or loss of menstrual periods can cause bone loss in women
Diet	Calcium and vitamin D are important for strong bones, but other nutrients also play a role
Lifestyle	Cigarette smoking and excess alcohol intake adversely affect bone mass
Bio-Replenishment	Can help restore metabolic homeostasis, and possibly repair or reverse bone dysfunction such as osteoporosis.

Overview

Since the introduction of synthetic chemicals a century ago, profound changes have occurred in the way humanity inhabits the planet. Population growth, incursion into previously uninhabited areas, rapid urbanization, intensive farming practices, environmental degradation, and the misuse of hormone-analogs have disrupted the equilibrium of the human metabolic homeostasis, including of the bone. With prolonged life expectancy and the increasing number of elderly, it is predicted that the bone metabolic disorders, osteoporosis, in particular, will reach epidemic proportions.

Fortunately, during the past few decades, our understanding of bone metabolism and pathogenesis of bone diseases has grown tremendously because of the improved technology in measuring BMD and in using the markers of bone turnover. With proper strategies, bone diseases can be prevented in the vast majority of individuals; also when identified early and treated effectively in those who contract them.

In 2000, the Human Genome Project unveiled a road map of the six billion chemical bases, or alphabet molecules, that make up the body's genetic structure called DNA. Now is the time to use new techniques in genomics to gather in-depth knowledge of the genes involved in the pathogenesis of various bone diseases. There are at least 30 genes associated with the development of osteoporosis alone. Such knowledge can be applied to develop new diagnostic, preventive and therapeutic approaches to improve bone health.

Maintaining a healthy skeleton depends on a number of factors, and diet, alongside an appropriate level of physical activity. The emerging evidence indicates that bone replenishment could initiate a new era in the management of bone health - globally. However, the biggest road block is a lack of awareness of recent scientific developments in bone metabolic research among both the public and health care professionals. The aim of this *Bio-replenishment for Bone Health* volume is to bring such public awareness in a user-friendly format.

Bio-Replenishment Theory

Bio-Replenishment is the innate ability of a living organism to continuously refill its expended (depleted) chemicals that are vital to maintain homeostasis and negative entropy, while aging.

LIFE is a self-regulating organization that responds to chemicals passing through its open system, in order to promote its own survival, growth and replication. *Energy* is the quintessential force that operates these self-regulating processes. Most of the energy is used in the making ('anabolism') of new molecules such as proteins and in the breaking ('catabolism') of large chemicals such as carbohydrates into simple sugars. These vital processes are collectively known as *metabolism*. Life regulates its metabolism within a narrow range of milieu conditions such as temperature, pH, ionic and molecular availability. Such innate ability to maintain balance (or equilibrium) in an open system and to operate self-regulating (automatic) mechanisms to counteract any influences that drive towards imbalance is called *homeostasis*.

Bio-Replenishment is the innate ability of a life form to refill chemicals that are vital for self-regulation and homeostasis of its open system on a regular-basis. Any breakdown in bio-replenishment process with no prospect of restarting, the open system will shut down. In other words life meets death.

Cell is the basic unit of life. Every cell is enclosed by membrane with an acid-polymer called DNA that carries all vital instructions to run its operations, maintenance and reproduction. Every living cell uses an exclusive operation manual, in which the *DNA makes RNA makes Protein*. There are billions of different proteins used by living organisms – all made from 20 amino acids, the *'building blocks of life'.*

Aging is the biological deterioration of a living system over the sequential passage of time. Aging increases susceptibility to disease and vulnerability to toxic environmental conditions. It also leads to deterioration in mobility and flexibility. Aging, in and of itself is not a disease; but a natural process characterized by a decline in the resilience of the body's organs, that some scientists refer to this process as "biological entropy".

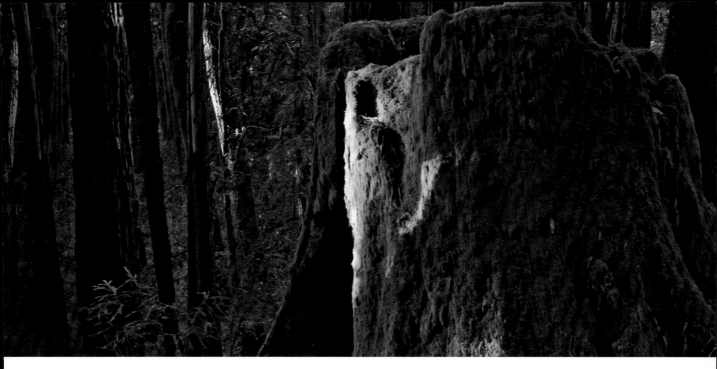

The body expends its internal chemicals during metabolism and eventually 'refills' those chemicals back. However, the overall concentration of vital (species-specific) biochemicals in the body stays about the same or changes only in a gradual manner (with aging). Such internal maintenance of vital chemicals at a steady state is referred to as *homeostasis* – the sign of a healthy body. Homeostasis is "round-the-clock" chemical monitoring that keeps life in check from the inside. Any significant deviation from the homeostasis, with chemical levels either above ('hyper') or below ('hypo') the steady state can trigger malfunction of several internal systems, which could lead to disorders, diseases or even death.

Bio-Replenishment Theory elucidates the intricate relationship between cellular homeostasis and entropy as a function of time (aging). Homeostasis is an integral part of the bio-replenishment process, which helps the body to achieve: i) proper amounts of gases, ions, nutrients, and water; ii) maintain the optimal internal temperature and; iii) sustain optimal fluid volume for the health of cells. However, the functional scope of bio-replenishment is beyond the homeostasis. Biological systems need repair, replacement and refurbishing of the worn out parts on a regular-basis to sustain life.

Bio-Replenishment Theory elucidates the nature of regulatory molecules in reversible and irreversible mode of metabolic activities. The reversible pathways in living organisms operate by feed-back mechanism(s) to maintain a steady-state metabolism as a function of optimal 'survival' mass (or concentration), the *homeostasis*. Aging and natural death probably first arose with the development of multi-cellular life.
A treatment for aging could result in delaying or relieving age-related diseases that now kill more than 80% of the people who die in the developed world and substantially extend the length and quality of countless lives.

Skeletal System

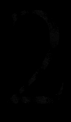

Skeleton derives its name from the Greek "skeletos," which means dry. Bones are anything but dry; they are dynamic living tissue that reinvent themselves in response to stress and repair themselves when broken.

Humans are vertebrates (with spine or backbone) and they rely on a sturdy internal skeletal frame centered on a prominent spine. Skeletal system makes a perfect combination of form and function: the S-shaped spine keeps the body upright and supports the head, while the pelvis balances the upper body over the feet. Like the framework of a house, skeletons form the internal structure that provides resistance to the force of gravity, move through space, and carry the physical body with grace and dignity. The male and female skeletons are similar in nature. However, the female frame is usually lighter and smaller than the male frame, and includes a wider pelvis for childbirth. Bones are rigid organs that form part of the endoskeleton of vertebrates. They come in a variety of shapes and have complex internal and external structures.

Bone is one of the hardest structures of the human body; it also possesses certain degree of toughness and elasticity. The primary tissue of bone is relatively hard and lightweight composite material; made mostly of calcium phosphate in the form of *hydroxyapatite*. While bone is essentially brittle, it has certain degree of elasticity mainly due to the presence of *collagen*. Bones contain several living cells embedded in the mineralized organic matrix. Bones are hollow, in order to provide the body with a frame that is both light and strong. *Cortical* bone, the outer dense shell, makes up about 75% of the total skeletal mass; and remaining 25% is a fine spongy network of *trabecular* bone inside the cortical shell.

Bones of the human body come in a variety of sizes and shapes. Accordingly, there are 5 different types of bones: *long, short, flat, irregular and sesamoid*. Surface markings and other characteristics make each bone unique. There are holes, depressions, smooth facets, lines, projections and other markings. These usually represent passageways for vessels and nerves, points of articulation with other bones or points of attachment for tendons and ligaments. Several bone components assemble to form an organ (eg. skull, vertebra, trunk, limbs, etc.) to accomplish a specific bodily function.

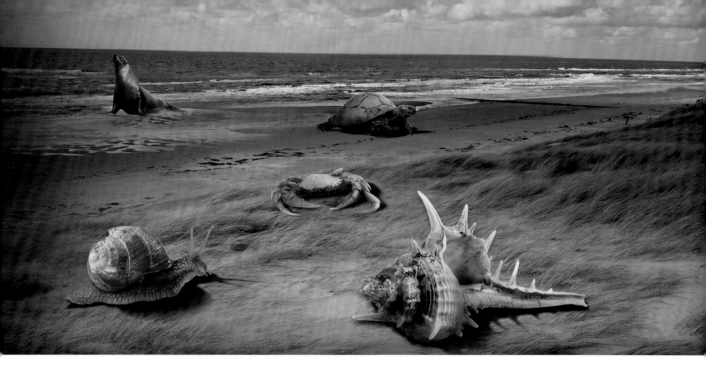

Human skeleton consists of bones, cartilage, ligaments and tendons that accounts for about 20% of the total body weight. Bones, muscles and joints work together to constitute the skeleto-muscular system. Muscles pull on the bone joints to facilitate the body movement. The human body has more than 650 muscles that make up 50% of the body weight. *Joints or articulations* provide flexibility and movement. The ends of bone are covered by cartilage to reduce mechanical friction or grinding of bone joints. The joint is surrounded by a protective capsule called *synovium*, which produces *synovial fluid*, a clear substance that lubricates and nourishes the cartilage and bone joints. Bone joints are vulnerable to injury and degeneration with aging. *Ligaments* connect bone to bone and *tendons* connect muscles to bone; with a purpose to transmit biomechanical forces. The fibers of both ligament and tendon are made of closely packed collagen fibers. These fibers are held together with other proteins, particularly with *proteoglycan* in compressed regions of the tendon. Tendons can passively modulate forces during locomotion, and provide additional stability to bone joints. It also allows tendons to store and recover energy at high efficiency. Mechanical properties of ligaments and tendons increase from early childhood to young adulthood; however, further aging process affects their stiffness. Immobilization of a joint for long periods of time is detrimental for joint structure and function, including decreased range of motion for the joint. *Cartilage* is a dense connective tissue that allows bones to slide over one another at all moveable joints with ease; thereby, reduces friction, and prevents damage. Any breakdown of cartilage in the bone joints leads to a severe bone disease – *osteoarthritis*.

Bone mass and its architecture or shape is influenced by the mechanical forces on the skeleton. Genetics and life style factors play a critical role in the structural outcome of a skeleton. Bone mass and architecture continuously change throughout life in response to mechanical stress and function.

Bones change in size, shape, and position by *modeling and remodeling* processes. In modeling, a bone is formed at one site and broken down in a different site, which changes its shape and position. In remodeling, the cellular activity of bone removal and replacement occurs at the same site. While remodeling is the predominant process during early adulthood – the bone forming years; modeling, however, continues throughout life, in response to weakening of the bone. As a result, most of the adult skeleton is replaced about every 7 years.

Bone is dynamic living tissue under continuous reorganization; however, the normal bone maintains equilibrium between the old bone being dissolved and the new bone being laid down. This process is called – *bone turnover*. Bone turnover ensures the mechanical integrity of the skeleton throughout life and plays an important role in calcium homeostasis. The processes of bone building and breakdown in response to internal and external signals are carried out by specialized cells that build or break down bone. The cells that form bone are *osteoblasts* and those breaks down the bone are *osteoclasts*.

Calcium is one of the abundant minerals in the human body, and perhaps the one with most direct impact on bone health. More than 99% of total body calcium is stored in the bones and teeth, providing vital support to the skeleton. A constant level of calcium is required in body fluids and tissues to perform vital body functions. The blood, the heart, the muscular system, the nervous system, the hormonal system, the kidneys, and the gastrointestinal system are all affected by calcium and demand a specific calcium balance. It should be noted that the physiological levels of calcium can be maintained only through diet and supplements, because the human body can not produce this bone mineral by itself. *Phosphorus* is also an essential element required for bone mineralization. Bone contains about 85% of the body's phosphate in the form of a calcium salt called hydroxyapatite *(HA)*, which is the major structural component of the bone. Phosphorus is critical for the making of adenosine triphosphate *(ATP)*, a molecule the body uses for storage and exchange of energy.

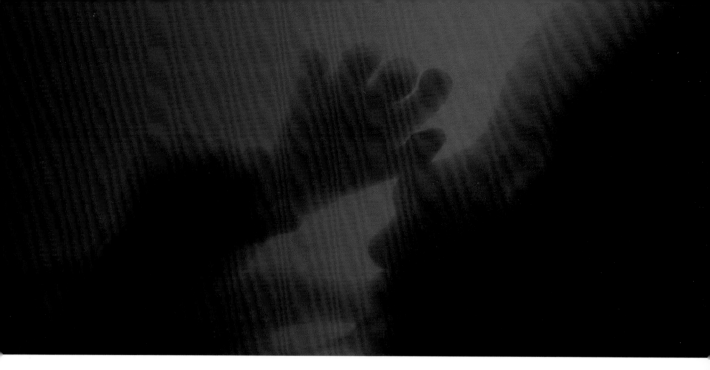

Calcium absorption in the gastrointestinal tract involves two specific cellular pathways: i) *trans-cellular*, an active transport that requires magnesium and vitamin-D; and ii) *para-cellular*, passive process that requires acidification of the calcium salts in the stomach. Factors that influence calcium absorption include age and health status of the individual, vitamin-D availability, calcium levels in food consumption, type and amount of fiber in the diet. It should be noted that all calcium ingested is not absorbed into the body. Calcium absorption begins in the stomach with its acid (hydrochloric acid), which dissolves, ionizes and facilitates mineral assimilation in the gut. However, secretion of stomach acid decreases gradually with age; up to 40% of post-menopausal women may be severely deficient in this natural stomach acid, with a predisposed risk of poor calcium absorption.

Several hormones affect calcium mineralization in the bone. The *parathyroid hormone (PTH)* transports calcium from the bones into the bloodstream. It also signals the kidneys to conserve calcium and other minerals from the urine. Additionally, PTH signals the kidneys to produce *calcitrol*, which is formed from vitamin-D that regulates the small intestine to absorb more calcium. The thyroid gland secretes *calcitonin*, which increases bone mineralization, and decreases the rate of bone breakdown.

Calcium homeostasis is a closely regulated process that maintains the levels of Ca^{2+} ions in the body within a tight normal range. During this process, calcium is removed from the bone and released into the blood circulation to maintain Ca^{2+} at 2.5 mmol/L (normal level). The typical calcium content of the adult human body is 1 kg, virtually all is found in the skeleton; the amount in body fluids and cells of the soft tissues accounts for the remaining for1% calcium reserve.

BONE is a remarkable organ that serves structural function; provides mobility, support, and protection for the body; and a reservoir function, as the storehouse for essential minerals. Though delicate in appearance, the bones in our skeletal system are ounce for ounce, stronger than "mild" steel. Skeletal bone framework is adapted to provide adequate strength and mobility to resist factures upon substantial impact, or during vigorous physical activity. Shape and structure of the bone are equally important as its mass in providing such strength.

Mineral Bank: The primary function of the skeletal system is to operate the deposits and withdrawals of minerals. The bone matrix is enriched with mineral salts, the most important being calcium phosphate. The dynamic process of withdrawal and storage of calcium is a multifunctional characteristic, which is critical for several vital functions, especially for the heart to beat, the nerve cell to flash an electric impulse, the muscle to twitch, the bowel to move and a kidney to filter. Maximum depository of minerals, defined as the 'peak bone mass', largely depends on genetics, environmental factors and diet.

Blood Production: Bone marrow is the body's designated manufacturing site for blood components. Bone marrow constitutes 4% of total body weight in adults. Bone marrow generates red blood cells *(RBC)* that oxygenate the tissues, white blood cells *(WBC)* that provide immune barrier against foreign bodies, and platelets that facilitate blood clotting.

Protection: Skeletal system protects the vital organs of the body. It provides a sturdy *'cage of bones'* that are designed to house the delicate internal organs and fragile body tissues. The fused bones of the cranium enclose the brain and make it less vulnerable to injury; the vertebrae surround and protect the spinal cord; and bones of the rib cage efficiently shield the heart and lungs.

Acid-base balance: Bone contains large stores of buffer, in the form of mineral salts to effectively balance the pH changes that occur in the body. Acid-base balance (or titration) in

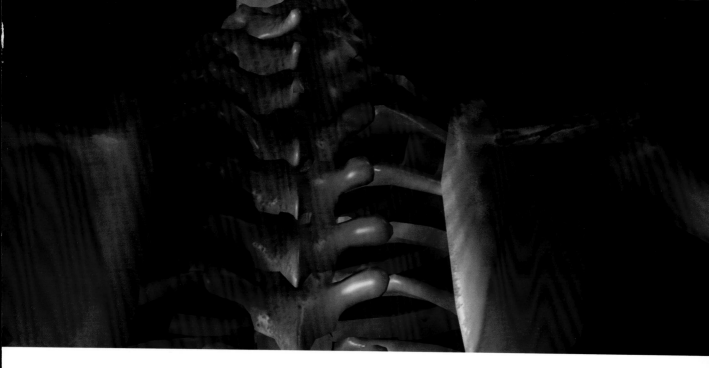

the body has a significant metabolic outcome on the bone turnover, especially on the rates of bone resorption and calcium mobilization.

Detoxification: Skeletal system is designed to scavenge several toxic chemicals, in particular, the heavy metal contaminants (i.e. lead, mercury) in body fluids and effectively dispose these artifacts via the circulatory route that runs through the skeletal matrix. Bone is also the major sink for vanadium heavy metal that enters the body.

Sound Management: The human auditory system is designed to detect several aspects of sounds, including pitch, loudness, and direction. Sound waves are acquired by the external ear and channeled through the ear canal to the eardrum. Three bones in the body, called as the *auditory ossicles*, help to convert the sound waves (vibrations in air) to mechanical (hydraulic) vibrations in tissues and fluid-filled chambers. Even the smallest vibration of the eardrum results in a significant amplification in the fluid chamber. This allows us to hear even the faintest of whispers

Movement is a basic function of the skeleto-muscular system, which manifests into postures and motions. This function is dependent on several muscles that attach to the bones through tendons, ligaments and cartilage. Muscle contraction, a familiar phenomenon that flexes the *'biceps'* or tightens the *'abs'*, is the quintessential force that enables mobility. Human evolution freed upper limbs from the burden of bearing body weight during locomotion; this enabled us to grasp and manipulate objects with precision.

Shape or figure of a human body is defined exclusively by the structural frame of the skeleton. Skeletal structure (or size of the bone) grows and changes only up to the point at which a human reaches the adulthood and remains essentially same for rest the life. Genetics, gender and lifestyle play a cumulative role in the overall development and appearance of the body shape. Finally, bones not only gave us a shape but a face to look into the mirror.

Genetics, diet, environment and lifestyle influence the outcome of bone structure and its function. Deficiency or dysfunctions of any above factors lead to *'metabolic bone disease'*. Bone disorders often result in weak bones that can lead to painful and debilitating fractures. The symptoms of bone disorders manifest as skeletal deformities, in some cases can be irreversible, affecting the posture and mobility of the body. Certain affected individuals can be seriously handicapped and confined to wheel chair. Some chronic bone disorders are extremely severe and life-threatening.

Osteoporosis is a skeletal disorder characterized by compromised bone strength, and increased risk of fracture. Once a bone fractures, osteoporosis is often extremely painful and crippling. A reduction in height or a fracture to hip or wrist may be the first sign of osteoporosis. Osteoporosis may significantly affect life expectancy and quality of life. This disease manifests due to an imbalance between bone formation and bone resorption. As a result, the bone mineral density *(BMD)* is reduced, bone architecture is disrupted, and the quality of bone matrix is altered. Advanced aging is the common underlying cause for the onset and progression of osteoporosis in both men and women.

Osteoarthritis *(OA)* is a degenerative bone disease, caused by the breakdown and eventual loss of the cartilage in one or more joints. In severe OA, complete loss of cartilage cushion causes friction between bones, causing pain during rest or pain with limited joint mobility. OA occurs more frequently with aging. Before age 45, OA occurs more frequently in males. After age 55 years, it is more common among females. *Rheumatoid Arthritis (RA)* is an inflammatory bone disease that causes pain, swelling, stiffness, and loss of joint function. RA is an autoimmune condition with several clinical features that make it unique from other types of arthritis.

Genetic Abnormalities can result in weak, thin or overly dense bones. The hereditary disease, *osteogenesis imperfecta* is due to abnormalities in the collagen protein, which

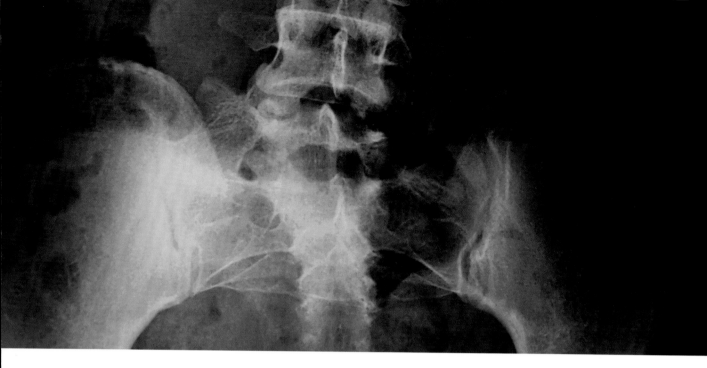

weakens the bone matrix and predisposes multiple fractures. Another congenital (hereditary) disorder, *osteopetrosis*, tends to make highly dense bone. Nutitional deficiencies, particularly of vitamin-D, calcium, and phosphorus, can result in the formation of weak, poorly mineralized bone. In children, vitamin-D deficiency causes *rickets*, with typical weak bones, bowing of the long bones and a characteristic deformity due to overgrowth of cartilage at distal ends of the bone. In adults, vitamin-D deficiency leads to softening of the bone (a condition known as *osteomalacia*), with increased risk of fractures and skeletal deformities.

Hormone Disorders can cause serious skeletal problems. Overactive parathyroid glands (or *hyper-parathyroidism*) can cause excess bone breakdown and increase the risk of fractures. Growth hormone malfunction can affect skeletal development, which may lead to short body stature. Loss of gonadal function (or *hypogonadism*) in children and young adults can set off severe osteoporosis due to loss of testosterone and estrogen. Blood sugar imbalance (e.g. diabetes) could affect bone health in different ways. Type 1 diabetes is associated with modest reductions in BMD. Altered bone metabolism in adolescents with type-1 diabetes may limit peak bone mass acquisition and increase the risk of osteoporosis in later life. Several factors including obesity, changes in insulin levels, high calcium and glucose excretion in the urine, reduced function of the kidneys and inflammation contribute to bone loss in diabetic adults. Also, diabetes is known to induce complications of capillaries (micro-vasculature) that reduce blood flow to the bone leading to bone loss and fragility.

According to the **American Academy of Orthopaedic Surgeons *(AAOS)*,** men are more likely to experience fractures than women until about age 45. After that, fracture rates (especially, stress factures) are higher among women. Prior to age 75, *colles fracture* (just above the wrist) is common; however, hip fractures become more frequent in the later years of life.

Bone Replenishment

Bone Replenishment is to maintain homeostasis of bone turnover (resorption vs. formation) in the skeletal system with relation to age and sex of an individual.

Bone Replenishment is the homeostatic management of bone metabolism. Multiple factors such as PTH and prostaglandin E, stimulate bone resorption as well as bone formation in tandem. Lactoferrin *(LF)* and ribonuclease *(RNase)* appear during the early embryonic stage (ossification and vascularization) and regulate bone metabolic homeostasis through each phase of human development. These vital factors are continuously depleted during bone metabolism; and their synthesis (levels) gradually decline with aging.

Given the dramatic increase in skeletal size during growth, and the need to preserve skeletal mass during adulthood, and to allow the bone "bank" to make mineral deposits and withdrawals – homeostasis takes the center stage. Internally, the metabolic pathway self-regulates in response to changes in the levels of substrates or products; for example, a decrease in the amount of calcium or phosphate can increase the flux through a pathway to compensate the loss.

Bone remodeling can be stimulated by *hormones* that regulate mineral metabolism, *chemical factors* (e.g. growth factors and cytokines) that control bone growth and *stress factors* (e.g. mechanical and weight bearing). Sex hormones – *estrogen (E)* made in the ovary of females, and *testosterone (T)* made by the testes in males, are important for bone strength. *Parathyroid hormone (PTH)* maintains the level of calcium and stimulates both resorption and formation of bone. *Calcitonin (CT)* inhibits bone breakdown and may protect against excessively high levels of calcium in the blood.

The inter-reliance between the cardiovascular and the skeletal system manifests as: i) the bones provide cellular machinery for the circulatory network, whereas, ii) the circulatory portal supports the bone metabolism with mobilization of chemicals to and from the skeletal tissue. Bone-replenishment plays a significant role in maintaining the fine balance between both systems. Malfunction or breakdown in bone-replenishment could impair several vital pathways and lead to homeostatic imbalance.

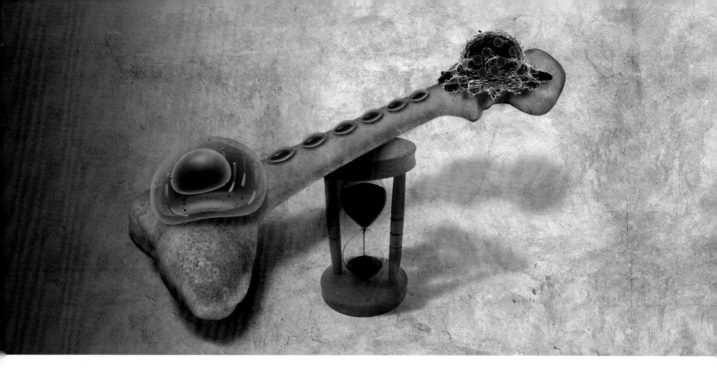

Abnormal or insufficient *angiogenesis* (formation of new blood vessels) is the cause of many bone disorders including *arthritis, synovitis, osteomyelitis* and *osteophyte* formation. Osteoporosis and impaired healing of bone fractures are linked to insufficient angiogenesis. Age dependent decline of angiogenesis leads to impaired bone formation, one of the risk factors for osteoporosis. Diminished angiogenesis due to chemical inhibitors prevent fractures from healing. Delayed bone healing and non-fusion of fractures are shown to be associated with low angiogenic activity. Ribonuclease (RNase), a class of angiogenins derived from milk has recently shown very promising results in promoting bone formation with age-related and post-menopausal bone loss. Bio-replenishment is a potent, physiological process that underlies the natural manner in which bones respond to any decline in nutrient supply through the circulatory transport. The production of new collateral vessels with RNase-replenishment could overcome the bone metabolic imbalance.

Transport and uninterrupted delivery of nutrients, vitamins, minerals, building blocks (amino acids, bio-polymers, etc) and regulatory molecules (enzymes, hormones, etc) to bone matrix is critical for homeostasis of the skeleto-muscular system. Therefore, gastro-intestinal health is of pivotal importance to facilitate efficient mineral transport and to maintain calcium homeostasis. Lactoferrin *(LF)* appears at early embryogenesis and plays a critical role in skeletal development and homeostasis throughout the life.

Anabolic Agents directly stimulate bone formation (distinguished from anti-resorptive agents that act by blocking bone resorption) thus, allows the endogenous rate of bone formation. The difference between the lowered bone resorption rate and the continuing intrinsic bone formation results in an eventual gain in bone mass. Both RNase and LF from milk have been proven to be potent anabolic agents for bone formation. A combination of *RNase-enriched lactoferrin (R-ELF)* could serve as an effective bio-replenishment to restore the balance of bone turnover and maintain homeostasis in skeletal metabolism.

Bone Health is dependent on several factors including, nutrition (e.g. minerals, trace elements, vitamins, and supplements), lifestyle (e.g. physical activity, hygienic practices, and addictive habits), environment and aging. Nutrition is a critical factor in the management of bone health. Among bone nutrients most attention has focused on the beneficial role of calcium and calcium-rich foods (e.g., dairy products); however, several macro-nutrients (eg. proteins, carbohydrates, fats) and vegetables are necessary for bone health.

Vitamins perform a wide range of biochemical functions, including acting as hormones (e.g. vitamin-D), antioxidants (e.g. vitamin-E), and regulators of cell and tissue growth (e.g. vitamin-A). Finally, the B-complex, the largest group of vitamins, acts as catalyst and substrate in metabolism. Folic acid supplementation reduces homocysteine levels in post-menopausal women, thereby reduces the risk of osteoporosis. Vitamin-K in combination with vitamin-D not only increases BMD in osteoporotic individuals, but also reduces the fracture rate. Vitamin-C is important for bone matrix formation through its role in collagen synthesis.

Minerals are integral part of bones, teeth, soft tissue, muscle, blood, and nerve cells. They perform several vital functions in the body - from building strong bones to transmitting nerve impulses. Minerals essential for bone health are of two types, (i) *Macro-minerals*, which include calcium *(Ca)*, phosphorus *(P)*, magnesium *(Mg)*, sodium *(Na)*, potassium *(K)*, and chloride *(Cl)*; (ii) *Trace elements,* which include iron *(Fe)*, copper *(Cu)*, zinc *(Zn)*, manganese *(Mn)*, selenium *(Se)*, iodine *(I)*, chromium *(Cr)*, cobalt *(Co)*, nickel *(Ni)*, molybdenum *(Mb)*, fluoride *(F)*, arsenic *(As)*, silicon *(Si)* and boron *(B)*.

Bioavailability and functionality of bone health nutrients are closely inter-related; the presence or absence of one may influence the uptake of another. *Inulin-type of fructans (ITFs)* are reported to increase the absorption of several minerals (calcium, magnesium, in some cases phosphorus) and trace elements (mainly copper, iron, zinc), thereby enhance bone health. Because of its potent anti-inflammatory properties, *curcumin* (from turmeric) has

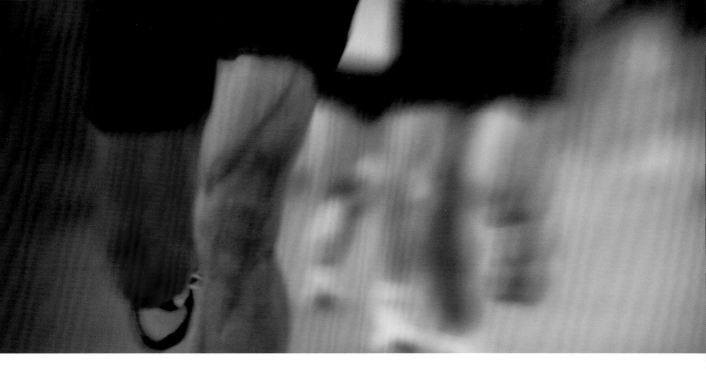

emerged as a natural treatment for osteoarthritis *(OA)* and rheumatoid arthritis *(RA)*. *Bromelain* (from pine apple) helps to alleviate the symptoms of OA, relieve joint stiffness in RA, ease the swelling associated with gout, and help sufferers of carpal tunnel syndrome. As an anti-inflammatory agent, bromelain is effective in treating sports injury, trauma, and other kinds of swelling.

Physical activity or routines that cause bones and muscles to work against gravity are called weight-bearing exercises. Resistance exercises such as weight training are also important to improve muscle mass and bone strength. Examples of weight bearing exercises are walking, running, dancing, aerobics and skating. Non-weight bearing exercise include swimming, cycling and water aerobics.

Bone Health Disruptors: Lifestyle, especially certain addictive habits, such as tobacco consumption, smoking, alcohol, drug abuse, extreme dieting and certain medications can adversely affect bone health. Dieting habits (e.g. weight loss diets, semi-starvation diets, crash diets) mostly among women, and also some men, attempting to be fashionably thin, can cause serious bone health problems. Chronic alcoholism leads to poor mineral absorption and increased excretion of important bone-building nutrients like calcium, magnesium, vitamin-C, zinc and copper. Bone-damaging effects of *nicotine* and other harmful chemicals in cigarette smoke include elevation of the *cortisol* levels (hormone that regulates bone breakdown); and slowing down the *calcitonin* (hormone that helps to build bones). *Caffeine* is often implicated in the development of osteoporosis, due to its effect on calcium absorption. It could temporarily increase calcium excretion and may modestly decrease calcium absorption. Soda drinks, high in phosphate content, are perhaps the most pervasive habit that promotes a calcium drain in the body. Phosphorus, an acid-forming mineral in the cola drinks, can interfere with calcium absorption by the bone and set off calcium loss through urinary excretion. Some studies have reported that high carbonated soda drink consumption either increased the fracture risk or decreased BMD.

Abbreviations

ACSM	american college of sports medicine
BAP	bone-specific alkaline phosphatase
BMD	bone mineral density
BMI	body mass index
BMR	basal metabolic rate
Cal	calorie
CLA	conjugated linoleic acid
CR	calorie restriction
CT	calcitonin
DHEA	dehydroepiandrosterone
DNA	deoxyribonucleic acid
Dpd	deoxy-pyridinoline
DRI	dietary reference intake
DV	daily value
DVT	deep vein thrombosis
DXA (or DEXA)	dual energy X-ray absorptiometry
E	estrogen
ECF	extracellular fluid
FDA	Food and Drug Administration
FNB	Food and Nutrition Board
FOS	fructooligosaccharide
Δ G	Gibbs Free Energy
HA	hydroxyapatite
HCl	hydrochloric acid
HDL	high density lipoprotein
HLA	hyaluronic acid
HRT	hormone replacement therapy
IL	interleukin
IOM	Institute of Medicine
ITF	inulin-type fructan
IU	international units
L	liter

Abbreviations

LDL	low density lipoprotein
LF	lactoferrin
MBD	metabolic bone disease
mcg	microgram
mg	milligram
mL	milliliter
NHANES	National Health and Nutrition Examination Survey
NIH	National Institute of Health
NSAID	non-steroidal anti-inflammatory drug
NTx	N-telopeptide
OA	osteoarthritis
OARSI	osteoarthritis research society international
OC	osteocalcin
OI	osteogenesis imperfecta
ONJ	osteonecrosis of the jaw
PPM	parts per million
PTH	parathyroid hormone
PUFA	polyunsaturated fatty acid
RA	rheumatoid arthritis
RANK	receptor activator of nuclear factor κ B
RBC	red blood cells
RDA	recommended daily allowance
R-ELF	ribonuclease-enriched lactoferrin
RNase	ribonuclease
SERM	selective estrogen receptor modulator
T	testosterone
TNF	tumor necrosis factor
UL	upper intake limit
UV	ultra-violet
WBC	white blood cells
WHO	World Health Organization

Glossary

Active Ingredient is the chemical in a drug or supplement that exerts desired action.

Adenosine Triphosphate (ATP), is a nucleotide (part of DNA, the genetic material) that occurs in living cells; and a major source of cellular energy.

Alkaline Phosphatase is an enzyme released by *osteoblasts* and an indicator of bone formation. This enzyme is responsible for removing phosphate groups from many types of molecules.

Amino Acid is one of the 20 building blocks of protein: alanine, arginine, asparagine, aspartic acid, cysteine, glutamic acid, glutamine, glycine, histidine, isoleucine, leucine, lysine, methionine, phenylalanine, proline, serine, threonine, tryptophan, tyrosine, and valine. Eleven amino acids are produced by the body and the remaining 9 (known as essential amino acids) come from the diet.

Anabolism is the phase of metabolism in which simple substances are synthesized into the complex materials of living tissue.

Andropause is a biological change characterized by a gradual decline in male sex hormones *(androgens)* in men during and after mid-life.

Anorexia is an eating disorder characterized by reduced appetite or total aversion to food.

Antagonist is an agent that acts against and blocks an action.

Arthritis is a group of clinical conditions that affect the health of the bone joints in the body.

Articular surface is the area of the joint where the ends of the bones meet, or articulate, and function like a ball bearing.

Assimilation is conversion of nutriment into the fluid or solid substance of the body, by the processes of digestion and absorption.

Atrophy is partial or complete wasting away of a body part. Causes of atrophy include poor circulation, malnutrition, hormone deficiency, reduced nerve impulse, or lack of exercise.

Autopoiesis is the process whereby a system, organization, or organism produces and replaces its own components and distinguishes itself from its environment.

Auditory Ossicles are tiny bones in the middle ear that transmit acoustic vibrations from the eardrum to the inner ear.

Basal Metabolic Rate (BMR) is the body's resting level of energy expenditure; the number of calories needed to sustain basic life processes during a 24-hour period.

Bio-Replenishment is the innate ability of a living organism to continuously refill its expended (depleted) chemicals that are vital to maintain homeostasis and negative entropy, while aging.

Bioavailability refers to the amount of an active compound in food, medication, or supplement that is absorbed in the intestines and ultimately available for biological activity in the body.

Bi-pedalism is walking upright on two feet instead of on four limbs. Bipedalism made the human form of birth possible.

Bisphosphonates are non-hormonal medications used to prevent and treat osteoporosis. Examples include etidronate (Didronel, Didrocal), alendronate (Fosamax), risedronate (Actonel) and zoledronic acid (Aclasta). Bisphosphonates can prevent bone loss, increase bone density and reduce the risk of fracture.

Body Mass Index (BMI) is a standardized ratio of weight to height, and is often used as a general indicator of health. BMI can be calculated by dividing body weight (in kilograms) by the square of body height (in meters). A BMI between 18.5 and 24.9 is considered normal for most adults.

Bone-specific Alkaline Phosphatase (BAP) is an enzyme found on the surface of osteoblast cells. BAP is a biochemical indicator of bone turnover.

Bone Formation is a process by which *osteoblasts* fish out the circulating calcium from the bloodstream and fix it in the bone matrix.

Bone Mineral Density (BMD) is the density of minerals (such as calcium) in bones, which is measured by using special X-ray, computed tomography (CT) scan, or ultrasound. This information is used to estimate the strength of bones.

Bone Modeling is a process in which bone is sculpted during growth to ultimately achieve its proper shape. During modeling, the bone resorption and bone formation occur on separate surfaces *(formation and resorption are not coupled)*.

Bone Remodeling is a continuous process throughout life, in which damaged bone is repaired, mineral homeostasis is maintained, and bone is reinforced for increased stress. It involves replacement of old bone tissue by new bone tissue *(formation and resorption are coupled)*.

Bone Resorption is the process by which *osteoclasts* break down bone and release the minerals from bone fluid to the blood.

Buffer is a chemical solution that resists change in pH by neutralizing both acids and bases to maintain the original acidity or alkalinity.

Calcification is the deposition of calcium salts in the body that occurs *normally* in teeth and bones but *abnormally* in injured muscles and narrowed arteries.

Calcitonin is a hormone secreted by the thyroid gland; available as a medication, in an injectable form and as a nasal spray; used to treat osteoporosis and relieve pain caused by spinal fractures.

Calcitriol is the active form of vitamin D3, which helps the body absorb calcium.

Calciuric effect relates to excretion of elevated amounts of calcium in the urine due to intake of medications or diet (e.g. consumption of high protein diet).

Calorie is a unit of measurement for the amount of energy that is released from food upon oxidation by the body. Carbohydrate, protein, fat and alcohol provide calories in the diet. Carbohydrate and protein have 4 calories per gram, fat has 9 calories per gram, and alcohol has 7 calories per gram.

Catabolism is breakdown of more complex substances into simpler ones together with release of energy.

Cartilage is a gel-like, porous, elastic, slippery tissue that coats the ends of the bone. Normal cartilage provides a durable, low-friction, load-bearing surface for joints.

Cholecalciferol is a form of vitamin-D, also called vitamin-D3. It is structurally similar to steroids such as *testosterone, cholesterol*, and *cortisol*.

Chondrocytes are basic cartilage cells, critical for balance and function of bone and joints.

Clinical Trial is a pre-planned study to evaluate the safety, efficacy, or optimum dosage schedule (if appropriate) of one or more diagnostic, therapeutic, or prophylactic drugs, devices, or techniques selected according to predetermined criteria of eligibility and observed for predefined evidence of favorable and adverse effects.

Collagen is the main protein found in *all* connective tissues of the body, including muscles, ligaments, cartilage and tendons. It provides the bone with a framework on which minerals can be laid down, most importantly calcium phosphate and hydroxyapatite.

Cortex is a tissue that forms the outer layer of an organ or structure. For example, *cerebral cortex* is a layer of neurons located in the cerebrum of the skull.

Cortisol, a hormone released by the cortex (outer portion) of the adrenal gland when a person is under stress; helps regulate blood pressure and cardiovascular function, as well as the body's use of proteins, carbohydrates and fats.

Cytokines are chemicals that are secreted by various types of cells and act on other cells to stimulate or inhibit their function.

Daily Value (DV) is a reference value used on labels for dietary supplements and are based on a 2000 Calorie intake for adults and children. DV is based on *Daily Reference Values* (that apply to fat, saturated fat, cholesterol, carbohydrate, protein, fiber, sodium, and potassium) and *Reference Daily Intakes* (of essential vitamins and minerals).

Deoxy-pyridinoline (Dpd) occurs mainly in Type I collagen of bone. In the process of bone degradation, Dpd is released into the blood circulation and cleared by the kidneys. Hence Dpd has been shown to be a biochemical indicator of bone resorption.

Dietary Supplement is any product taken by mouth that has a *'dietary ingredient'*, which may include vitamins, minerals, herbs, and amino acids, as well as substances such as enzymes, organ tissues, metabolites, extracts or concentrates. Dietary supplements can be found in many forms such as pills, tablets, capsules, liquids or powders.

Diuretic agent or compound increases the flow of urine from the body.

DNA *(or deoxyribonucleic acid)* is a nucleic acid that contains the genetic instructions used in the development and functioning of all known living organisms and some viruses.

Dosage is the total amount of a dietary supplement given to, taken or absorbed by a person.

Double-blind study is when neither the patient nor the doctor knows whether the patient is receiving the study drug or a placebo.

DXA (previously DEXA), dual energy X-ray absorptiometry measures bone mineral density (BMD) to provide evidence of osteoporosis (or when there is loss of bone mass).

Efficacy is capacity or power of a drug or dietary supplement to produce a desired effect or to affect a claimed health condition.

Endocrine is the system of glands that regulates a person's mood, growth, sexual function, reproductive processes and metabolic activity. The endocrine system includes the pituitary gland, thyroid, parathyroids, adrenal glands, pancreas, ovaries (in women) and testes (in men).

Entropy is the quantitative measure of disorder in a system. The concept comes out of thermodynamics, which deals with the transfer of heat energy within a system.

Enzyme is a protein that speeds up chemical reactions in the body.

Epiphyseal Plate, also known as the *growth plate* or *physis* in a long bone; and a thin disc of hyaline cartilage. In the long bones, the epiphyseal plate disappears by 20 years of age.

Estrogen is a female sex hormone essential for the development and functioning of the female reproductive system, including menstrual cycles and pregnancy. It has a key role in maintaining strong and healthy bones.

Fibrous dysplasia is a developmental anomaly of the skeleton, usually during childhood. Bone lesions usually stop developing at puberty. This condition is a hereditary disorder.

Free radicals are highly reactive molecules in the body that can destroy tissues by oxidizing cell membrane lipids and damaging DNA. Free radicals are produced through the body's normal process of metabolism.

Glycosaminoglycan (GAG) is a type of long, polymer of amino-sugars. GAGs form viscous solutions with good lubricant characteristics and support the major structural components of cartilage and connective tissue.

Growth Factors are vital for bone formation, bone repair and bone remodeling.

Growth Hormone (or somatotropin) is a powerful anabolic hormone that affects all systems of the body and plays an important role in muscle growth.

Hematopoiesis is the formation of blood cells in the body. All blood components derive from the hematopoietic stem cells located in the bone marrow.

Homeostasis is the physiological capacity of an organism to regulate itself by rapidly restoring internal conditions in response to sudden changes in the external environment.

Hormones are chemical messengers that transport signals from one cell to another in different parts of the body. Only a small amount of hormone is required to alter cell metabolism.

Hormone Replacement Therapy (HRT) is the administration of exogenous hormones to replace those the body is unable to produce; HRT most often refers to the replacement of estrogen and progesterone following menopause.

Hydroxyapatite or 'HA' is a hard substance that gives weight-bearing capacity to the bone. It 'glues' the collagen fibers to the bone and provides a strong matrix or framework.

Hyperparathyroidism is excessive activity of the parathyroid glands (located near the thyroid gland in the neck), which results in the excessive production of parathyroid hormone (PTH) .

Hyperthyroidism is excessive activity of the thyroid gland (found in the neck), which results in the excessive production of T3 and T4 hormones.

Hypogonadism is decreased activity of the sex organs – in men, the testes; and in women, the ovaries.

IU (International unit) is a unit of measurement of vitamin activity determined by biological methods rather than by direct chemical analysis.

Lactoferrin (LF) is a protein found naturally in milk, saliva, tears, blood, *synovial fluid in bone joints, sperm*, various secretions, tissues and other parts of body. LF is credited with numerous functions including metal regulation, antimicrobial, antioxidant, immue modulation, and anti-inflammatory effects. LF is a quintessential bio-replenishment for mammalian development and growth.

Lactose intolerance is the inability to metabolize lactose, a sugar found in milk and other dairy products, because the required enzyme lactase is absent in the intestinal system or its availability is lowered.

Ligament is a cord made of collagen fiber that supports numerous internal organs (e.g. breasts); it also attaches to the bones on both sides of a joint to provide strength.

Mcg (Microgram) is equal to one millionth of a gram.

Menopause is the time in a women's life when menstruation permanently stops. Sometimes referred to as the "change of life", occurs due to decrease in production of estrogen and progesterone by the ovaries.

Metabolism is a set of chemical reactions that occur in organisms to sustain life. These processes allow organisms to grow and reproduce, maintain their structures, and respond to their environment.

Mg (Milligram) is equal to one thousandth of a gram.

Milk ribonuclease (RNase) is a protein molecule involved in the formation of new blood vessels. Milk contains RNase types 2 and 4.

Mineral is a naturally occurring, inorganic substance with a definite chemical composition and a crystalline structure. Minerals are generally classified into the following chemical classes: silicates, carbonates, sulfates, halides, oxides, sulfides, phosphates and metals.

N-telopeptide (NTX or NTx) is a cross-linked protein fragment of type I collagen and a specific breakdown product of bone cartilage. NTX is used as a marker of bone turnover and measured in the urine or serum. Urine NTX levels >40 nmol/L indicate excessive bone turnover and is a sign of osteoporosis.

Ossification is the process of bone formation, in which connective tissues, such as cartilage are turned to bone or bone-like tissue.

Osteoarthritis (OA) is a non-inflammatory degenerative joint disease that occurs mostly among the elderly. The cartilage in joints breaks down; as a result, the joint becomes irritated and swollen (inflamed).

Osteoblasts are cells responsible for making new bone, maintaining the balance of calcium in the blood and bone. They form new bone tissue in response to increasing demands of the bone turnover.

Osteocalcin is a non-collagenous protein found in bone and dentin. It is secreted by *osteoblasts* and plays a role in bone mineralization and calcium *homeostasis*.

Osteoclasts are cells that break down the bone, release minerals into the blood stream, to serve various functions in the body. They dissolve bone tissue by secreting enzymes and regulate calcium and phosphate levels in body fluids.

Osteocyte is a star-shaped cell, abundantly found in the bone; with a function to sustain bone as living tissue.

Osteogenesis Imperfecta (OI) also called the "brittle bone disease", is a hereditary disorder caused by a genetic defect that affects type 1 collagen. OI results in extremely fragile bones that are easily broken even by touch.

Osteomalacia is softening of the bone caused by vitamin-D deficiency or problems with this vitamin metabolism. Decreased mineralization leads to low bone density that cause folding fractures and bowed bones.

Osteomyelitis is infection of the bone, usually by pus-forming bacteria. Most bacterial osteomyelitis starts as acute infection or sepsis that eventually spread to the bone.

Osteopenia refers to a decrease in bone density that, although too low to be called normal, is not low enough to be considered *osteoporosis*.

Osteopetrosis also known as *'marble bone disease'*, is a hereditary disorder of excessive bone mineralization, resulting in altered stature, frequent fractures, lack of bone marrow function, and severe *osteomyelitis* of the jaws.

Osteophytes are bony outgrowths or lumps, especially at the joint margins. They develop in order to offload the pressure on the joint by increasing the surface area on which your weight is distributed.

Osteoporosis *(porous bone)* is a skeletal condition that develops when bone is no longer replaced as quickly as it is removed. Abnormal loss of bony tissue results in fragile bones due to low BMD; most common in postmenopausal women.

Paget's disease is a chronic disorder in which bones become enlarged and deformed. Bone may become dense, but fragile, because of excessive breakdown and deformation.

Para-cellular transport is the second major mechanism for calcium and other minerals to mobilize from the intestinal lumen into the blood circulation. It is dependant on acidification, solubility, gut permeability and sojourn time.

Parathyroid glands are round bodies, about 1/4 to 4/5 inches in size, located in the neck near the thyroid gland. These glands regulate the use of calcium and phosphorus

Parathyroid hormone (PTH) is a protein hormone secreted by the parathyroid gland which regulates calcium and phosphorous levels in the body.

pH (potential of hydrogen) is the measure of the acidity or alkalinity of a solution. The pH scale ranges between 0 and 14. Water with a pH of 7 is neutral; a pH of less than 7 is acidic; a pH greater than 7 is alkaline.

Phytate is an acidic chemical found inside the husk of whole grains and cereals that binds certain minerals and makes them unavailable.

Prebiotics are indigestible carbohydrates that stimulate the growth and activity of beneficial bacteria *(probiotics)* that reside in the gastrointestinal tract.

Probiotics (meaning *'for life'*) are live micro-organisms, when ingested can have beneficial effects on the gut, boost immune system, and contribute to general health and wellbeing (e.g. *Lactobacillus acidophilus* in the yoghurt).

Proteoglycans are large molecules that build cartilage. They are important due to the ability to bond with water, which helps high water retention in cartilage.

RANK-Ligand (also known as osteoprotegerin ligand) is a local paracrine factor that originates from osteoblasts and mediates the effects of most, if not all, agents that are known to impact osteoclast development in bone.

Recommended Daily Allowance (RDA) is the average daily dietary intake level that is sufficient to meet the nutrient requirement of nearly all (97 to 98 percent) healthy individuals in a particular life-stage and gender group.

Rheumatoid Arthritis (RA) is an autoimmune disorder where the body attacks itself; the inflamed lining of the joint *(synovium)* progresses to severe damage and in few cases, deformity. Inflamed joints are painful and stiff.

Rickets is an abnormal bone formation in children due to inadequate calcium supply to the bone; consequently, a failure to mineralize bone. Bowing of the long bones, sometimes severely deformed long bones, is the most common outward sign.

Selective estrogen receptor modulators (SERMs) are a class of medications that have estrogen-like effects. The SERM raloxifene is used to prevent and treat osteoporosis.

Senescence is the organic process of growing older and showing effects of increasing age.

Synovium is the fluid-filled lining of a bone joint. It secretes *synovial fluid* that lubricates tissues where friction would otherwise occur and also supplies nutrients and oxygen to the cartilage.

Tendon is a fiber made of collagen that secures muscle to bone and muscle to muscle.

Testosterone is a sex hormone secreted by the adrenal glands in both males and females . This anabolic steroid plays an important role in immune function and libido.

Trans-cellular transport is specific for calcium absorption, which requires vitamin-D and magnesium. Calcium crosses the cell through calcium channels.

T-score is a measuring system used to compare the bone density of an individual to that a group of young adults of the same sex. A T-score indicates the number of units (standard deviations) a person's bone density is above or below the standard. The higher the T-score, the denser the bone. According to the WHO, a T-score higher than -1 is considered normal; a T-score between -1 and -2.5 indicates osteopenia; and a T-score below -2.5 indicates osteoporosis.

Vitamin is an organic substance essential in small amounts to support growth and activity of the body. Vitamins can be obtained from plant or animal sources.

Z-score is a measuring system used to compare the bone density of an individual to the average bone density of a group of the same age, weight, sex and race. A Z-score below -2.0 indicates that the individual's bone mass is lower than expected for someone of that age.

Index

necrosis of the jaw (ONJ) 204
Ossification 67
Osteoarthritis 61, **114, 115**, 138, 148, 150, 151, 198, 199
Osteoblast 44, 67, 70, **71**, 78, 125, 137, 148, 153, 167, 208
Osteocalcin 44, 71, 155
Osteoclast **70**, 125, 148, 167
Osteocyte 46, 61, **71**
Osteogenesis **67**, 71
Osteoporosis 33, 77, 94, 95, 100, **111-113**, 122, 126, 138, 184, 194, 200, 204, 210, 218
    DXA **112**
    fracture 113, **122**, 140, 202, 211
    GIO 71, 110
    treatment 79
    T-score **112**, 122
Oxidation (oxidative damage) 18, 31

P
Paget's disease 33, **118**, 138
Parathyroid 71, 127
    hormone 70, 71, 77, 84, 85, 125, 127, 129-131, **136, 137**, 192, 194
    gland 87, 109, 136
    therapy 137, 153
Peridontal diseases 204
Phosphorus **76**, 126, **186, 187**, 211
    deficiency 76
    dietary source **186, 187**
    metabolism 76, 126, 210
Phytates 83
Post-menopause 77, 79, 84, 111, 138, 183, 194
Precocious puberty 206
Probiotics 197
Proteoglycan 60, 61, 71, 148

R
RDA (recommended daily allowance)
    amino acids 25
    calcium 166, 182, 184
    chromium 193
    folate 175
    magnesium 188, 189
    phosphorus 186, 187
    vitamin-C 177
    vitamin-D 172, 211
    vitamin-K 179
    zinc 191
R-ELF **154, 155**, 211
Rheumatoid arthritis (RA) 110, **116, 117**, 148, 190, 198, 199

Ribonuclease (RNase) 125, **140, 141**, 154, 155, 166

S
Schrodinger, Erwin 5, 9
Selenium **25**
Senescence 14
SERM **156**
SKELETAL SYSTEM **39-64**, 102, 103, 129, 147, 222, 223
SOD 78
Soda **210**
Soy **167**
Spinal cord 43, 48, 50, 51, 93
Strontium **79**
Synovium 116
    cavity 58
    fluid 58, 116, 149, 151
    transport 148

T
Telomere (telomerase) 14
Tendon 24, 47, 58, **60**, 102, 116
Teriparatide 137, **153**, 156, 211
Testosterone 84, 109, 130, 131, **133**, 144
Thymus 22
Thyroid 25, 33, 87
Thyroxine 20
Turmeric (curcumin) **198**
Trabecular **45**, 67, 110, 197, 202, 204

V
Vascular 61, **140-142**
Vertebra 49, **50**, 93, 98
Vitamin-A 78, 164, 167, 168, 170, 181, 211
Vitamin-C 25, 170, **176, 177**, 181, 211
Vitamin-D 77, 79, 81-83, 86, **134, 135**, 168, 170, **172, 173**, 194, 200, 211, 218
    hormone 134
    metabolism 134
    homeostasis 126
    dietary source 164, 172, 173
    drug interactions 172, 186
    deficiency 109, 118, 119, 134, 135
Vitamin-K 153, 164, 170, **178-180**, 211
    dietary source 178-180
    adverse effects 179
    drug interactions 179

Z
Zinc 25, 78, 168, **190, 191**

Image Credits

Note: The artist, photographer or copyright holder name is followed by a parenthesis (which refers to the page number in the book with the corresponding image).

Digital Spice team: Reshma Mallecha, Amol Sondekar & Sameer Nigudkar (58, 59, 69-72, 97, 103, 112, 113, 115, 124); and Alan Chan (Dr Naidu image)

The following copyrighted images were licensed from Shutterstock:

Medical illustrations from Sebastian Kaulitzki (7, 22, 39, 47, 52, 53, 65, 87, 91, 100, 107, 114, 124,128, 142, 145, 154, 161); hkannn (20, 101, 112, 204); Linda Bucklin (46, 49, 53); Chepe Nicoli (54, 55); Patrick Hermans (51, 52); Michael Taylor (8, 12) and James Steidl (47, 51). **Histological sections** from Jubal Harshaw (18, 82, 85, 128); **Molecular structures** from Stanislaff (150, 151, 171) and **Chemical illustrations** from Fabrizio Zanier (73, 76-79, 82).

Front pages: Igor Bliznyuk (ii); Tono Balaguer (v); Janaka (vi) and Tischenko Irina (x)

Chapter-1: Ostill (1); phdpsx (2); Sharon Day (4); Nik Niklz (5); Oleinikova Olga (7); S-Oleg (9); Digitalife (10); Antonis Papantoniou (11); Jarrod Erbe (14); Yellowj (15); MilousSK (17); Michal Szczepaniak (19); Bruce Rolfe (22); Paul Cown, Hakimata Photography & Mark Lorch (25); Christian Darkin (27) and Reeed, POMAH (30).

Chapter-2: Deviation/Edwin Verbruggen, Michael Zysman, Eric Isselee, twobluedogs, Tomo Jesenicnik & Dmitry Petrenko (40); JaBa, Brad Thompson, Bruce MacQueen, Ewan Chesser & Frederick Matzen (42); R McKown, Antonio Petrone (43); Roberto Sanchez (44); Denis Pepin (45); higyou (48); AYAKOVLEVdotCOM (58); Aaliya Landholt (60); and Judex (61).

Chapter-3: Ramzi Hachicho, Fanfo, Ostill, Jarno Gonzalez Zarraonandia, Galyana Andrushko, Soundsnaps, David Mckee, kirych & Cristi Bastian (74); Benjaminet, Saiva-I & Franck Chazot (76); Matthew Cole (78); and Viktoriya Popova, Flipchuk Oleg Vasiliovich & Federov Oleksiy (84).

Chapter-4: Chris Harvey (92); Robert Pernell (95); Olivier Le Queinec (99); AXL (101); and Bob Ainsworth (102).

Chapter-5: Lauren Dambies (108); Vadim Kozlovsky (109); Martin Vonka (113); Gordon Swanson (116); Laurin Rinder (117); and Eduard Cebria (119).

Chapter-6: Alin Andrei (124); Shebko (128); moxduul (132, 133); Aleksandar Todorovic (134); OPIS (142); cbpix (150); Lim Yong Hian (151); and forbis (152).

Chapter-7: Stephen Strathdee (162); Andresr (165); Vlychko & Andrjuss (166); Igor Dutina (167); Gladkova Svetlana (168); Denis Vrublevski (171); Jovan Nikolic, bravajulia, Michael Nguyen & Stephen Finn (173); Victor Burnside, Microgen & Jovan Nikolic (175); Elenamiv, Olga Langerova, Shi Yali & Shkind (177); Newton Page, Elenamiv, Eric Gevaert & Yana Petruseva (180); Frances Fruit, digitalife, Geanina Bechea & crolique (185); Peter Grosch, SunLu4ik, Osmozist & Jacek Chabraszewski (187); George Bailey, Tatiana53 & plastique (189); M Dykstra, Valentyn Volkov (191); Roman Sigaev, Elena Kalistratova, Rey Kamensky & Sergei Didyk (193); Whadener Endo, Dhana Shekar & Ilja (195); Elena Moiseeva & Elena Schweitzer (198); Sandra Caldwell (199); Emin Kuliyev (201); Rene Jansa & Rafa Irusta (202); Jiri Vaclavek (204); Stefan Glebowski (207); Sandiren (209); and Kathy Burns-Millyard (210) and robybret (218).

Notes